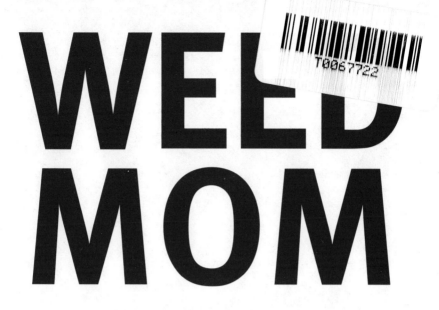

# WEED MOM

### The **Canna-Curious** Woman's Guide to Healthier Relaxation, Happier Parenting, and **Chilling TF Out**

**Danielle Simone Brand**

Published in the United States by:
ULYSSES PRESS
P.O. Box 3440
Berkeley, CA 94703
www.ulyssespress.com

A longer version of the preface originally appeared in 2019 in the cannabis publication, *Civilized*.

ISBN: 978-1-64604-121-3
Library of Congress Control Number: 2020936172

Printed in Canada by Marquis Book Printing
10 9 8 7 6 5 4 3 2

Acquisitions editor: Ashten Evans
Managing editor: Claire Chun
Editor: Renee Rutledge
Proofreader: Kate St.Clair
Front cover design: Lilith Stepanyan
Artwork: Marijuana leaf © Sergejs Makarovs/shutterstock.com; page 34 © Ralph Hallowell Rogers III; page 36 © Roxana Gonzalez/shutterstock.com; page 287 © Mountain Tree Studio
Layout: Jake Flaherty

NOTE TO READERS: This book has been written and published strictly for informational and educational purposes only. It is not intended to serve as medical advice or to be any form of medical treatment. You should always consult your physician before altering or changing any aspect of your medical treatment and/or undertaking a diet regimen, including the guidelines as described in this book. Do not stop or change any prescription medications without the guidance and advice of your physician. Any use of the information in this book is made on the reader's good judgment after consulting with his or her physician and is the reader's sole responsibility. This book is not intended to diagnose or treat any medical condition and is not a substitute for a physician. The author and publisher disclaim liability for any medical outcomes that may occur as a result of applying the methods suggested in this book.

This book is independently authored and published and no sponsorship or endorsement of this book by, and no affiliation with, any trademarked brands or other products mentioned within is claimed or suggested. All trademarks that appear in this book belong to their respective owners and are used here for informational purposes only. The author and publisher encourage readers to patronize the quality brands mentioned in this book.

# CONTENTS

# PREFACE

Dear Alcohol,

I have some difficult news. Deep breaths. Here it is: I'm breaking up with you.

We've had plenty of good times together—believe me. You were there for me in my twenties when I wanted you. You helped me through those (let's be honest, completely asinine) college parties and awkward holiday rituals. It's true that you and I *seemed* like a good couple in those times.

I used to enjoy my time with you while writing or doing creative work and thought you helped me express myself better. But now I realize that I didn't sound smarter or more well read at those times, just buzzed.

Alcohol, I'm sorry to tell you like this, but I've found someone else. Someone who meets my needs as a grown woman. My new someone goes by many names: weed, marijuana, pot, ganja, green, cannabis.

I love hanging out at home with my kids and my new friend. Cannabis helps soothe my anxiety about to-do lists or getting the littles to bed at 8 p.m. sharp. I can read bedtime stories for a good while when I'm hanging out with cannabis—and then deliver the requested hundred kisses.

On New Year's Eve, I told you I was just gonna chill at home, but I actually went to a party with cannabis. I hate to tell you this, alcohol, but I didn't miss you at all. Cannabis is just more sophisticated, more varied, and frankly, more interesting than you are. I can microdose for a calm, focused feel. I can soothe my nerves and sleep well with the right strain. Or, I can get energized for running around the park with my kids, pulling weeds (actual weeds, not *weed* weeds), or one of those Sunday night laundry-folding marathons. Plus, in many states, I can now find cannabis whenever I want—legally, and with ease. Cannabis will come to my doorstep 24/7 if I ask.

I particularly enjoy long walks with cannabis. Traversing the urban canyons that dot my neighborhood, I revel in the scents of sage and juniper and fathom my family's place under the endless blue skies. I like to let my thoughts meander down any course they care to, and this has led to the kind of insights that I've never had with you. I feel so much more *stimulated* with cannabis.

Speaking of stimulation, we have to talk about sex. I don't want to embarrass you, but sex with cannabis is better. I feel more in tune with my senses and my sensuality. My orgasms rock. I'm sorry, alcohol, that's just the way it is.

And before you ask—no, alcohol, I don't want an open relationship. Thing is, aside from liking weed better, I have some legit issues with your behavior. For instance, after we spend the night together, I feel like death warmed over the next day. Lately, alcohol, even when I partake in you very sparingly, it doesn't feel good. I wish I could say differently, but my body doesn't lie.

I did a little digging about you online, alcohol, and found some disturbing things. A recent study from the University of Colorado found that, over long-term use, you're more damaging to the brain than cannabis.[1] Plus, everyone knows your hangover symptoms: fatigue, nausea, vomiting, headache, dizziness, concentration problems, and mood instability, among others. They're no picnic. Apparently, there are even consortiums on hangover research, and a doctor in Las Vegas who provides a medical hangover cure for $160. I mean, damn.

Also, I have to be honest: I don't really like your friends. I mean, some of them are fine. But others are obnoxious and rude. They don't have good boundaries. They tend to pee where they shouldn't, and sometimes, puke. Some of them have even tried to feel me up when they've been hanging out with you, and that's not cool. Friends of cannabis don't do that.

And another thing: I have spent way too much money on you. With my friend cannabis, I can chill all night for the price of a drink. Just think about what I could do with all that money saved—like take a vacation (with cannabis!).

Truthfully, I deserve better. I'm a working mom with many interests who's also trying to maintain a modicum of a social life. (Like I said, a grown woman.) Alcohol, I held onto you for far too long. If I see you at the holiday table, I'll say hey, but don't expect me to change my mind.

Sincerely,

Your ex

# INTRODUCTION

I wasn't the kind of little girl who dreamed of having children of her own. I dreamed of traveling the world as a translator for the UN or swinging from vine to vine while rescuing valuable artifacts à la Indiana Jones. Though I married young, my husband and I didn't think about children for several years. We were too busy going to grad school, traveling, and having lots of (non-procreational) sex.

As our thirties approached, we debated the question of parenthood. Then my body issued her own statement on the matter while on vacation in a little seaside Mexican town, precisely—I kid you not—on my thirtieth birthday. Her answer? *Get pregnant this fucking instant.* My husband, accommodating guy that he is, agreed to help out.

Born the next year, our son soon became the center of a new kind of love that bowled us both over with its immensity. Two years and ten months later, our daughter was born. And though it doesn't seem possible to love your second child as much as you love your first, if you have more than one kid you can attest to the fact that it *is* possible. Your heart just grows.

By the time this book picks up *circa* 2016, I was in my mid-(ish) thirties and had lived in about fifteen different cities before ending up with my family in San Diego. And my husband and I had recently been through a big old mess in our marriage—more on that later.

Along the way I'd earned two degrees and worked as an academic researcher, a yoga teacher on Capitol Hill, an adjunct professor, an essayist and journalist, and a full-time stay-at-home mom (the hardest of all those jobs by a million). I loved all things healthy and yoga-y, and cared very much about the environment and peaceful parenting. I'd never been arrested and never done much in the way of drugs. I was pretty much on the straight and narrow. Yeah, I liked wine. But weed? Not so much.

So how on Earth did someone like me become a cannabis writer, somewhat of a lay cannabis expert, and a genuine weed enthusiast? And why the heck am I writing a book on parenting and cannabis, of all things? That's a thread we'll follow throughout this book, but the short answer is because I found out, a bit late perhaps, that I actually *love* weed. And as soon as I introduce you properly—I think you and a ton of other moms out there will, too. Cannabis helps in so many ways that we moms really need. I'll tell you all about the ways in these pages.

Evidence of a cultural shift from the "wine mom" to the "weed mom" is everywhere. And why wouldn't it? These days, with a little education on the subject, it's easy to calibrate your dose and tailor your experience. Cannabis makes most people, most of the time, feel happier, or more relaxed, or both. It enhances creativity, parallel thinking, and—with the right strain in the right amount—focus. For many, it eases nausea, reduces pain, or helps control seizures. Certain strains can help you sleep through the night. Unlike alcohol, weed doesn't cause a hangover, and there is a fairly low risk of developing dependence or addiction.[2] People who consume cannabis are found to exercise more and have more sex than those who don't. And it's a substance with a long history of interaction with *Homo sapiens*. Some people even say we humans coevolved with the plant.

Weed is legit awesome.

So of course moms are gonna be into the stuff. You can find all kinds of opinions on the internet about how smoking pot makes you a better parent, or about what it's like coming out of the "weed closet." You'll even find a segment on *Good Morning America* called "Weed Moms Are the New Wine Moms." Cannabis is becoming a normal and everyday part of contemporary family life. It's finally *happening*.

But what, you might ask, are the consequences? Will consuming cannabis hinder your ability to function as a parent? Will you be stigmatized by peers and family? Will your kids experiment with pot earlier if they know their mom is a consumer? Even if these questions *don't* provoke an anxiety attack, you may wonder how to even start down the skunky-sweet yellow brick road to your own personal happy place. You may not know the first thing about researching, shopping for, and consuming cannabis.

That's why I'm here: to answer your questions, allay your fears, and inform you about the newly emerging world of legal cannabis and what it means for moms. Nearly every day, I talk to other moms in my community and online who are curious but cautious. They ask me questions like: Should I try CBD? How do I choose the best product if I don't want to get too high? What if I *do* want to get high? How can I talk to my kids about cannabis? What should I know before hitting up a dispensary?

And if you have these questions, too, I'm well positioned to understand where you're coming from: just a few short years ago, I could pack every single thing I knew about weed into a one-hitter.[3] But, after reading and writing extensively on the subject and enjoying a ton of weed, I now know a bunch of things about cannabis that I'm incredibly excited to share with you. In my career and personal life, I'm already on the frontlines of this cultural sea change that's normalizing cannabis—rendering it nearly as ordinary, but arguably healthier than alcohol—certain pharmaceuticals, and even some products born of the wellness industry. Because I know cannabis *and* I know the challenges and opportunities of parenting, I'm writing this book to help moms like you, your neighbor, your hairdresser, your contractor, your financial planner, your colleague, your friend—all of us—embrace this moment.

Today, my kids are seven and ten years old. Yours may be older or younger than mine. You may have one kid, or two, or more. You may be bio-momming, adoptive momming, step-momming, or momming under any number of other circumstances. Whatever your situation, whatever your background or skin color or sexual orientation or gender identity, if you identify as a mother and are curious about cannabis, this book is for you. I seek to present this subject with clarity, honesty, respect, and love.

I also want to make super clear that, even though certain stigmas remain for white moms who admit to loving weed, the consequences are so much greater for moms of color. In seeking to provide moms with useful information about cannabis and help break down stigmas, I acknowledge that I come at this subject from a place of privilege. There are still too many Black and brown women in this country, many of them mothers, in prison for marijuana-related offenses. There are also those who have had their children taken away for the same thing—all facts that remain ludicrous to fathom, given that millions of Americans can now access a Nordstrom-level weed shopping experience with minimal risk to them or to the person behind the counter.

Yes, it's true—and wrong—that immaculate stores run by kind and knowledgeable people can cater to a customer's every taste for edible, smokable, vaporizable, or topical applications of THC, when many people of color still languish in jail for small marijuana offenses. And, to top it all off, those Nordstroms of weed charge a pretty penny for the good stuff and tack on a whole bunch of taxes. Eleven states, including the large and populous state of California (where I lived for about half my adult life), have deemed cannabis safe enough to be legal for anyone over the age of twenty-one. Marijuana has many known medical applications as well as a host of other potential ones. Based on all that, marijuana prohibition—and its racist application in this country—simply doesn't make sense. Prohibition needs to, and will, end soon.

Ahem—so to step down from my soapbox—point is, I love my kids. I love my husband, my family, my life. And I also happen to love the shit out of weed. And that's totally okay. If you're tired of feeling crappy after drinking alcohol, or if you're looking for a way to sleep better, have amazing sex, or ease pain and inflammation—or if you're just looking for a way to maximize quality time with your family—you might be a weed mom like me. Maybe you just don't know it yet.

In this book, you'll learn about the new landscape of cannabis: how, when, and why to use it; how to talk about it with kids, spouses, and friends; and how to integrate it into a healthy lifestyle. Because there are also some risks and downsides to cannabis, I will present those fairly, too. It's my hope that reading this book will feel like a long conversation with your smart (if I say so myself), funny (ditto), cannabis-loving ('nuff said) mom friend.

Here's an overview of what you'll find in this book:

Chapter 1 introduces you to my own unlikely journey with the plant and how I became a cannabis-loving mom. In Chapter 2, we get into the science behind cannabis, or why and how it does what it does. Chapter 3 tells the story of *Cannabis sativa* and how we humans have long enjoyed and tended it. Chapter 4 drills down into THC, CBD, and all kinds of other good stuff you'll find in cannabis, and Chapter 5 is a close look at how to consume. In Chapter 6, I address concerns about parenting and cannabis by answering questions like, "In what ways might cannabis make you a better parent?" and "What are the appropriate ways and times to partake?" I also address what's known about pregnancy, breastfeeding, and cannabis.

Chapter 7 is an overview of cannabis and young people, including medical uses for kids and teens, and what studies show about teen development and recreational marijuana consumption. In Chapter 8, I dissect "the talk" you might have with your kids and teens about cannabis, including how to share information and help young people make healthy choices. Chapter 9 is about when things go off course. Recognizing the signs when you or someone you love has an unhealthy relationship with the plant is important for savvy moms.

In Chapter 10, I explore the ways that cannabis can enhance sex and intimacy. Many moms struggle with sex after kids, and cannabis can help in a variety of ways if you take the time to understand your body, consume the right stuff, and communicate with your partner. In Chapter 11, I turn the spotlight on socializing with cannabis where, in addition to "weediquette," I talk about the cultural shifts around weed that are happening *at this moment*. In Chapter 12, I touch on how cannabis can help our parents' generation with some of the common conditions and symptoms of aging. Because, as moms, we often mediate the cultural divide between older and younger generations, I also discuss how you might talk to older adults in your life about this versatile and helpful plant.

Chapter 13 focuses on self-care from the perspective of wholeness in body, mind, heart, and spirit. You won't find body-shaming or promises to lift your ass here—instead, it's all about nourishing yourself on a deep level so you can shine in whatever way you were meant to.

In the last chapter, I indulge in a little fortune-telling to envision what humans and cannabis might be up to next by addressing questions like, "How is the political, cultural, and on-the-ground cannabis landscape changing?" and "When will marijuana finally be legal in the United States and worldwide?" Answer: June 18, 2025. Just kidding. No one knows, but we do have some educated guesses, precedents, and room for hope.

Throughout this book, I weave my experiences with the plant into the narrative. I also interview doctors, cannabis scientists, entrepreneurs, educators, therapists, and lots and lots of mothers. Bear in mind that I'm a mom and a journalist, but I'm *not* a credentialed expert in cannabis science. I'm here to start you on your journey of asking questions and contemplating the ways cannabis might enhance your life, but I am not you, nor am I your doctor, your mother, or your elected representative. I *can't* tell you what's right for you and your family, but I *can* tell you what's worked for me. Thank you for buying a ticket to this wild tour of the brand-new world of legal cannabis.

You may not be as in love with the plant as I am—yet. But read on, and I think you will be. The bottom line is that you can, of course, choose to embrace it or abstain from it, but cannabis is here to stay. It's the right and privilege of us mothers to take good care of ourselves and our families—possibly with a little help from *Cannabis sativa*—and to educate and uplift others along the way. This book aims to help you do just that.

## CHAPTER 1
# ROOTS

My happily-ever-after cannabis story began in a most unlikely place: a rehab center. More precisely, it started soon after I dropped my husband off at one so he could recalibrate his relationship—not to pills or powders or booze—but to *weed*.

"Wait, what?" you ask.

You may've thought this guide was a straight-up cannabis love story—and that'd be a good guess. But my weed history's a bit more complex than that, and to show you how I came to adore the plant, I have to first tell you about how and why I hated it. Let me explain.

When I said goodbye to my husband and drove away from the rehab center, where he would spend the next five weeks, my only thought was, "I sure as hell hope this works." I wasn't yet thinking about the long days and nights of solo parenting ahead of me. I wasn't yet thinking of the many, many times I'd have to explain to our children—who'd only just turned four and seven—where Daddy was. I wasn't thinking about our long-term future, whether financial or relational, or if my husband and I would make it as a couple. All I really knew that windy, blue-sky February 2017 morning in Southern California was that weed called the shots in his already turbulent brain, and he and I both desperately needed for him to be free.

Eyes darting back and forth between the road and the rearview, I recalled a big guy smoking a cigarette and talking to my husband. He looked like a bouncer, though he'd introduced himself as the treatment center's residential coordinator when we had walked up the gravel drive carrying my husband's duffel bag and backpack just a few minutes before. I wondered whether he acted as a kind of reverse bouncer—keeping people *in* the facility instead of out. "I'll look out for your man," he had told me. It was an oddly perceptive comment given that I had recently felt like it was my job to take care of my husband—to talk him out of his most egregious departures from reality and convince him that there was plenty of good in his life to live for.

Tears probably flowed as I accelerated, watching the rehab center grow smaller and smaller in my rearview like the zoom-out function in Google maps. But I can't quite remember whether or not I cried because at that period of my life, crying felt as normal and involuntary as breathing, my cheeks more often streaked and salty than smooth. I had recently cut off my long hair into a severe bob, the whole thing shot through with swaths of pink. I had also just sat for my first and only tattoo—three dahlias that covered my left shoulder and upper back. The pink hair and tattoo were conspicuous markers that met a need to redefine what I had believed myself to exclusively be for the last many years: mother—safe and present and endlessly giving—and wife. I rolled down the car windows even as I merged onto the six-lane freeway, letting the air wrap its cold arms around my neck and whip the strands of pink hair in my eyes. In the abandonment of that gesture I felt a deep sadness, a kind of relief, and the resignation of having little to lose.

In that moment I hated weed. Hated that something everyone seemed to think was either harmless or could do only good had taken my husband's brain—already prone to dark, twisty turns—and fucked it up so badly. Never in a million years would I have thought that one day *I'd* be the one to embrace cannabis. I'd seen this substance erode my husband's sense of self-worth and drive its dank tendrils deep into his body and psyche. It was *not* good, *not* health-promoting, and most certainly *not* for me. This I knew.

But, as with so many other things in life, the line between abhorrence and acceptance is much finer than we all might like to think. We humans are *sure* that we're sure about so many things. Until we're not.

For me, cannabis was one of those things.

🌿 🌿 🌿

Interestingly, I had had the opportunity to vote on pot legalization in California just a few months before. Prop 64 was presented to voters in November 2016. One evening, once the dishes were scrubbed and the kids tucked in, I sat at my kitchen table to fill out the mail-in ballot. After carefully darkening the bubble corresponding to my choices for president and the congressional seats, I considered the language, and the possible repercussions, of the measure.

Surely no one should go to jail for marijuana, I thought, though I vividly remembered my husband's longtime struggle with the stuff—a struggle I believed then was already over—and wondered if legal pot would tempt him. Though medical marijuana had been quasi-legal in the state since 1996, it seemed clear to me that recreational use would render it even more ubiquitous and mainstream. I wasn't sure how I felt about that. Though I had no interest in pot myself, legalizing it for recreational use nonetheless seemed like the right thing to do. I voted yes.

Weeks later, my husband confessed to the addiction he'd been hiding for years. It would be the capstone of a period of utter tumult that started when weed had become more important to him than sleeping. Maybe it had started when we left Washington, DC, to follow my fantasy of a DIY life and spent our savings on a failed homestead before fleeing back to the city. Maybe it started in the early years of parenting our two little ones, providing all the messy, exhausting care they require without an extended family to lean on. Maybe it started when I found myself a stay-at-home mom—

something I'd never intended—covered in baby and toddler effluvia for days on end, giving little to myself and believing that's just what mothers did. Maybe it started when I grew weary of all that and had a brief but terribly destructive affair.

Or, perhaps, none of those problems were the real root of our marital breakdown. Perhaps our troubles were embedded in my DNA and his—my thirst for connection, and his need to escape his own brain with the substance that proved creative and euphoric in small amounts but destabilizing in large quantities. The truth is that I don't know when exactly it started. But I do know that things began going very badly for us, and then they got worse.

After my husband confessed his secret addiction, it took another several weeks for us to find him a spot in rehab. As I dropped him off that February morning, I would have cursed myself for voting yes on cannabis legalization if indeed I had remembered doing so in that moment. But though Prop 64 had passed, it hadn't yet gone into effect, and I had much bigger fish to fry.

✹ ✹ ✹

When I first laid eyes on my future husband—bursting with energy, crowned with shoulder-length, curly black hair, and wearing round, bookish glasses—I thought, with equal intensity, *I want him* and *I should probably keep my distance*. The wanting him won out, of course.

Our differences were numerous: his olive skin and dark eyes contrasted with my fair skin and blue eyes; his tall, lanky frame made me seem even shorter and curvier; his cynical skepticism accentuated my idealism. We were opposites and, yet, we would soon fit together like yin and yang. Within a week of our first date we were officially a couple, and a little more than a year later, I converted to Judaism and we were married.

For him, weed was always there. Though I was never a big fan of the stuff myself, in the early days of our relationship, I accepted pot as part of what made my husband who he was. Love it or not, I reasoned, it wasn't *so* bad.

My husband's indulgences didn't run toward the alcoholic, or the cheating. So the musky smell of charred buds permeated our everyday lives, just like the lingering aroma of fried tofu or our commingled scents in the sheets.

About the time we started grad school, I noticed my husband's moods grow dark and deep—inscrutable morasses for which I had no map or timeline. In those long periods, he was walled off—metaphorically—from meaningful connection. Then he'd come back, and things would be good again. He was already medicated for a mental health condition, so more than anything else, I believed weed was to blame for my husband's emotional absences.

I begged him to quit, or at least slow down. I monitored his stash and sniffed him suspiciously. Even when he swore he wasn't using, I'd interrogate and lecture, thinking that if only I could show him how much he was hurting himself and me, he'd stop.

That continued until finally, he did stop—except, not really. He did what addicts do: he lied. And I did what spouses of addicts do: I half-believed.

We finished grad school, moved around, had kids. By the time I dropped him off at rehab in early 2017, we were once again living in California—this time in San Diego—and he and I had just walked through a veritable hellscape of bitter separations and joyful reunions that spanned several months and left us both with emotional whiplash.

🌿 🌿 🌿

While my husband was getting right in his brain so that a day without getting high could feel possible, I considered all my options. I had owned a successful yoga business before kids but scaled back on work after becoming a mother. It felt natural at the time; the beings I had gestated and nursed needed me nearly all day and night. And I needed them, too: their warm milk breath, the brush of their fuzzy peach heads against my lips.

But my closeness with them came at a price. My skills had languished over a few years, and as a mother of young children, I lacked the stamina and time I once had to run a business in my industry. There was a new crop of teachers whose bellies weren't stretched by pregnancies and whose faces did not bear the worry lines from pacing dark corridors with a colicky baby at 3 a.m. They taught yoga and meditation in booty shorts.

I had a master's degree but it was years since I'd worked in the conflict resolution field. In the meantime, trying to paper over years of scant paid work on my resume felt taxing and disingenuous. Sure, I was a smart and educated person who had honed many skills as a mom, such as organization, management, decision-making, multitasking, and buttloads of patience. Unfortunately, recruiters weren't impressed that I could pay the electric bill while changing a diaper.

Having long put pen to paper to funnel the chaotic world around me into a comprehensible shape, I was already a writer—just not a paid one. So I tried my hand in the freelancing world and, before too long, some of my pitches were actually landing. Wellness and parenting became my most natural beats in the form of "tips for your yoga practice" and essays about navigating contemporary life with little ones.

And then there was cannabis. In the early days of legal weed in California, cannabis-slanted stories were in crazy high (lol) demand, and I—a one-woman freelancing machine—was happy to supply some of them. At first, I wrote about weed while not caring for it much at all. But the more I learned, the more curious I became. Cannabis snuck up on me and then legitimately captured my fascination with its many points of intersection between science, health, policy, education, and culture.

🌿 🌿 🌿

The worst of the turbulent times in my marriage passed. I had ended the affair weeks after it had begun, and my husband—on a new regimen of meds—was clean from weed. We rebuilt our trust in each other very slowly. I still often wondered whether he could hide his addiction from me again, and he wondered what it would take for someone else to pry me away. But we learned to accept uncertainty as part of the deal in love, which, despite everything, we still had.

❋ ❋ ❋

Double-checking that my husband wasn't looking over my shoulder, I cautiously googled "legal cannabis near me." Half-amused and half-alarmed that I'd been writing more and more frequently about weed, he'd already agreed for me to give it a whirl and make up my own mind as long as he didn't have to see it.

By then, signs and billboards advertising a dozen recreational dispensaries peppered the freeways in and around San Diego. Buying weed had, from my observations, long been a shady process with buyer and seller exchanging little information. But as of January 1, 2018, anyone in California over the age of 21 with a valid ID could purchase or possess up to an ounce of cannabis and grow six plants for personal use. And, presumably, such a person could ask any kind of question he or she wanted to in the process.

People were no longer talking about pot, grass, ganja, or even marijuana. Now, it was "cannabis," which seemed different somehow—untethered to the couch-locked and tie-dyed stoner stereotypes of the pot I was used to frowning upon my husband for using. Before recognizing it as a problem in his life and well before kids, I had on occasion smoked with him and felt disoriented and lost in my own thoughts, or hungry, or nothing at all. A strange substance, it seemed to me, with little rhyme or reason to its effect.

But as the legal regime progressed in the nearby states of Colorado, Washington, and Oregon, and as mainstream publications began running stories about its many uses, the aura of cannabis was changing in the public eye, and, slowly, in my own. What I read promised a more predictable experience, a tailored one. Women I knew, other moms included, had started experimenting with cannabis or talking more openly about their longtime enjoyment of it.

Driving around town, my family began noticing all kinds of advertisements for dispensaries with names like Urbn Leaf and Golden Greens. "What's cann-a-bis?" my older child asked as we pulled into the Trader Joe's parking lot. And I hadn't a clue how to answer.

Was cannabis something good? Something bad? A medicine that helps people with chronic pain, or migraines, or cancer? Or the substance that made Daddy's brain spiral down such a dark path that he had to leave us for five weeks to "go to the program," as we referred to rehab in our house? Was it a harmless plant, or an insidious and habit-forming drug?

My husband had once believed it to be the former and now felt strongly that it was the latter. He had told me that he wished he had never picked up a pipe, bong, or joint, and I agreed. But others, I knew, felt that cannabis enhanced their creativity, brightened their outlook, or helped them get a good night's sleep with no adverse effect. With all these conflicting messages, I didn't know what to think or how to answer my kids' questions.

So perhaps it was curiosity—the need to know, pure and simple—that led me to place that first order. Not yet ready for a dispensary experience, I studied the dizzying array of products available on the online menus and chose delivery from a dispensary whose web copy felt wellness-oriented. I was pot-illiterate, so, with a pang of guilt, I ordered what seemed easy and discreet: cookies and a vape pen.

I received my first cannabis delivery while my husband was at work and my kids at school. The delivery guy inspected my ID and handed me an innocent-looking white paper bag with a receipt stapled to the top—as if it contained items as ordinary as toothpaste and gum. I paid cash, wondering all the while if I was doing something wrong. I sure hoped my neighbors hadn't seen me standing at my front gate and handing the nice, non-stoned-looking driver a wad of bills.

There I was: a suburban mother of two, a hardworking writer, and a wife still struggling in some ways to put her marriage back together, holding a white paper bag full of weed. Errr, cannabis. I didn't know what to do with it, so I stuffed it in my sweater drawer and tried to forget about it.

But I didn't forget.

On an evening alone, I cautiously opened the drawer and inspected what I'd bought. The vape pen enticed me with its clean lines and promise of precisely 2.25 mg of THC per pull. I read the packaging from cover to cover then pried the thing from its case and held it in my palm. Such a light instrument, holding a substance both maligned and revered. Which would it be for me?

No matter what else is going on in life, a yoga mat has long been a place for me to come back to myself, so I decided to put cannabis to the test on that familiar, purple turf. I rolled out the mat, my heart beating fast. I sat in the middle of it, closed my eyes, put the vape pen to my lips, and inhaled.

At first, all I wanted to do was sit there. *Stoner* my mind shouted. *You're wasting a perfectly good evening to yourself!* But those thoughts quieted in time, and I found myself pleasantly altered. Sitting segued into a flow of spinal undulations. I languorously moved my spine in the six directions: forward bends, backbends, left- and right-side bends, twists. Alternating between organic movements and longer holds seemed like the way to meet my body exactly where it was in the moment. Vocalizations and sighs escaped my lips, though normally I would have felt too inhibited to allow that particular kind of release. I was alone, and it felt good. More than good—it felt *great*.

Next, I lay down on my mat and was enraptured by movement that hardly resembled the more classic postures I usually practiced. My lower body felt alive and glowing, and I didn't want to get up for a long while.

When I finally stood, I practiced sun salutations, lunges, warrior poses, and squats, finding the same satisfying ease between movement and long holds. Even as my legs began to shake in horse pose, I didn't stop immediately, as I might otherwise have done; instead, I rode out what felt like a powerful movement of energy. My teachers' voices played in my head around clearing emotional residue through movement and careful attention. The synchrony between body, heart, and mind felt clear and palpable. I was a goddess—purely and simply—on my mat, thinking, *why the hell haven't I done this before?*

From the spread of each toe to the workings of individual muscles as I lengthened and contracted according to what the postures required, I truly inhabited my body. And while I can't report any profound insight from that night, I embodied what so many of us who practice yoga hope for. When I noticed the question "What's next?" growing in the back of my mind, I recognized the thought and, with deliberateness, set it aside. On a yellow notepad alongside my mat, I scrawled: NOW. THIS. THAT'S ALL. And it felt true.

✿ ✿ ✿

From that evening, a short jaunt down cannabis lane transformed me from worried newbie to full-on enthusiast. I learned that, contrary to what I'd long believed, cannabis *can indeed* be used responsibly to promote health, well-being, and optimal functioning. I learned that, with the right intention, dose, and product, cannabis is a tool for self-care and self-awareness; quite simply, I learned that cannabis is *wonderful*.

So I dove in, researching all I could about cannabis; talking to anyone who would listen about my newfound love of the plant; trying tons of products (many of which I liked, and others I didn't); getting super-comfortable with browsing a dispensary and chatting up the budtenders; learning how to talk to my kids, friends, and parents about cannabis; and becoming a cannabis journalist. Along the way, I had to readjust my own assumptions and stereotypes about a million times. And I had to talk to my husband over and over again about what all this meant for me, for him, and for us.

I've learned more about cannabis, and about myself and my family, in the past few years than I could have ever anticipated. And I'd love to help you learn, too. Let's get down to it.

# CHAPTER 2

# SUN, SOIL, WATER, AND AIR: THE BASICS OF CANNABIS

Today, cannabis goes by all kinds of names: weed, marijuana, pot, ganja, Mary Jane, 420, skunk, chronic or—quite simply—green. In decades past, names like reefer, grass, tea, and even muggles were more common. (Does J.K. Rowling know?)

But whatever you call it, it's clear that the subject of cannabis is a vast one. Let's talk terminology first.

## CANNABIS TERMINOLOGY

### *CANNABIS SATIVA* L.

Cannabis belongs to the species *Cannabis sativa* L., a giant umbrella term for the myriad varieties of the plant out there today—including types that *won't* get you high and are instead used for things like the materials or food industries, as well as THC-rich types that *will* get you high.

It's pretty well settled that cannabis originated in Central Asia and adapted to new environments in varied ways as it was introduced and enjoyed by travelers, traders, and farmers of all stripes. Genetically varied descendants of those original cannabis plants would eventually thrive throughout Asia, Africa, Europe, and, eventually, the Americas and the entire Pacific region. In warmer climates, cannabis plants have evolved to produce more THC, and in cold climes, they generally produce less. But for a very long time, people have been breeding plants for their specific needs and wants, too, thereby shaping the morphology (appearance) and attributes of the plant. Some, like Michael Pollan in *The Botany of Desire*, say that cannabis and humans "coevolved" as each party took turns molding and accommodating the other in mutually beneficial ways. How freaking cool is that?

As mentioned, many varieties, aka subspecies, of *Cannabis sativa* L. don't contain enough THC to get anyone high. In fact, the first human uses of the plant were likely less about altering consciousness and more about accessing the plant's fiber for rope, clothing, and (later) ship sails, as well as for its nutritive value; hemp seeds and oil are both highly nourishing suppliers of essential fatty acids like omega-6 and omega-3,[4] along with significant protein, minerals,[5] and every single amino acid necessary for human life.[6]

These low-to-no-THC varieties of cannabis are commonly known today as hemp or industrial hemp and were grown in vast, vast quantities in the Old World and in the colonial New World. Hemp was one of the first crops cultivated by English colonists in the Americas and, in 1619, the Virginia colony passed a law *requiring* farmers to grow hemp because of its many material uses.

We'll talk about subvarieties of cannabis in a bit; but for now, you just need to know that the species *Cannabis sativa* L. encompasses three subspecies: *Cannabis sativa*, *Cannabis indica*, and *Cannabis ruderalis*. (Believe me, I can appreciate that the name game's more than a little confusing when it comes to cannabis!) *Cannabis sativa* and *Cannabis indica* are the two subspecies we'll concern ourselves with; *Cannabis ruderalis* is generally very low in useful cannabinoids and doesn't figure into the consumables market—so don't worry about that one!

# HEMP

Hemp has multiple uses as material, food, and medicine. Its stalks can be used to make paper, clothing, shoes, packaging, and biofuel. Hemp seeds and hemp seed oil can be found in nutritional products like protein shakes, breads, milks, and bars.

Hemp also provides the raw material for much of the CBD on the market today. Hemp-derived CBD contains 0.3 percent THC or less, and—let me assure you—ain't no one getting high on 0.3 percent.

The term "industrial hemp" simply refers to hemp that comes in under that 0.3 percent THC threshold. This product was legalized with the 2018 Farm Bill—meaning that it can now be grown, processed, and transported freely within the US. While some states (I'm looking at you, Idaho) were slow AF in implementing the new law, it's finally safe to say that hemp—which I repeat, *can't* get you high—is wholly legal in the US. *About freaking time!*

# MARIJUANA

This Spanish colloquialism used to describe THC-rich varieties of cannabis was adopted in the US during a particularly nasty moment in the 1930s when white Americans' fear-driven, racist ideologies toward Mexican migrants equated the plant with crime, degeneracy, and the corruption of American youth. Harry Anslinger, America's first anti-cannabis crusader, worked tirelessly to demonize the plant and sway lawmakers' opinions in favor of prohibition. Today, the word "marijuana" is still commonly used on the medical side, though many people on the recreational side of the market have consciously dropped it from the lexicon.

## MEDICAL VS. RECREATIONAL CANNABIS

While these two categories are both the same thing (cannabis, duh!), medical marijuana typically has higher potency (particularly when it comes to edibles) and costs less than recreational (aka "adult use") cannabis. That's in part because patients pay out of pocket for medicine that insurance companies don't cover, and states set lower taxes on the medical market.

In states where both medical and recreational cannabis are legal, some dispensaries might serve both kinds of consumers; others just choose a lane and stick with it. And even though medical and recreational are distinct markets with different trends and demographics, there's certainly crossover between the two: a survey of current US cannabis consumers found that over half of those asked say they use cannabis in both medical and recreational ways.[7] So, clearly, the two buckets are not mutually exclusive.

I dislike the terms "recreational" and "adult use" for cannabis because they obfuscate the many ways cannabis can help. Cannabis is enjoyable and makes you feel good, but it's really so much more than that. It's a better night's sleep, an antidote for anxiety, and a means to nurture creativity. It's better orgasms and an aid to yoga and mindfulness. Some have used the crossover term "recredicinal" to connote that middle space between rec and med; "wellness-oriented use" is another way to describe it, but you may agree that the term *wellness* is a bit overplayed.

I use cannabis for better health *and* because it produces a mellow euphoria and sustained focus that I enjoy. Touting cannabis only for "wellness" downplays the fun and pleasure of it—as if pure enjoyment were a mark of degeneracy. It isn't. I claim *all* the things: healing, self-care, pleasure, and transcendence—and so can you.

# THE COMPONENTS OF CANNABIS

## THC, CBD, AND CANNABINOIDS

THC, tetrahydrocannabinol, is the psychoactive molecule that's present in many varieties of cannabis. Once you activate it with heat, THC is the substance that gets you high, or elevated, or enhanced, or baked, or stoned. To backtrack just a sec, it's technically THCA (tetrahydrocannabinolic acid) that occurs naturally in cannabis and becomes THC once heated. THC has several known medical uses and many more hypothesized ones. More on that in a bit.

CBD, or cannabidiol, on the other hand, is the nonpsychoactive molecule present in some varieties of cannabis that's currently all the rage in the health and body-care industries. CBD has some known therapeutic benefits and other potential benefits.

Some cannabis plants have been bred to express high concentrations of THC; others contain mostly CBD; other varieties feature both. Both THC and CBD are known as cannabinoids, or cannabis compounds that interact with our bodies in numerous and awesome ways. Cannabis contains a little more than a hundred other cannabinoids—like THCV, THCP, CBG, CBN, and CBC—many of which we're only beginning to understand. For now, you just need to know about the two biggies: THC and CBD.

Knowing how much THC and CBD you're consuming is crucial to having a safe and responsible cannabis experience; but, until recently, you could only guess at the THC and CBD content of whatever weed or edibles were out there. Today, all products in legal dispensaries are labeled (either in percentages or grams, depending on the form of the product), so it's easy to know how much of each you're getting. That, in itself, is a huge advantage offered by the legal marketplace.

# "BUD" OR "FLOWER"

These terms refer to the actual flowers of female plants that contain THC and/or CBD.[8] After being harvested by the grower, trimmed of stems and leaves, and properly dried, this is the product you may have bought from the guy in a Baja hoodie in college.

If you were unlucky, "shake"—or scraps and bits of flower ubiquitously sold on corners and college campuses all throughout the 1990s—was all you could find. You may have also come across "brick weed," which is, as it sounds, a heavy block of compressed, low-quality weed that was trafficked from south of the border for decades. I've never actually seen the stuff, but it's legend.

Even if what you got back in the day was actual bud, it was probably puny and smelled like hay—a far cry from the richly aromatic and Rubenesque buds you'll be able to get your hands on today. If that's the case, prepare to have your mind blown: flower sold on the legal market is big, beautiful, and glistening with sticky-icky, cannabinoid-carrying resin. A pure delight.

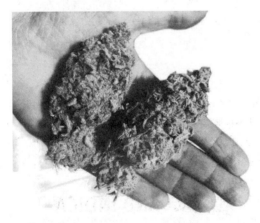

*Of the two terms, "flower" feels a little fresher than "bud" and is more frequently used in the legal market.*

I love to smell, handle, and smoke flower in all its earthy, rooty, spicy, skunky greatness. I don't often smoke joints because they give off a lot of, well, *smoke*, but there are other ways to smoke cannabis that don't produce as much. There's also a lot more you can do with flower besides smoking it—details in Chapter 5.

I should mention that I didn't start my cannabis journey loving flower, and you may not, either. It's all good! Still, I recommend handling or sniffing flower at least once to acquaint yourself with the purest form of this amazing plant.

Oh, and you *can't* get high from touching, smelling, or even eating buds. Cannabis flower must be heated to the point of decarboxylation ("decarbed") in order to convert the cannabinoids into a psychoactive form. The decarb process is accomplished by smoking, vaping, baking, or otherwise heating it. I repeat: plain flower is *not* psychoactive until it's heated to at least 220 degrees Fahrenheit.

## SINSEMILLA

Spanish for "without seeds," this term, though not as frequently used today, actually applies to most of the commercial flower on the market. It reflects a more contemporary approach used from the 1970s onward, where cultivators separate the flowering, female plants from the male ones, essentially preventing the females from being pollinated.

As a result of this sexual frustration, female plants generally produce flower that's richer in all the good stuff—cannabinoids, terpenes, and the rest—in an effort to get pollinated already (like me on my thirtieth birthday). Sinsemilla is now considered top-notch, gold-standard cannabis.

## SATIVA AND INDICA

You've probably heard that there are two basic varieties of cannabis flower you can buy in a dispensary: indica and sativa. There are also hybrids, which are a mix between them—so I guess that's three.

Indica plants are usually described as short with broad leaves—the J. Lo of pot—while sativa plants are tall and willowy, with slender leaves—more like Kate Moss in the nineties. Indica plants are said to produce flowers that, when smoked or consumed, favor the user with a mellow, soporific, pain-relieving kind of experience, a "body high." Indica is jokingly referred to as "in da couch," for this reason; it can make you want to chill, binge Netflix, and eat a pint of Ben & Jerry's.

Sativa plants, on the other hand, are said to feature flowers with perkier effects that move you to clean the house, talk a blue streak, or compose poetry with lots of exclamation points—a "head high," as it were.

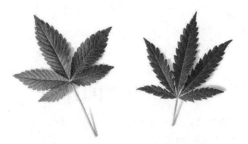

*Indica (left) vs. sativa leaves (right)*

Spoiler alert: today, the distinction between indica and sativa is essentially a fiction.[9] New Jersey cannabis nurse and founder of MarijuanaMommy. com, Jessie Gill, says a lot of what's sold as indica or sativa comes down to marketing hype and shorthand.

Close to a hundred years of prohibition drove cannabis cultivation under-ground, where growers cross-bred to produce literally thousands of strains and record-keeping was minimal. So we don't really have any pure indicas or pure sativas out there anymore, folks, despite what the labels on the jars say.

What we *do* have is plenty of flower that produces a more chill, indica-like "body high," and plenty of flower that will uplift you like a sativa. Also, we have plenty of in-between flower that could give you some of both. But it's *not* because of those plants' ancient genetic lineage or the appearance of the plants themselves (e.g., short or tall). Instead, the effects of a flower or a cannabis product have more to do with the total THC content, the ratios of THC to CBD (if applicable), and their terpene makeup (covered in the next section).

Also, I'd be remiss if I didn't add—and reiterate frequently—that each person is somewhat different when it comes to the effects of cannabis. Our unique endocannabinoid system, or ECS, along with our set and setting (i.e., mood and location) have a lot to do with how we experience the plant. In this book, you'll learn how to gauge your individual needs and consume for specific effects.

# STRAIN

A pretty simple one here. Strain, also known as cultivar, indicates a specific variety of cannabis, each with a slightly different look, smell, taste, and feel. Classic strains like OG Kush, Northern Lights, and Granddaddy Purple have provided genetic material for dozens, if not hundreds, of offshoots and crossbreeds on the market today.

Newer strains include Purple Urkle, Zombie Killer OG, and Alaskan Thunder-fuck. If you're chuckling, now's a good time to share that prohibition helped create a culture of rule-breakers and renegades with colorful personalities and a certain flair for the absurd. For years, many of those unconventional sorts did the cultivating and naming of strains. Some of them are still in the business of growing weed—in and out of the legal market.

But behind the fun strain names, these cannabis OGs experienced real risks to life and freedom. White growers, sellers, and cannabis advocates suffered plenty, but those with Black or brown skin suffered much worse. Many people of all backgrounds and ethnicities were pushed around and harassed—and had their grows and their lives literally uprooted—by cops and Drug Enforcement Agency (DEA) agents[10] trying to enforce the outdated, and frankly idiotic, War on Drugs. Consequently, many of the people who grew and named the weed we enjoy today gave absolutely zero fucks about decorum. Bless them.

When it comes to strain names, here's a parting thought: chuckle at the fun monikers, but take them with a healthy grain of salt. Today, some say strain names are wholly unreliable, while others claim that—accounting for outliers—they're *more or less* accurate. I'm in the latter camp. Still, I wouldn't bet my life on a strain name, and I know better than to assume that Dog Walker OG will always produce the same effects for me as it does for my weed mom friends. Cannabis is just a bit more complex than that.

# TERPENES

Terpenes are the compounds that give cannabis flowers their distinctive aromas; these are basically essential oils produced by the tiny "hairs," or trichomes, on the flowers themselves. Cannabis features a number of terpenes (and similar compounds called terpenoids) that tons of common plants also have. **Limonene**, for instance, is a terpene found in lemon and orange peels that exudes the fresh, citrusy scent. Limonene is present in some varieties of cannabis, too, and if you train your nose, you can detect a bright, lemony smell coming off of strains like Strawberry Banana, Do-Si-Dos, and Wedding Cake.

Though it's not yet proven, many people find that terpenes influence the direction or mood of the cannabis experience. Limonene, for instance, is most associated with perky and upbeat (so-called sativa) highs. Incidentally, limonene is often found in lemon-scented cleaning products, which (if it's real limonene) may put a spring in your step while you tackle housework. So think about *that* next time you're scrubbing toilets. Or, better yet, toke up with a limonene-dominant strain before you start. You'll be glad you did.

The most common terpene found in commercial cannabis is **myrcene**, also found in plants as diverse as mango, hops, thyme, and lemongrass. Unlike limonene, myrcene isn't easily identifiable across all these plants. When it is present in cannabis, people generally describe it as musky, earthy, and "skunky." It's the dominant terpene in an estimated 20 to 40 percent of the strains out there today and is most associated with a deeply chilled-out, pain-relieving kind of experience (in other words, more of a so-called indica feel). It might also have cancer-fighting properties. Strains like OG Kush and Granddaddy Purple are high in myrcene.

## COMMON TERPENES

| Terpene | Scent | Possible Effects | Sample Strains |
|---|---|---|---|
| Limonene | Citrusy | Relieves anxiety and depression, elevates mood | Strawberry Banana, Wedding Cake |
| Myrcene | Earthy and skunky | Provides pain relief, relaxation, and possible anticancer benefits | OG Kush and Granddaddy Purple |
| Pinene | Pine | Cultivates focus and clarity | Blue Dream, Jack Herer (while pinene-dominant strains are rare, these common strains have significant pinene content) |
| B-caryophyllene | Peppery, spicy, or fuel-like | Reduces stress and inflammation | GSC and Bubba Kush |
| Linalool | Lavender, floral | Promotes relaxation, is associated with the "rest and digest" response | Kosher Kush and Zkittlez |
| Humulene | Woody or hoppy | Provides anti-inflammatory, antibacterial, and possible anticancer benefits | Gelato, Sherbet (while humulene-dominant strains are rare, these common strains have significant humulene content) |

**Pinene**, also present in pine needles, is associated with a focused and clear kind of high. The strain called Jack Herer, named for the late legalization activist and author of the pro-cannabis manifesto, *The Emperor*

*Wears No Clothes* (1985), features significant pinene. It also may provide bronchodilation, or opening of the airways, which may be helpful for people with asthma and other respiratory issues.

> **FUN FACT:** it's a cannabis-lover's urban legend that eating mango just before smoking or consuming weed will intensify your experience, presumably because of the myrcene in mango. I can't say definitively whether it's true, but it does sound like a delicious experiment.

The weird thing about **b-caryophyllene**, another terpene, is that it kinda-sorta acts like a cannabinoid in your body. I'll cover what that means in the next section, but for now just know that b-caryophyllene is a shapeshifting trickster that has anti-inflammatory properties and a number of potential medical benefits, like reducing the stress response on genes and potentially promoting longevity.[11] It's pain-relieving, anxiolytic (combats anxiety), and may also be therapeutic for people with addiction. In nature, b-caryophyllene is found in black pepper, cinnamon, oregano, and basil. It's most often described as "peppery" and can be found in higher ratios in strains that have a spicy or a fuel-like smell, such as GSC (formerly known as Girl Scout Cookies) and Bubba Kush—two of my faves!

**Linalool**, also found in lavender and birch bark, gives off a light, floral scent and has been studied for its soothing influence. Few strains feature linalool as their dominant terpene, but Kosher Kush and Zkittlez usually have enough to be detected in a sniff test. Linalool is thought to activate the body's parasympathetic nervous system—nicknamed the "rest-and-digest" system—because that's exactly what your body does when you're at ease: it rests and it digests. When you're stressed, on the other hand, your body tenses, your breath gets shallow, and your digestive process effectively ceases as you get ready to fight, flee, or freeze. So linalool—much like yoga—may help turn off the flood of stress-related chemicals like cortisol and adrenaline.

**Humulene** is one more terpene worth mentioning; though it's found in small quantities in cannabis, this hoppy or woody-smelling terpene is noteworthy for its potential as an anticancer, anti-inflammatory, and antibacterial agent.

✿ ✿ ✿

While I recommend getting to know your terpenes, unfortunately, most states with legal weed don't yet *require* labeling for terpene content the way they do for THC and CBD. Some companies include terpene lab results anyway, and I encourage you to inquire about them when you're in the market for flower; the industry is consumer-driven all the way, so keep asking for what you want.

Until labeling for terpene content is required, use your nose when choosing flower (if your dispensary allows it, of course!)—not to discern specific terpene ratios exactly (though you may well identify citrus, pine, floral, fruity, skunky, and fuel scents) but to determine whether that particular flower supports your health and happiness.

Trust your body. Take a deep sniff and let the scent hit your limbic system, the emotional center most connected with your sense of smell, and see how you feel. If you *feel* good and if the flower smells delicious, chances are it's a good one for you. On the other hand, if it smells gross, or weird, or otherwise unappealing, keep looking.

It's okay if terpenes still seem a little vague at this point; get to know your cannabis smells and they won't be a mystery for too long. Some say that terpenes are the next frontier in cannabis research and consumer experience—definitely worth exploring, if you ask me.

# CANNABIS AND YOU

## ENDOCANNABINOID SYSTEM

If you ever go down the rabbit hole of online cannabis research, you're bound to come across this term. (But I'm writing this book so you don't have to do that!) It's pronounced *end-o-can-AB-in-oid*, and it's a super-cool thing that you should run out and buy immediately. Just kidding, you already have one.

Your endocannabinoid system (ECS) lives primarily in your nervous system and is a complex bunch of interrelated chemicals, receptors, and enzymes that researchers are deep in the process of learning about. Interestingly, our bodies actually produce two cannabinoids (known as "endocannabinoids" because they are endogenous, or naturally occurring), called anandamide and 2-arachidonoylglyerol (2-AG), which bind to receptors found in various parts of the body. Cannabinoid 1 (CB1) receptors, as part of the body's endocannabinoid system, are found mostly in the central nervous system (brain and spinal cord), while cannabinoid 2 (CB2) receptors hang out in the peripheral nervous system (scattered throughout your body) as well as in the brain, GI tract, immune system, and other spots.

When you take in plant-based cannabinoids (from cannabis, of course!), THC will bind to those CB1 and CB2 receptors—causing a cascade of effects in the body and mind. And that's because the job of the ECS is to help us with homeostasis, or physiological equilibrium, so that we can eat, rest, procreate, and live healthfully. The ECS, as it turns out, is really important in that it influences such functions as appetite, sleep, mood, pain signals, memory, stress, and inflammation, among other things.[12]

I spoke about the ECS with Emma Chasen, a cannabis educator and consultant with a science background, tons of industry experience, and a special knack for distilling cannabis concepts for laypeople. She tells me that, whenever one or more of the basic functions I just mentioned get out of whack, the ECS starts whirring and humming to bring it all back into balance. It does that by releasing anandamide and 2-AG, which help the body find homeostasis and, interestingly enough, make you feel good, too. If you're hungry or tired or in pain, your endocannabinoids are meant to engage and help your body come back to a physiologically sound place. But when a higher volume of endocannabinoids gets released in your system, you'll get a temporary lift, or elevation.

The term anandamide comes from the Sanskrit word *ananda*, or bliss. When you feel great after working out (the "runner's high" that you can also get from a flow yoga class or an exhilarating hike), you're feeling the effects of lots of anandamide circulating in your system.

Additionally, 2-AG, which interacts with both your CB1 and CB2 receptors, helps bring your immune system back into balance. This is especially important for people with autoimmune disorders, whose immune systems are not functioning optimally.

Even beyond the ECS, cannabinoids interact with a number of different systems. For instance, they can stop and dally with capsaicin receptors, which regulate the way we respond to pain. CBD is known to engage with vanilloid receptors; that may be another key to how CBD seems to help with pain. Indeed, cannabinoids are "promiscuous," says Chasen, because of how much they get around with different receptors and systems all over the body.

But what if your ECS isn't functioning well? Cannabis researcher Ethan Russo, MD, has suggested that, because of chronic stress, a bunch of us are probably going through our lives with insufficient amounts of circulating endocannabinoids. It's called the theory of endocannabinoid deficiency, and Chasen explains it for us:

"The enzyme that's produced as a result of us being stressed degrades anandamide. When we're stressed, we make this enzyme and store it in our cells. That enzyme from stress is so accumulated in all our tissues because we're all so chronically stressed because the world is *crazy*, and it immediately degrades our endocannabinoids before those endocannabinoids can complete any kind of systemic change or have therapeutic value."

And that, says Chasen, is where plant-based cannabinoids come in. Yes, THC binds to CB1 and CB2 receptors and causes its own cascade of homeostasis-promoting, feel-good effects, but THC and CBD *also* help the body accumulate its own endocannabinoids by preventing their degradation. THC and CBD jump on fatty acid–binding proteins (FABPs), which Chasen says "are responsible for picking up anandamide and transporting it to its demise." With the FABPs otherwise occupied, she says, "anandamide can still hang out and do its thing." In other words, part of the reason we feel good when we use cannabis is that THC and CBD help our naturally occurring, feel-good molecules hang around just a bit longer.

Conventional medicine doesn't have a great track record with treating migraines, fibromyalgia, IBS, and certain other conditions related to pain and inflammation—and that could be, hypothesizes Dr. Russo, because pharmaceuticals temporarily dull the pain but don't address the underlying ECS deficiency. But guess what does? Cannabis, of course!

CBD doesn't have much affinity for CB1 or CB2 receptors and, instead, seems to do other helpful things like activate serotonin receptors—which help support some of the same functions as the ECS, like appetite, sleep, mood, and memory. In addition to helping prevent the brain from clearing out its store of anandamide, CBD works in so many other cool ways in the body. For a close look at CBD science, check out an online resource, Project CBD.

# SESH

This is the moment you use cannabis, of course! Your session, or sesh, is when you get together with your weed mom friends—or cozy up on your own—and elevate. Maybe you're smoking a bowl (consisting of a bit of ground-up flower in a glass pipe) or rolling a joint (aka a "jay"). Maybe you're munching on a brownie or a gummy, or dosing with tincture. Or, perhaps, you're just taking a moment for a few draws from your favorite vape.

Whichever mode of consumption you're employing, and whether you're smoking socially or flying solo, this, weed moms, is your sesh. My advice? Take a couple of deep, slow breaths. Sense your body—the air on your skin, the touch of your clothes, your feet on the floor. Remind yourself of what you seek from cannabis, the *why* behind the choice to use this plant. Inspiration? Self-care? Relief? Pleasure? You may want to offer a quick blessing or expression of gratitude at this moment—if that's the kind of thing you like to do. Feel your body and your mind start to relax. Enjoy your sesh.

## ENTOURAGE EFFECT

As the guy who discovered the molecular structures of THC and CBD back in the sixties, Raphael Mechoulam, PhD, of Hebrew University in Jerusalem is often called the father of cannabis research. In 1998, he introduced the theory of "the entourage effect," the idea that the various compounds in cannabis work better together than apart. They boost one another's signals, so to speak.

Extrapolating, some say that products with exclusively THC or CBD won't bring the full suite of therapeutic benefits the way whole-flower products do. The latter naturally include an array of the major cannabinoids (THC and CBD), some of the minor ones (like THCV, CBG, and CBN), and terpenes. The problem is, medical research methods are best suited to studying individual compounds, and consequently, three of the four cannabis-based medications that have so far been approved (Cesamet, Epidiolex, Marinol) contain only single-molecule—in some cases synthetic—versions of THC or CBD. And though the medications *do* provide relief for patients, they may not be as effective as whole-plant medicine.[13]

What does all this mean for you? Honestly, no one can say with total certainty, but my money is on the value of whole-plant medicine over partial plant medicine. That's why I prefer full-spectrum cannabis—like flower is, naturally. But you can also find a wide array of full-spectrum manufactured stuff, from tinctures to oils to vapes to edibles.

# THE LEGAL CANNABIS MARKETPLACE

## BUDTENDER

Finally, an easy one! Budtenders are the people working at dispensaries. Their job is to help you decode the dispensary and find what you want. They'll meet you where you are—whether you're walking through the dispensary doors as a complete newbie or an OG cannabis consumer. Just be honest about what you're looking for and what you know and don't know. Ask them lots of questions. I find budtenders are often both friendly and knowledgeable. And, if they're not, find another dispensary.

That being said, you may run into budtenders who don't know as much as they probably should. Many—though not all of them—are really young because 1) if you were born in the late nineties you probably have fewer weird hang-ups about the plant, and 2) budtending is a retail job that's better suited to people whose college loans aren't yet in repayment status.

Because budtending gigs have the lowest barrier to entry in the industry, be aware that in newer markets you might find people who insist the indica/ sativa dichotomy is totally real. But in more mature markets, like Portland, Oregon, and California's Bay Area, you'll likely encounter extremely cannabis-savvy folks working as budtenders. So it varies. But, honestly, all budtenders I've ever encountered have been kind, at the very least, and that ain't nothing.

# DISPENSARY

So what, exactly, is a dispensary? It's a retail shop that's licensed by the state to sell medical or adult-use cannabis, or both. If you're in a state with legalized medical marijuana only, you'll first need a recommendation from a doctor (more on that in a moment), but if you're in a state that allows both, you'll only need a valid ID showing that you're over 21 to access recreational weed.

Usually, you'll enter the building via a reception area, where your ID will be checked and a guard may ask to peek inside your bag—standard compliance and security stuff. After that, you may have to wait in the lounge area for a bit if they're busy, or you may get buzzed in to the retail area right away. Some dispensaries feature a "boutique style" layout, where you can stroll and peruse the pretty displays at your leisure, while others are more "pharmacy style," which means that you'll need to wait in line to talk to, and then make your purchase directly from, the budtender.

If you're in a medical-only state, start by researching the qualifying conditions. Some states have restrictive parameters that seriously limit medical marijuana access, while other states are more open-minded toward medical Mary Jane for conditions like migraines and anxiety. If you think you may qualify based on a health concern, you'll need to plan for how you'll get your recommendation. Since legal dispensaries have to comply with all state and local regulations, there are a number of variations on how it's done. Some states allow medical marijuana doctors to write recommendations right from the store, while others require that you meet with a doctor beforehand or make an appointment just to come into the dispensary. Best bet is to call your closest dispensary and ask how it's done there. There are also numerous online sites that help you locate a practitioner with a few clicks.

Like all retail, dispensaries feature gradations of posh. Some have the streamlined look of an Apple store and others feature a Nordstrom-like swank. There are also middle-of-the-road dispensaries, holes in the wall, and everything in between. In addition to looks and price points, dispensaries do vary when it comes to the subtleties of vibe. For decades, cannabis culture in the US has been stoner culture, and stoner culture can feel very bro-centric and possibly unwelcoming, if you're not a bro. Some of the pot-related marketing campaigns of days past relied on juvenile and sexist tropes like "stoner babes" in skimpy bikinis posing on the hoods of cars with penis-shaped bongs. Yep, sex has always sold, and stoner culture is no exception. (Commence deep eye roll.)

And while this kind of nonsense can *still* be found, the alternatives are growing more widespread. Yes, some dispensaries burst at the seams with a *duuuuude* vibe, but others are more neutral, or wellness-oriented. Veronica Castillo, a cannabis writer who's visited dozens of dispensaries in multiple states, told me that each one reflects the culture of the place and the people who live and work there. In the Oregon and Washington beach communities, for instance, Veronica says that the dispensaries tend to project a laid-back hippie feel resplendent with tie-dye and sixties rock posters that appeal to anyone who remembers that era fondly. And while she enjoys those kinds of dispensaries, those spots don't reflect the same diversity that Veronica, a woman of color, finds in Portland, for instance— where the staff as well as the consumers come from all places and all walks.

"Las Vegas dispensaries are larger than life—which is totally in line with Vegas," Emma Chasen tells me. She describes huge facilities and mountains of merch. On the opposite end of the spectrum, some Eastern states with established medical programs that are just opening up to the adult-use market have a more clinical, doctor's office kind of feel to their dispensaries.

And while I prefer dispensaries with a laid-back, craft vibe, it's still kinda cool to see the many incarnations of canna-retail out there. Western states, in Chasen's view, lead the pack with longstanding cultural norms around cannabis. "The West Coast had a leg up when it came to legalization because people already had a lot of ideas on how to operate comfortably in that space," she says.

Veronica notes that dispensary employees in some states check your ID only once when you walk in, while others—like in Colorado and Nevada—seem a little OCD about the whole thing and insist on verifying your identity every time you move one foot to the left. When comparing dispensary experiences across states, Chasen tells me that, because of the lack of a coherent federal system, there are definite differences right now when it comes to compliance and that impacts how dispensaries can display their product, and how customers can interact with that product.

In Washington, for instance, state law requires that all flower be pre-packaged. But in Oregon, "the capitol of craft cannabis," smelling and admiring flower before it's measured out for you is not only permitted, but encouraged. California varies more than most states, but it's still possible in many spots to feast your eyes on the mounds of unpackaged bud and really get your smell on.

All these factors and more influence how you're going to feel while shopping and will also help determine whether your dispensary feels merely transactional or like a community space. Your city and state, the part of town where the dispensary is located, and what its founders and employees bring to the table are all factors here. Point is, dispensaries are not all alike. Shop around if you can.

Just please, please, *pretty* please, patronize a legal dispensary and not a fly-by-night that's parading as one. In some markets (LA is notorious for this), illegal operators set up shop in brick-and-mortar storefronts that lend them the air of legitimacy. You shouldn't assume that it's a legit and licensed shop because there's an "open" sign in the window or they advertise on the internet.

So how do you identify unlicensed cannabis retail? Look for red flags like failing to check IDs, handing out weed in plastic baggies, or using packaging that looks flimsy, counterfeit, or reused. There's a good deal of counterfeit product on the illegal market—so keep your eyes out.

If you're in California, you can use the Bureau of Cannabis Control's license search tool, available on their website or as an app, to make sure you're patronizing a licensed dispensary. But the most direct way to ascertain your shop's legal status is to ask an employee, "Is this dispensary licensed by the state and compliant with all regulations?" and "May I see your license?" Considering the risk you, or any consumer, would take by patronizing an illegal dispensary, it's not a big ask. If they're operating legally, they'll be happy to prove it.

I won't lie—taxes at dispensaries are, ummm, *high*, and not in the good way. But as a point of comparison, I want to clarify that moderate cannabis use—even if you patronize the Nordstrom of dispensaries—is still *way* cheaper than moderate alcohol use. Sure, I can drop a chunk of change at a dispensary, but it'll provide me with a month or more of daily elevation. And since I spend, let's see—*nothing*—on alcohol and pharmaceuticals, I see my dispensary habit as a worthy investment in well-being.

The licensed market offers protections you just can't find on the illicit market. Products are tested and labeled for THC and CBD content (and terpenes, too, if you're lucky). Suppliers for the legal market need to pass all sorts of regulatory hurdles, comply with safety standards, and ensure that products are free from contaminants and dangerous fillers like those first discovered in illegal vapes in 2019. Plus, when you buy legally, you can trace where your product was grown and what the companies you're supporting are up to. If you buy on the illicit market, it's a total crapshoot, and even though you'll save money, it just isn't worth it.

In case you need another incentive to buy on the regulated market: legalized cannabis will only work on a large scale if we support the fledgling industry with dollah bills, y'all. We wanted it. We voted for it. And I say this with much love—time to pony up.

# WEED MOM Q&A

**Q: So what's it like to get high?**

**A:** If you've somehow managed to get through adolescence and young adulthood as a total cannabis virgin, know that you may not actually get high the first time. This happens to a subset of people and theories on the phenomenon range from "you *are* high, you just don't know how to recognize it" to "your ECS is parched and needs to be replenished with phyto-cannabinoids first." If this happens to be you, be patient, and don't worry. Keep trying—you'll get there eventually.

For me, feeling high is *awesome*. I can access the fabled flow state, when I feel aware but not self-conscious, creative yet relaxed, and totally functional while unencumbered by the repetitive, often anxious habits of ordinary mind. And, yet, enhancing with cannabis is a subjective experience that's mediated not only through the peculiarities of each person's ECS, but also through their expectations and the cultural norms they've internalized around the use of weed. It also depends on the user's mood before they consume and the setting, or locale, in which they do so.

All that said, most people who've consumed the right dose of cannabis experience "elevation," or being high, as a mellow kind of euphoria. With the right partner—or solo—sex can unfold at a *where have you been all my life* kind of level. For many of us, appetite and gustatory pleasure are also enhanced, though the munchies get kinda a bad rap. In my experience, eating a nourishing, homemade meal while high is *way* more satisfying than scarfing down a bag of Cheetos.

People describe getting high as slowing down to appreciate each moment in its entirety instead of perpetually leaning into the next one. Things like watching the way light filters through a window or inhaling the fresh scent of earth after rain can feel sensuous, satisfying, and even transcendent, like a drop of grace from the Universe or from God, if that's the sort of thing you believe. Indeed, spiritual experiences are often reported by cannabis lovers who spend time in nature, prayer, and meditation. It's also a powerful tool for self-reflection, as Bob Marley famously pointed out: "When you smoke the herb, it reveals you to yourself."

Depending on the consumer's personality and the strain they use, elevating with cannabis can bring on free-flowing thoughts and associations, fanciful imaginative meanderings (I mean, what *is* the deal with UFOs?), and occasional big breakthroughs. A 1975 study found that low doses of THC may promote something called "divergent thinking,"[14] which is one measure of creativity that consists of a kind of nonlinear, "outside-the-box" approach that helps in brainstorming, problem-solving, and unconventional solutions.

For some people, the right strain and dose of cannabis is an incredible focusing tool, helping hone attention to tasks as varied as composing music, gardening, solving equations, performing Shakespeare, and surfing. Other strains, or heavier doses, can engender a to-the-bones kind of *settling* that does wonders to ease aching bodies and harried minds.

## Weed Moms Speak on What Elevating Feels Like

"Like a hot blanket fresh out of the dryer giving my brain a hug."
—*Sierra, mom of 2, Massachusetts*

"It puts you in more of a childlike state—like when you would color just because you got new crayons." —*Toni, mom of 2, Massachusetts*

"It's like your senses are enhanced, and everything around you is magical. You just genuinely feel great and happy. Almost like looking at everything with 'new eyes' and then ending with a strong need to eat (cue the munchies!)." —*Anonymous mom*

"Your mind is completely unloosed, freely associating ideas and presenting you with totally new ways of looking at the world. It's just utter freedom and bliss." —*Georgia, mom of 3, Massachusetts*

"It's like listening to your favorite song...you hear it and it comes over you and fills you up with happiness, wakes you up, literally, and to your surroundings. It makes you think about what that song means to you, broadens your mind as to what it means to someone else...The groove is right and the sun is shining, you're smiling and alive and present and ready, and you know it'll be a good day." —*Rachel, mom of 2, Massachusetts*

"Meditational, euphoric, creative... My kids used to say, 'mom smokes happy grass.'" —*Celeste, mom of 2 and grandma, Massachusetts*

"Psychotherapy with God." —*Jill, mom of 5, Massachusetts*

"I get a powerful sense of connectedness. How people are connected to each other. How society is connected, how nature is connected, how we are connected with nature... The smallest of details can house an entire world." —*Jennifer, mom of 1, New Hampshire*

"I really hear song lyrics and understand them. Music in general is just amazing. I feel like I'm floating instead of dragging through life. And I just want to hug everything." —*Erica, mom of 1, Massachusetts*

"It adds rose-colored glasses to life." —*Julie, mom of 3, Massachusetts*

"It feels like the weight of the world is lifted and the stress melts away. Getting high connects me to the spirit of my inner child: imaginative, positive, curious, and present. It's downright liberating." —*Kristin, mom of 1, stepmom of 1, Connecticut*

**Q: Isn't it bad/unhealthy/morally wrong to take a drug?**

**A:** Americans (including yours truly), in the words of cannabis writer Sophie Saint Thomas, have "hang-ups about pleasure."

"It probably goes back to the seven deadly sins and the Puritan foundation of this country," Jennifer, a cannabis-loving mom from New Hampshire told me. Meaning anything that doesn't fit neatly into the buckets of hard work, self-restraint, and thrift—is suspect. Meaning it's still hard for some people to wrap their heads around sex for pleasure, not procreation. Meaning that, to many Americans, recreational drugs, which exist to help people *feel* good, must *be* bad.

Here's my two cents: humans have been deliberately altering consciousness in some way or another for basically—well for a very long time. Thirteen thousand years ago, semi-nomadic peoples were brewing beer[15] in the Middle East. Indigenous Amazonians somehow figured out that if you scrape a small amount of toxic substance from the back of a giant leaf frog, you can experience different dimensions of your own mind and possibly even break your worst habits, like addiction.[16] There are countless other examples of tools employed to temporarily alter the way we see the world and ourselves. From alcohol to caffeine to opium to sugar to coca to antidepressants, attempting to influence ordinary waking consciousness toward the joyful, mystical, creative, revelatory, or peaceful side of our natures is a basic impulse that's found in people everywhere.

Even beyond both licit and illicit drugs, if you put everything people spend money on to expand consciousness or change the way they feel into one category, you'll find trillions of dollars spent globally on the "altered states economy" each year.[17] Drugs are in there, yes, but personal growth, media, and recreation also fit the category. If you've ever paid for a yoga class or a cocktail or a self-help seminar, that's all part of it. We as a species are on a constant search to change the way we feel for the better. It's utterly human.

Dr. Andrew Weil, whom many people know as a complementary and alternative medicine guru, wrote on this issue back in 1972. In *Natural Mind: A New Way of Looking at Drugs and the Higher Consciousness*, Weil revisited the foundational "hierarchy of human needs theory" by Abraham Maslow and took it a step further to argue that altered consciousness in some form or another may be a basic human need. While taking a drug to alter consciousness *isn't* the need, doing so is *one way* to meet the need. As long as those who alter their consciousness with psychoactive substances do so responsibly and cause no harm to others, the behavior needn't be judged or maligned.

In my view, there's nothing inherently wrong with trying to alter your state of mind or being. Yoga is one way I do this. Meditation is another. Being thoughtful about my food choices, the media I consume, and the amount of exercise I get all come into play here for me—and I'd guess for you, too. I see little distinction between these things and cannabis; when used thoughtfully, all are pieces of self-care that alter my ordinary state just enough to help me function optimally and feel great.

Do I like to feel great? Hell yeah! And is it okay for a responsible adult to take a drug to help bring that about? I think so—as long as you can reflect on your decisions while honestly observing the consequences. Ask yourself questions such as:

◊ How often do you want to take this drug, and how often do you actually take it?

◊ What are its impacts on your health—both short and long term?

◊ Do you feel like yourself when under the influence, or do your thoughts, feelings, and behavior change significantly?

◊ How do you feel when you stop using the drug?

◊ How does using this drug affect your important relationships? What about your work?

◊ Do you feel happier, healthier, and more at peace in your own skin with this drug in your life?

For me, cannabis use is absolutely compatible with being a good mom, having a career, and making health a priority. I don't use more of it than I plan to, and I feel better—not worse—the moments and days afterward.

You may have grown up on the DARE program and Just Say No campaign, like I did. You may have been force-fed all the fear-mongering about how marijuana is an addictive gateway drug that will turn you into a braindead loser. But I'm smart enough to observe the real-world effects of using cannabis for wellness and fun, and to make my own good decisions—and so are you.

Personally, I choose not to medicate pain with opioids or NSAIDs, or to seek help for anxiety in a bottle of benzos. I choose, for the most part, not to drink alcohol because it makes me feel sleepy while imbibing and something akin to roadkill the next day. Cannabis helps me feel healthy, happy, and well, while also giving me—here's that word again—*pleasure*. And I, for one, am straight-up owning it.

# CHAPTER 3

# BEYOND REEFER MADNESS: A BRIEF HISTORY OF HUMANS AND CANNABIS

## THE LONG LOVE AFFAIR

From its home in Central Asia, cannabis has, umm, *flowered* into an incredibly successful and varied species. Today, thousands of domestic and wild cultivars thrive in indoor and outdoor environments as diverse as the people who use and love them. Humans probably first cultivated the plant for its fibrous stalks and nutritive seed oil, but medical, spiritual, and euphoric uses didn't wait long in the wings. Evidence for early cannabis use pops up in many ancient texts, like Herodotus's fifth-century BCE work, *The Histories*, which detailed the practice of burning and inhaling cannabis smoke for recreational and spiritual purposes.[18]

In 2008, the excavation of an archaeological site left by the Jushi people in northwestern China dating from twenty-seven centuries ago was found to contain a quantity of THC-rich cannabis. Because it was flower, not hemp fiber, found in a shaman's gravesite, researchers believe this is the first material evidence of the plant's use as a ritualistic aid.[19] In 2019, an analysis of the Jirzankal Cemetery site, also in western China, yielded wooden braziers (pipes, essentially) and the charred remains of psychoactive cannabis that was thought to be burned and consumed in 500 BCE.

References to cannabis in traditional Chinese medicine (TCM) date from around 200 CE, and some researchers have proposed that the psychoactive properties of the plant were known and utilized by that time.

On the Indian subcontinent (from which we—and the Jamaicans—borrowed the name *ganja*), cannabis has long been associated with Shiva, god of meditation, yoga, and the arts. It figures in Ayurvedic medicine as a remedy for anxiety, sleep, fever, appetite, and depressed mood—a suite of psychopharmacological uses that sounds familiar, given today's most common wellness uses for the plant. And there's a long and venerable tradition in India of wandering, mendicant holy men known as *sadhus*, who smoke hashish (a potent cannabis concentrate) and imbibe a milky, cannabis-infused preparation called *bhang* to reach new heights of spiritual adeptness.

Psychoactive cannabis and its derivatives have been smoked and treasured for hundreds, if not thousands, of years in Asia and the greater Middle East, from Afghanistan to Nepal to Morocco to Persia, and those traditions persist in many places, despite heavy penalties.

Hemp, as we know, was grown all across Europe and the early American colonies for use as a fiber in paper, ship sails, rope, and textiles. And while Europeans and American colonists, including George Washington himself, grew hemp, it's unlikely that they knew anything about its psychoactive properties. The hemp they were growing probably had very little THC, anyway, as THC-rich varieties tend to thrive in warmer climates (or indoors).

# PUFF, PUFF, PASSED AROUND THE WORLD

It wasn't until the 1800s—after learning from colonized Indians about the therapeutic and psychoactive qualities of THC-rich cannabis—that Europeans began using the plant as medicine. By the 1850s, cannabis tinctures were a staple in European and American apothecaries, marketed as a remedy for a wide variety of ailments, including nausea, low appetite, tremors, and epilepsy. And hashish-eating as a form of recreation for artists and bohemians became a thing in Europe after the Napoleonic wars, when French soldiers brought the habit home from Egypt.

But the heyday of cannabis medicine in the West eventually faded as those crude cannabis formulas were replaced by early pharmaceuticals such as barbiturates, aspirin, and morphine. That's possibly because many pharmaceutical drugs are actually far less complex and varied than cannabis medicine. While cannabis works through more targeted and specific pathways, morphine "is more like a machine gun," Isaac Balbin, PhD, owner of a cannabis software company called Parsl, tells me. But without the scientific means to investigate its complexities, cannabis medicine was considered less effective than the newer, bigger guns.

Indigenous Africans had known about the psychoactive properties of cannabis for hundreds of years by the time untold numbers of them were kidnapped and forced into slavery by Europeans. People from places as far apart on the African continent as equatorial Guinea and traditional Zulu lands knew how to prepare and inhale cannabis smoke from clay pipes, bamboo stalks, or earthen mounds; in fact, it's likely that enslaved Africans brought the first psychoactive cannabis seeds to the New World aboard European slave ships, and that some of the first cannabis in the Americas was tended in Brazil by those slaves and their descendants.[20]

Climate conditions in parts of Central and South America favored THC-rich strains; some of this new kind of weed grew wild, and some was deliberately cultivated by slaves and former slaves. Indigenous peoples in the Americas probably learned from Africans about the plant's euphoric properties and how it could help soothe the pains of physical labor.

Even back then, big business was involved in the movement of cannabis around the world. Barney Warf, PhD, professor of geography at the University of Kansas, tells me that the British East India Company played a role in establishing cannabis in the Caribbean. Indentured Indian servants may have already been in the habit of consuming, and the company imported the products to sell in the Caribbean and appease the underclass. Indeed, as Warf told me, there were probably "multiple entry points" of cannabis to the New World. Eventually, it spread to Mexico, which is where the American cannabis story heats up.

"Evidence suggests that the large-scale entry of cannabis occurs after the Mexican Revolution of 1910," Warf tells me, "when there were lots of Mexican refugees fleeing the violence and moving into Texas. And, almost immediately thereafter, you start getting backlash against it because it was seen as a brown people's drug."

It may shock you, but up until the early 1900s, the federal government wasn't in the business of regulating drugs—whether for medical or recreational purposes. Picture a moment when cocaine was part of the Coca-Cola recipe, opium dens flourished in San Francisco, and heroin injection kits could be purchased at Sears. Few people then gave any thought to the legal status of cannabis. In fact, by 1920, alcohol was considered a much more pernicious substance when the Eighteenth Amendment—outlawing alcohol's production, sale, and consumption—went into effect. Alcohol prohibition lasted a tumultuous thirteen years; by the time it was legalized again, the demonization of cannabis was well underway.

At the time, smoking weed—often known as reefer—was common among Black jazz artists such as Louis Armstrong, Ella Fitzgerald, and Cab Calloway, who felt that cannabis helped loosen inhibitions and spur their improvisational musings. Cannabis forged social bonds between people of the counterculture, Black and white, and its social consumption in jazz clubs in New Orleans, Chicago, and New York helped create an unusually integrated subculture. "When the African American community picked up on it," says Warf, "especially jazz musicians in New Orleans, it became known to the federal government as a brown and Black people's drug."

Meanwhile, the decades-long migration of Mexicans to Texas and the Southwest motivated some particularly angry white people to scapegoat them for all kinds of things—in ways that eerily mirror some of the anti-immigrant rhetoric today. This is when the term "marijuana" (rendered as "marihuana" at the time) became part of the American lexicon and was invoked in race-baiting smear campaigns that perpetuated outright lies and fanned xenophobic hysteria.

William Randolph Hearst, newspaper magnate and famously rich asshole, had a personal vendetta against Mexicans and marijuana because some of his vast holdings in northern Mexico were overrun by Pancho Villa's army during the war. Hearst directed writers to engage in anti-Mexican and anti-marijuana slander. He created the kind of fact-free newsroom environment that gave rise to the term "yellow journalism," perfectly described by historian and journalist Frank Mott as relying on "crime news, scandal and gossip, divorces and sex, and stress upon the reporting of disasters and sports,"[21] while ignoring the most pressing social and political issues of the day.

# ORIGINS OF AMERICAN PROHIBITION

Enter Harry Anslinger, an ambitious and prejudiced federal employee who was appointed director of the brand-new Federal Bureau of Narcotics (FBN) in 1930. At first, the FBN (precursor to the DEA) ignored cannabis, but within a few years Anslinger—nearly single-handedly—managed to orchestrate a total one-eighty when it came to federal policy on the plant. A concentrated campaign of propaganda and fear-mongering morphed marijuana into public enemy number one. Anslinger used any means necessary to defame the plant and the people who partook of it—denouncing it as "the Devil Weed," which would cause innocent (white) youth to descend into insanity, murder, and rape. This was the "Reefer Madness" era, which predated—and set the scene for—the American War on Drugs.

Though a few states had already banned it, the Marihuana Tax Act of 1937 was the first national legislation aimed at the plant; it effectively outlawed cannabis, including hemp, by rendering it prohibitively expensive through taxation and by a weird catch-22 that made registering to even pay the tax a self-incriminating act. (The law was found unconstitutional by the Supreme Court in 1969.) Apparently, the feds and Anslinger chose taxation as the smoothest road to cannabis prohibition because the Federal Bureau of Narcotics was housed in the Treasury Department. Weird times!

At any rate, the Boggs Act, signed into law in 1951, explicitly set criminal parameters for marijuana—succeeding and outpacing the prior act.[22]

A number of theories swirl around the origins of prohibition. Cannabis activist Jack Herer embraced the notion that the Mellon family, owners of DuPont, pressured the feds to penalize all hemp and marijuana in order to protect their own profits. Martin A. Lee, author of a book on cannabis social history called *Smoke Signals* (2012) and director of Project CBD, tells me, "It's not implausible. There's just no evidence."

Lee confirms what I've heard from many quarters: when it comes to cannabis prohibition, "it's about racism, first and foremost."

Professor Warf also emphasized the racist roots of prohibition. "As soon as white law enforcement authorities found that they could weaponize cannabis against Latino and Black communities, they began to enact laws against it—first in El Paso and then elsewhere—never based on any scientific evidence." In fact, Warf tells me, "so much of the War on Drugs from the beginning until today is based on racism."

It's easy to point out the ridiculous histrionics of Reefer Madness, but many people were convinced that cannabis made you both irreconcilably crazy and violent. Some saw through the false narrative, however, leading to one of the biggest ironies around pot prohibition in this country: when Anslinger began his anti-marijuana campaign, it's estimated that only about 50,000 Americans—mostly Black and Latinx people—were smoking it. After ten years of "Reefer Madness" type propaganda, the number was probably closer to 100,000.[23] As it turns out, prohibition does not just fail to squash demand; it may even encourage people to consume.

Worth mentioning is the fact that Anslinger's Reefer Madness rhetoric was later flipped on its head; by 1948, Anslinger preyed upon Americans' Cold War–era fears about the spread of communism in declaring to Congress that "marijuana leads to pacifism and communist brainwashing." The plant he once described as "the most violence-causing drug in the history of mankind" was now painted as the ultimate drug of idleness, which would render American masses lazy and utterly unable to stave off the Red Army.

Interestingly, few lawmakers in Anslinger's day were even familiar with the intoxicating uses of the plant, though "cannabis" was known to them in hemp form as an industrial crop. By calling it "marijuana," Anslinger was conferring "other" or "foreign" status on the plant and also confusing a good number of people who had no idea that marijuana was no more than a variation of hemp.

In the 1950s, Beat writers, poets, and activists took on the mantle of cannabis as a tool for creativity and nonconformity. Many beatniks saw pot as a political issue, a means to preserve the essential freedom of one's own mind. Allen Ginsberg and other members of the Beat scene were famously surveilled and harassed by cops and the FBN, who feared their ilk as a fundamental threat to the emerging consumption-oriented, law-and-order ethos of the 1950s.

Those fears were confirmed when hippies took up not only pot-smoking, but psychedelics like LSD. In the 1960s, hundreds of thousands of young people showed up for anti-Vietnam war protests, civil disobedience, and music festivals like Woodstock, where weed and LSD were as commonplace as tie-dye and hairy armpits. Many American soldiers in Vietnam smoked marijuana for the very first time while on active duty, and some of those young men continued to use the herb to ease post-traumatic stress and physical pain once they returned.

Within a few decades of prohibition, weed had suffused American pop culture. Bands like the Beatles (and later, Jimi Hendrix, Bob Marley, Willie Nelson, and the Grateful Dead) helped introduce their huge international fan bases to "grass," and by 1979, 51 percent of American high school seniors partook.[24] Meanwhile, millions of ordinary Americans were realizing that smoking pot was not a slippery slope to ruin.

# NIXON, REAGAN, AND THE WAR ON DRUGS

In the early 1970s, as the government grew increasingly uneasy about rebellious youth and their pot-smoking ways, the modern incarnation of the drug war came into being. Under Nixon, the Controlled Substances Act set the parameters for cannabis and other drugs we still live with today. Marijuana was temporarily classified as a Schedule I drug, indicating that it has a "high abuse potential with no accepted medical use"[25] and the DEA was formed just a few years later.

Nixon commissioned a special report by Pennsylvania governor Richard Shafer. In two-hundred-plus pages, *Marihuana: A Signal of Misunderstanding*,[26] recommended that marijuana be reclassified and decriminalized, as there were—even then—known medical uses and little evidence of harm. Weirdly, cannabis was never rescheduled, while far more dangerous drugs like morphine, oxycodone, and fentanyl—which, along with other opioids, accounted for 47,600 deaths in the US in 2017[27]—appear on the supposedly *less* dangerous Schedule II.

For a while, Mexico was the source of most of the weed sold in the US, but, eventually, the hills of northern California—a near-perfect environment for growing cannabis—became the heart of American cultivation. The primo weed grown in this area, known as the Emerald Triangle, found its way all over the country and the world. A self-reliant, largely off-grid kind of outlaw community developed over the decades there, and these folks revolutionized and refined the art of growing with specialized techniques for separating male and female plants, cloning, cross-breeding, and controlling light, nutrients, and temperature—all with the aim of developing the world's best weed.

Journalist Michael Pollan claims that the most talented horticulturists of the Baby Boomer generation put their skills to use up in the hills of northern California where, over the decades, they created modern, commercial cannabis. The Netherlands, too, became a place of cannabis innovation from the 1970s onward; while it's true that the Dutch government still hasn't fully legalized the plant, cannabis cafes operate openly in Amsterdam and weed botany is practically a Dutch cottage industry.

Under Nixon, penalties for growing, possessing, and dealing grew stiffer and stiffer. The 1970s were the beginning of the era of mandatory minimum sentences—a criminal justice policy that, over the next decades, led to an explosion in the US prison population with a hugely disproportionate impact on communities of color. Sometimes those serving time for drug offenses received harsher sentences and worse treatment than convicted murderers.

John Ehrlichman, a top Nixon aide and Watergate coconspirator, admitted in 1994 that the administration knew they were hyperbolizing the dangers of marijuana to justify warrantless searches, property confiscation, forfeiture, and harsh sentencing. In Ehrlichman's words, the Nixon White House:

"...had two enemies: the antiwar left and black people... We knew we couldn't make it illegal to be either against the war or black, but by getting the public to associate the hippies with marijuana and the blacks with heroin and then criminalizing both heavily, we could disrupt those communities. We could arrest their leaders, raid their homes, break up their meetings, and vilify them night after night on the evening news."[28]

And though Ehrlichman's statement has been challenged as an oversimplification of Nixon-era policy, it's still clear that the drug war—as initiated by Nixon and carried out by future presidents (Reagan, in particular)—came down particularly heavily on Black and brown people. Michelle Alexander, formerly of the American Civil Liberties Union (ACLU), argues in her book, The New Jim Crow (2020), "Nothing has contributed to the mass incarceration of people of color in the United States more than the War on Drugs."[29]

## The War on Drugs at a Glance

» The US has spent about a trillion dollars on the drug war.[30]

» One-fifth of the US prison population is serving time for a drug charge.

» The US incarceration rate far surpasses every country on the planet at 655 per 100,000; by comparison, Russia incarcerates 363 per 100,000, and England incarcerates 140 per 100,000.[31]

» According to the ACLU, Black Americans are four times more likely than white Americans to be arrested for cannabis possession,[32] despite stats showing roughly equal usage among Blacks and whites.

» People of color are much more likely than white people to be stopped, searched, arrested, convicted, and sentenced harshly.

# HOW WE GOT LEGAL WEED

Oh my gosh, there are so many people who worked tirelessly and sacrificed their freedom, property, livelihood, and reputation to get us this far. The Bay Area was the epicenter of the legalization movement, where "compassion" advocates had been selling or giving cannabis at low cost to people with HIV/AIDS, cancer, and other debilitating conditions at least as far back as the early 1990s. It's perfectly logical to approach legalization through the medical pathway because alleviating pain and nausea are two things cannabis does extremely well. Plus, it's a lot simpler to convince canna-skeptics of the rights of dying patients to feel *a little bit better* than it is to convince them of healthy people's rights to pleasure. (Thanks, Puritans!) Across the US, medical programs have pretty much always predated rec programs for these reasons.

Prop 215, also known as the Compassionate Use Act, was the landmark ballot initiative passed in California in 1996, stating that patients and their caregivers could legally possess and cultivate cannabis for medical use, and that doctors could not be punished for recommending cannabis to their patients (though this would be challenged over and over by the state and federal governments).

Prop 215 marked the beginning of a new era; cannabis enthusiasts and weed moms everywhere owe a debt of gratitude to people who made this possible. Here's a whirlwind look at some of those people:

**Allen Ginsberg:** Spearheaded the first marijuana legalization organization

**Jack Herer:** Authored the classic *The Emperor Wears No Clothes*; big-time marijuana activist

**Dennis Peron:** Founded the San Francisco Cannabis Buyer's Club (CBC), the first marijuana dispensary in the US; provided compassionate access for HIV-positive folks in the gay community; coauthored Prop 215

**Mary Jane Rathbun, aka "Brownie Mary":** Baked and delivered homemade cannabis edibles for HIV patients at San Francisco General for years and was involved in Peron's CBC as well as Prop 215

**Tod Mikuriya, MD:** Resurrected the science of medical cannabis; the first physician to recommend the plant to his patients; helped author Prop 215

**Debby Goldsberry:** Cannabis activist and early dispensary operator; in the eighties, Goldsberry's Cannabis Action Network helped change ordinary Americans' minds about medical marijuana

**Valerie Corral:** Founder of the collective Wo/Men's Alliance for Medical Marijuana in Santa Cruz in the early nineties; provided compassionate access to marijuana for seriously ill and injured people almost continually since then; involved in the passage of Prop 215

# LEGAL STATUS OF CANNABIS

According to a 2018 Gallup poll, 66 percent of Americans favor all-out cannabis legalization.[33] A 2019 Pew Research poll found similar results: 59 percent of US adults think cannabis should be legal for both recreation and medicine, and an additional 32 percent say that it should be legal for medicine only.[34] Combined, that means 91 percent of American adults approve of some form of legal marijuana! Decades of incrementally growing acceptance, along with the cascade of state-by-state legalizations, have finally resulted in a sharp upward tick in support of the herb. It's official: the cannabis train is moving in one direction, and that's toward *more* openness, *more* acceptance, and *more* access.

So far, progress has come from state-level initiatives led by voters and legislators, not from the federal government. As of this writing, cannabis is legal for adult use in eleven states and the District of Columbia. The states are:

- Alaska
- California
- Colorado
- Illinois
- Maine
- Massachusetts
- Michigan
- Nevada
- Oregon
- Vermont
- Washington
- Washington, DC

The pioneers here are Colorado and Washington, which both legalized cannabis for adult use by ballot initiative in the 2012 election, though it's worth mentioning that Alaska had decriminalized long before legalizing. After having been a medical-only state for twenty years, California jumped on the adult-use train in 2016, with actual sales starting in January 2018. And as of this writing, Illinois is the most recent to jump on the canna-bandwagon, with a few dozen of its formerly medical-only dispensaries having opened their doors for adult-use sales in early 2020.

As you can probably see, there are 420-friendly[35] clusters in the West and the Northeast, along with a smaller Midwestern cohort. Some suggest a "domino theory," where if one state legalizes, its smarter neighbors gear up for legalization, too.

It's worth noting here that, on the spectrum of legal weed, each of these states exists on a slightly different point. For instance, Colorado, Oregon, Washington, and California have robust, well-developed programs featuring the most consumer-friendly dispensaries anywhere. But even in these 420 havens, some cities still forbid dispensaries or delivery services.

Vermont and Washington, DC, are the adorable, fussy infants of legalization, prohibiting retail sales while allowing personal growing and gifting. (This, however, is likely to change quickly in both Vermont and DC, where retail-friendly tweaks are in the works.) And then there are the toddlers, like Massachusetts and Illinois, who, after establishing medical programs, are dipping their tiny toes into the rec world. Come on Massachusetts and Illinois—you can do it!

# LEGALITY OF MEDICAL MARIJUANA

Hemp-derived CBD is theoretically legal everywhere in the US (see Q&A on page 72), so this section addresses the legality and accessibility of medical THC. California paved the way for what is now an impressive and growing list of states that allow some form of medical access to THC-rich cannabis.

As of this writing, thirty-three states and several territories have medical marijuana programs; numerous states have also enacted decriminalization, meaning that possessing a small amount for personal use will land you a fine instead of jail time.

Because medical initiatives have been fought on a state-by-state level in a similar way that adult-use ones have, there's a good deal of variation when it comes to what exactly qualifies you as a patient. For example, before adult-use legalization in California, my husband got a medical cannabis recommendation in the back room of a hole-in-the-wall dispensary by claiming "chronic joint pain." Uh-huh. By 2016 this was, quite honestly, as common as Brussels sprouts at a gastropub; everyone knew that adult use was just a short jaunt down the road. But that kind of thing would never fly in some of the more conservative medical states, where you'd practically have to be on death's door to get any legal weed.

It's unfortunately true that legal access is all over the map, depending on—umm—where you live on the map. If you live in a medical-only state, it's worth looking into the qualifying conditions—not because you're going to make shit up but because you may legitimately have a condition that's recognized, like anxiety or migraines. Know, too, that laws are changing quickly and access is improving.

You can get involved in advocacy efforts by supporting the work of organizations like the National Organization for the Reform of Marijuana Laws (NORML) and Marijuana Policy Project (MPP). I encourage you to use the tools provided on their websites to lobby your lawmakers in favor of sane cannabis policy with a couple of clicks. And for an entirely up-to-date look at where each state stands vis-à-vis medical and recreational cannabis, check out the MPP's guide, found at www.mpp.org/states/.

# WHAT'S NEXT FOR LEGALIZATION? STATE-BY-STATE INITIATIVES

In November 2020, voters in New Jersey, Arizona, and Montana will vote on recreational cannabis; South Dakota voters will vote on both medical and recreational legalization at the same time, while Mississippi is looking to okay medical use only. Activists and lawmakers in other states seek to legalize cannabis through state legislatures, where dozens of decriminalization and/or legalization bills have been introduced. For the latest, use MPP's online tool to help you track the evolving legal situation across the U.S.: www.mpp.org/issues/legislation/key-marijuana-policy-reform.

# FEDERAL CHANGES IN 2020

To say that COVID-19 fucked a lot of shit up is a gigantic understatement. But there's still hope for two silver linings on the federal level. The Marijuana Opportunity Reinvestment and Expungement (MORE) Act calls for removing cannabis from Schedule I classification and sets aside a portion of cannabis tax revenue for a trust fund benefiting communities of color. That fund would pay for expunging criminal records, reentry programs for those leaving prison with cannabis offenses, and substance abuse treatment programs. The fund would also establish an agency to encourage minority participation in the legal cannabis industry. The MORE Act could really help where a lot of harm was done, and it deserves our support. As of this writing, it has passed through the House Judiciary Committee and is awaiting a full vote on the floor. If you favor cannabis reform at the federal level, let your representatives and senators know.

The second piece of legislation, The Secure and Fair Enforcement (SAFE) Banking Act, would allow marijuana businesses to access banking services (and enable cashless transactions at dispensaries!) without changing cannabis's federal legal status. The act passed the House in September 2019 and sits in a Senate committee as of this writing.

# WEED MOM Q&A

### Q: Is CBD legal everywhere in the US?

**A:** Yes, but it's confusing. The 2018 Farm Bill legalized hemp cultivation and transportation in all fifty states. Remember, hemp contains low levels of THC to begin with. But the law stipulated that all legal hemp under this bill must contain .3 percent THC or less. And while hemp that comes in under .3 percent is now federally legal, states still have some leeway in deciding whether any cannabis products can be grown, transported, or sold in their territory. Some states have been slow AF in accepting and implementing the 2018 Farm Bill.

Ironically, a few months before signing the contract for *Weed Mom*, I moved with my family to a prohibition state. Not only is recreational and medical use currently illegal where I live; until recently, even CBD was considered suspect. But less than a year later, the nonpsychoactive cannabinoid is sold openly in my city, hemp retail shops have popped up, and I can get a CBD-enhanced massage within a mile from my house. So, despite the lag in official policy, even people in prohibition states are finding ways to welcome and normalize cannabis.

# INTERNATIONAL STATUS

On the world stage, attitudes and policies toward medical marijuana are progressing. In 2018, Canada became the second country (after Uruguay) to federally legalize cannabis for adult use. Mexico and New Zealand may both legalize in 2020, and medical programs currently operate in Argentina, Colombia, Croatia, Germany, Greece, Italy, Jamaica, Peru, Poland, and Portugal.

🌿🌿🌿

Thousands of years of human-cannabis interaction comes down to this: we *really* like weed, and it's useful. Twentieth century prohibition was more like a weird blip in our shared history with the plant, because *Cannabis sativa* L. has endured and—thanks to tireless advocates, activists, and renegades—it's thriving. Year by year, access is improving all across the US, just as it should. So let's say we collectively chill TF out about this plant and welcome a new era of cannabis-human love. After all, as I learned from Ricardo Cortés's children's book on medical marijuana, *It's Just a Plant*.

## CHAPTER 4

# BEYOND GETTING HIGH

This is a book about the fun and wellness uses of cannabis for us moms, but because there's so much that cannabis *can* or *may* do, I must at least touch base on the medical side of things. Besides, as I've mentioned before, wellness uses of cannabis do seem to straddle that gap between med and rec—that so-called recredicinal space.

But first, a disclaimer: What's shared below is for informational purposes only. Nothing here should be taken as medical advice. I am not a doctor nor do I advocate self-administering medical cannabis without the guidance of a practitioner.

Okay. I'm back now.

The six most common reasons people use medical cannabis are: pain (61.2%), anxiety (58.1%), depression (50.3%), headache/migraines (35.5%), nausea (27.4%), and muscle spasticity (18.4%).[36] And, like I've said before, many of us aren't medical patients per se, but we use cannabis "recredicinally" to relieve pain or anxiety *while* feeling good.

# COMMON MEDICAL USES OF THC

One of the many bummers about federal prohibition is that it creates an environment where getting approval and funding to study cannabis is really tough. As a result, there's a lot we still don't know. But as cannabis is legalized on a state-by-state basis, some of those restrictions are changing, and new cannabis studies are teaching us a lot about what this plant can do.

## PAIN RELIEF

In the right quantities, THC is pretty much guaranteed to do two things: 1) get you elevated, and 2) relieve pain in some way. Some find the pain-relieving properties of cannabis so effective that they're able to taper and even quit opioids. A 2019 Canadian study found that, of 2,000 medical marijuana patients, 35 percent had chosen cannabis *instead* of opioids to manage pain.[37]

Most people find that cannabis doesn't annihilate pain the way opioids do (of note: opioids become less effective with chronic use). Instead, people report a "quieting down" or "settling" of their pain. (Like when your kids are watching a show without fighting or whining—but they still ask you for snacks every ten minutes. *That* kind of quieting down.)

I asked Jordan Tishler, MD, a Harvard-trained medical marijuana doctor practicing in Massachusetts and director of Inhale MD, about what THC can do.

"I think we can say that pain is pretty well settled," he tells me. "People try to split hairs about whether it's cancer-related pain or neuropathic pain," he adds. "But the data are good for both of those. There was even a study that came out recently that looked at acute traumatic pain—say, you fall off your bike—and cannabis is good for that as well." He points out that the National

Academy of Sciences, Engineering, and Medicine published a report in 2017 supportive of THC's capacity to treat pain.[38]

I also spoke with Rav Ivker, DO, an osteopath in Boulder, Colorado, who recommends medical marijuana to patients with qualifying conditions. Along with patient success stories, in his book, *Cannabis for Chronic Pain* (2017), Ivker described his own medical marijuana experience when treating pain caused by shingles.

Several moms I interviewed for this book use cannabis for some kind of pain, even if they also use it for fun. Jennifer, a New Hampshire mom and functional nutritionist, finds that nightly cannabis tinctures help ease the chronic pain of fibromyalgia. Kristin, an ex-cop from Connecticut and mother to a five-year-old, uses cannabis instead of Vicodin to cope with pain following a bad car accident and spinal fusion surgery. Diana, a writer in Maryland and mother to a toddler, tells me she's found enormous benefit from the pain-relieving properties of cannabis for both endometriosis and Crohn's disease.

I, too, use cannabis for pain; following a five-year wackadoodle rollercoaster of continuous pregnancy and breastfeeding, hormonal migraines began ruining my life for about four out of every twenty-eight days. When I use cannabis moderately and regularly, my headaches are less severe and mostly treatable with a quick sesh. And even though it's a medical use, I never applied for a medical card because I was a late bloomer—products on the rec market meet my modest needs.

# MUSCLE SPASTICITY

So what else can THC do? Dr. Tishler tells me that we have conclusive evidence backing up medical marijuana for spasticity associated with multiple sclerosis (MS) and amyotrophic lateral sclerosis (ALS).[39] These uses don't get a lot of press, he says, because MS and ALS aren't common—but cannabis can improve the quality of life for those who have them.

# NAUSEA AND VOMITING

A large scale review of the scientific literature found THC-rich cannabis more effective at relieving nausea and vomiting in chemotherapy than at least seven common antiemetic (anti-vomiting) drugs.[40] HIV/AIDS, too, often comes along with appetite loss, nausea, and vomiting—and the first real movement on medical marijuana legalization in the US centered on severely ill HIV patients in San Francisco in the 1990s.

# ANXIETY AND DEPRESSION

For anxiety and depression, the two most common mental health diagnoses in US adults to the tune of roughly 19 percent[41] and 7 percent[42], respectively, cannabis appears to have a strongly dose-dependent kind of benefit.

"A little bit of cannabis can be helpful," Dr. Tishler tells me, "but more than a little bit can be harmful." For people with anxiety or depression who use cannabis heavily, he says productivity tends to go down while symptoms might even worsen.

An Italian study on rats found that while low doses of THC reduced anxiety, higher doses had the opposite effect.[43] And though we should be cautious applying animal studies to humans, this kind of dose-dependent effect—for THC, in particular—appears consistent with a lot of anecdotal evidence and clinical practice.

"If we have lower, more meticulous exposure," says Dr. Tishler," and it's timed in a way that doesn't interfere with the activities of daily life, then it can be very helpful." For patients with anxiety and depression, he recommends low doses at bedtime and finds that people get relief lasting well beyond the euphoric or high feeling.

# INFLAMMATION

Inflammation is a necessary immune response that sometimes gets out of control and can contribute to arthritis, skin conditions, ulcerative colitis, and all kinds of other pain. Dr. Ivker calls cannabis a "terrific anti-inflammatory," and many cannabis users find relief from conditions related to inflammation.

This probably has to do with the fact that the ECS plays an important role in immune function and regulation. Cannabinoids are shown to help calm an overactive immune system in mice by reducing the prevalence of two inflammatory proteins known as cytokine and chemokine; though these processes haven't yet been proven in humans, cannabinoids show real promise as anti-inflammatory drugs.[44]

## The 6 Most Common Uses of Medical Cannabis[45]
*(Survey respondents could report medical cannabis use for more than one reason.)*

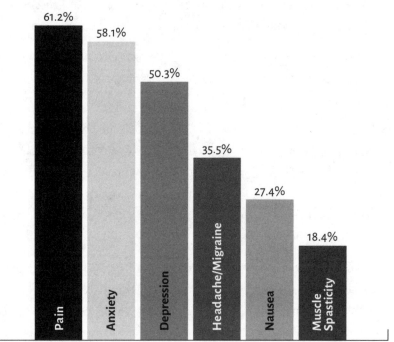

| | |
|---|---|
| Pain | 61.2% |
| Anxiety | 58.1% |
| Depression | 50.3% |
| Headache/Migraine | 35.5% |
| Nausea | 27.4% |
| Muscle Spasticity | 18.4% |

## OTHER POTENTIAL USES

There's a long list of other conditions that THC may help. We don't have a ton of rock-solid evidence about them yet, but we have some preliminary evidence and plenty of stories from people who swear up and down that THC-rich medical marijuana can be helpful for people with the following conditions:

- ◊ autism
- ◊ Crohn's disease
- ◊ eating disorders
- ◊ fibromyalgia
- ◊ glaucoma
- ◊ insufferable basic-ness (jk—that one's treatment-resistant)
- ◊ low sex drive/lack of sexual enjoyment
- ◊ post-traumatic stress disorder (PTSD)
- ◊ rheumatoid arthritis
- ◊ Tourette syndrome
- ◊ traumatic brain injury

For a full accounting of what qualifies for medical marijuana access in your state, visit: https://www.leafly.com/news/health/qualifying-conditions-for-medical-marijuana-by-state.

Some health professionals in the cannabis space stick to the well-researched medical uses of cannabis, pointing out that people are using and claiming benefit from cannabis for all kinds of symptoms and conditions that we don't have clinical trials to validate. But the fact remains: people *are* getting relief.

Martin A. Lee, director of Project CBD, talks about the different kinds of evidence we have about cannabis. While the double-blind, placebo-controlled standards are valid measurements, Lee tells me, "There are other valid criteria for assessing whether something is effective. Historical evidence, preclinical evidence, animal studies, molecular research, and anecdotal evidence can all contribute."

Cannabis educator Emma Chasen also argues that with cannabis, we should be looking at what she calls "aggregate anecdotal evidence" in addition to scientific evidence. That doesn't mean you should jump up and buy an ounce of Tahoe OG because your cousin's brother-in-law swears it'll heal a broken leg. It does mean that if a large number of people find cannabis helps a particular condition, there may be some validity—even if research isn't there yet.

"We need to think about plants as medicine in a different way," Chasen tells me. "The way that we use to determine whether a drug has medicinal value maybe isn't the right way to determine if a plant does."

For instance, if you suffered from Crohn's disease and taking pharmaceuticals knocked you on your ass, wouldn't you try plant-based medicine if you thought it *might* help and at the same time carried little risk of harm? It's true that we don't know THC can help with every condition found on states' qualifying lists yet. But we don't know it *can't.*

# SO WHAT ABOUT CBD?

In case you haven't noticed, CBD is trending in a big way. From bath bombs and infused coffees to tinctures, flower, vapes, salves, gummies, sprays, lubes, and everything in between, if you can think of it, someone's found a way to put CBD in it. (CBD toothpicks, anyone?)

But, seriously, does it work?

Depends on whom you ask. That's in part because quantifying CBD's effects, which are subtler than THC's, can be tricky. And while there are certainly faddish elements to the CBD craze, it's also clear that many people are getting benefit—particularly from full-spectrum CBD that contains a full array of the plant's compounds, including a small amount of THC. "A lot of studies are looking at CBD as an isolate," Patricia Frye, MD, Chief Medical Officer at Takoma Park Integrative Care in Maryland, tells me. "As an isolate you need a lot more CBD to be effective."

Personally, I've had success with CBD for anxiety and sleep. I've also found it helpful for pain—but only alongside THC. On the other hand, I sometimes feel lethargic when using CBD and find that my most beneficial dose is on the low side.

So while CBD isn't a cure-all and we still have a lot to learn, here's a look at some of the ways people are using—and loving—the stuff.

## EPILEPSY

The most well-studied and substantiated benefit of CBD is in the case of two rare seizure disorders, Dravet syndrome and Lennox-Gastaut syndrome (see Charlotte Figi's story starting on page 135). In 2018, the FDA approved a CBD-based pharmaceutical called Epidiolex for those specific uses.

## ANXIETY

A 2015 literature review published in the journal *Neurotherapeutics* found "considerable potential" for CBD to treat multiple anxiety disorders.[46] And a survey from 2019 found that 79 percent of people with anxiety being treated in a clinical setting showed improvement when taking 25 to 75 mg of CBD daily.[47] Anxiety relief was sustained for the subjects during the three-month duration of the study—which is absolutely encouraging. However, because the research was observational, it's considered preliminary evidence.

## SLEEP

The same study I just cited also looked at CBD and sleep, finding short-term improvement for almost 67 percent of participants after one month of use. The success rate of participants, however, fluctuated over time. A 2017 review of existing studies found that CBD might help people with REM sleep disorders and excessive daytime sleepiness.[48] And, anecdotally speaking, many people find that they go to sleep more quickly, stay asleep longer, and wake up more refreshed if they've taken the right dose of CBD. But whether those benefits last in the long term is not entirely clear.

In addition, Dr. Frye tells me that CBD doesn't negatively affect the deep-sleep patterns that are vital for the body to restore itself.

## DEPRESSION

A 2009 study showed that CBD alleviated depression in rats by interacting with serotonin receptors.[49] There's a good deal of anecdotal evidence about CBD and depression, too, but if you have clinical depression (as with any medical condition you'd like to treat using cannabis) it's best to seek help from a practitioner who's knowledgeable about both cannabinoids and pharmaceuticals. Cannabis-friendly psychiatrists are a thing now, and some do telemedicine—you can start the process with a simple online search.

## PAIN AND INFLAMMATION

Dr. Frye tells me that CBD, which she calls "more anti-inflammatory than prednisone," can help reduce pain that's caused by inflammation. Her patients' experiences with CBD—when taken either internally or topically—backs this up. Several animal studies have also been done on pain and CBD: in 2017, CBD was shown to relieve pain by altering both the sensory perception of it and the affective, or emotional, response.[50] Another model showed CBD improved symptoms of pain and inflammation related to arthritis.[51] And yet another study showed that CBD helps relieve neuropathic and inflammatory pain.[52]

Bill Code, MD, a Canadian doctor specializing in integrative medicine and author of *Solving the Brain Puzzle*, tells me that, in his clinical experience, CBD augments the effectiveness of painkillers such as OxyContin by four to ten times. This means that, under the care of a health professional, tapering down or quitting pain meds with the help of CBD may be possible without dipping into the pain zone. And though CBD may have pain-relieving potential on its own, doctors find that CBD and THC work best for pain relief when combined—particularly in a 1:1 ratio. Michelle Weiner, DO, an osteopath and pain specialist who recommends medical cannabis in Florida, also often recommends 1:1 products for pain, adding that "cannabis works synergistically with pain medications."

## PTSD, NIGHTMARES, AND PSYCHOSIS

A small study from 2019 found that ten out of eleven patients with PTSD experienced significant symptom relief with regular doses of CBD; a subset of this group also reported relief from nightmares associated with PTSD.[53] For people with psychosis, CBD may help promote more ordered brain activity.[54]

## NAUSEA

THC is the better-known player here, but CBD may have some benefit, too. People do self-report improvements in nausea symptoms with CBD, and a 2001 animal study seems to back that up.[55] Like we covered in Chapter 2, the endocannabinoid system is meant to bring us to homeostasis, and therefore helps regulate essential functions like appetite, sleep, mood, memory, pain, and—you got it—nausea and vomiting.

## SOS FOR THC

If you unintentionally get too damn high, adding CBD may be able to help tame the side effects and smooth out the experience. See Chapter 9 for more.

## SKINCARE AND BEAUTY

CBD is antibacterial and anti-inflammatory, so it's no surprise that skincare and beauty lines have started to incorporate it for everything from acne to psoriasis to wrinkles. There isn't a lot of science yet about CBD skincare, but it's fun to think that this lovely plant may have yet another use.

## Most Common Reasons Consumers Use CBD[56]

*(Survey respondents could report CBD use for more than one reason.)*

- Pain 40%
- Anxiety 20%
- Sleep/Insomnia 11%
- Arthritis 8%
- Migraines/Headaches 5%
- Stress 5%
- Muscle spasms/Soreness 4%
- General health (nonspecific) 4%
- Mental health/PTSD/ADHD/Neurological disorders 4%
- Recreational 4%
- Depression 2%
- Skincare 2%
- For pets 1%
- Gastrointestinal/Digestive issues 1%
- Inflammation 1%
- Other 7%
- No opinion 1%

# CHOOSING QUALITY CBD

Considering the incredible array of "it's possibles" when it comes to CBD, there's really no wonder it's such a thing. But a quick caution here: The CBD market is hardly well regulated (yet). One study found that the majority of consumer CBD products are mislabeled.[57] Quality and sourcing both matter when it comes to CBD, and it's absolutely true that you can find top-tier products alongside brands of low or questionable quality.

So how do you get your hands on quality CBD? First, buy from a licensed dispensary or a reputable online source. Rule out all your fly-by-nights, your pyramid schemes, and your gas station elixirs. Next, read the label. It should clearly state the total milligrams of CBD (and THC, if applicable) and that the product is lab-tested, preferably in a facility that meets the ISO 17025 standard (an international designation of technical competence). With quality brands, you should easily find info on the website about when and where products were tested, as well as the specific potency data for each "batch." The bottle itself should reveal a batch number. You can also talk to your budtender about sourcing quality CBD and check this book's appendix for recs.

You may want to seek out CBD that's sourced from domestically grown hemp; Colorado, Oregon, and Kentucky have robust hemp programs. And, in most things cannabis, full-spectrum or broad-spectrum CBD probably provides more benefits than what's known variously as "single-molecule CBD," "CBD isolate, or "CBD-only" products. Martin A. Lee compares full-spectrum CBD to fresh squeezed orange juice; of course, you can still get vitamin C from a pill, but you'll miss the rich matrix of other compounds that make the fresh, whole product better than the isolated molecule.

## A NOTE OF CAUTION ABOUT CBD

CBD utilizes the same group of liver enzymes, cytochrome P450 3A4, that're also responsible for helping metabolize up to 65 percent of pharmaceutical meds. Dr. Tishler tells me that, simply speaking, because CBD "occupies" those enzymes for a time, prescription meds may not work optimally if taken alongside CBD. The meds most likely to be disrupted include benzodiazepines, blood thinners, cardiac medications, seizure drugs, and immunosuppressants, like those cancer patients might be taking.

Some practitioners recommend avoiding the potential conflict by taking pharmaceuticals and CBD at different moments in the day, but you should consult with a cannabis nurse or doctor if you're taking any of the abovementioned meds or, of course, if you're looking to treat *any* medical condition with cannabis.

# WHAT THE HECK DO THE MINOR CANNABINOIDS DO?

Of more than a hundred cannabinoids found in flower, these are the most notable supporting cast to our costars, THC and CBD:

**CBG** (cannabigerol): nonpsychoactive; antibacterial; anti-inflammatory; may inhibit growth of cancer cells; may help with glaucoma; destroys methicillin-resistant *Staphylococcus aureus* (MRSA) in mice[58]

**CBN** (cannabinol): nonpsychoactive alone; boosts euphoria in the presence of THC; antibacterial; anti-inflammatory; appetite stimulating; may have a sedative effect (particularly in combo with THC)

**CBC** (cannabichromene): nonpsychoactive; pain-relieving; has potential as anticancer agent; may help treat acne; may contribute to the effectiveness of THC and CBD for depression

**THCV** (tetrahydrocannabivarin): psychoactive when present in higher quantities; appetite-suppressing; may help manage blood sugar

**THCA** (tetrahydrocannabinolic acid): nonpsychoactive precursor to THC; anti-inflammatory; possible neuroprotectant; antiemetic (for nausea and appetite loss); potential anticancer

**CBDA** (cannabidiolic acid): nonpsychoactive precursor to CBD; anti-inflammatory, possible antiemetic and anticonvulsant; may help with depression

**THCP** (tetrahydrocannabiphorol): potentially similar therapeutic benefit as THC; could be much more psychoactive than THC (though it appears in very small quantities, if at all, in commercial strains)

It's worth noting that, until cannabis science has a lot more research under its belt, you'll hear a lot of *coulds* and *mights* and *mays*. Indeed, as Dr. Frye says, "We're at the tip of the iceberg in terms of understanding all the compounds in this plant." I'm hopeful we'll know more soon and look forward to a day when cannabinoids, terpenes, flavonoids, and other compounds in cannabis become well known for their uses in medicine, wellness, and fun. But even now, you'll find commercial formulas featuring some of these other cannabinoids. Have fun with them, by all means, but take the packaging's claims with a grain of salt.

# CHAPTER 5

# BUD AND FLOWER: THIS AIN'T YOUR MAMA'S WEED (OR IS IT?)

> "A lot of women say to me, 'I don't like cannabis. I don't like the way it makes me feel.' And I say, 'Well, if your first-time drinking was doing a line of shots, you wouldn't like the way it makes you feel, either. You just didn't do it right.'"
> —*Shannon Chiarenza, founder of WeedMama.ca*

As we saw in Chapter 2, there's a hell of a lot of choice out there today. So say goodbye to the dime bags of unknown origin, and say hello to options, variable price points, and transparency—a smorgasbord of cannabis! Embrace the plethora of products you can eat, drink, vape, smoke, or rub on your skin!

Say hello to legal weed.

Some people like to point out that the legal marketplace overvalues increasingly potent THC products; they say that there's just too much highly concentrated stuff out there today and that we don't know the long-term effects of consuming massive quantities of THC.

It's true. The weed of today is not the weed of your mama's day and isn't the weed of your college days, either. A study showed that, in 1995, the average potency of cannabis seized by DEA agents was in the range of 4 percent THC.[59] Even if that seems like a really lowball number, it's undeniable that the weed of yesteryear was mostly inferior-quality, low-THC stuff—not the aromatic, voluptuous, and potent sinsemilla of today.

"Back in the nineties," says Jennifer, a mom in New Hampshire, "I was smoking shitty ditch weed that was full of twigs and seeds—but we were grateful for it anyway! That stuff was probably 5 to 10 percent THC." She remembers when *High Times* published a story about a strain called White Widow, with a "mind-blowing" 15 percent THC. "Nowadays," she says, "that's like nothing."

Indeed, you can find flower with upwards of 30 percent THC content today—which is really high and *will get you really high*. Don't start there. Honestly, you needn't ever go there unless you're medicating under a doctor's care. Emma Chasen says that, aside from treating for severe pain, there's no reason to consume massive quantities of THC, and I fully agree.

# RESPONSIBLE USE

If you use cannabis responsibly, the risk to your health and safety is very low; the vast majority of bad weed experiences come from irresponsible or uninformed use.

So what *exactly* is responsible use? One piece, of course, is correct dosing—we'll get to those details soon. But, first, I want to bring in a list of recommendations, adapted from a seminal work on responsible use by David F. Duncan and Robert S. Gold called *Drugs and the Whole Person* (1985).

In order to use cannabis responsibly, it's important to:

◊  Understand the health and safety risks (see Chapter 9)

◊  Make sure you trust your source (i.e., shop at a legal dispensary or grow your own)

◊  Develop awareness of your own tolerance levels and consume within those limits

◊  Use the smallest amount to achieve your desired effects, aka your minimum effective dose

◊  Determine safe settings and situations, and use cannabis only in the appropriate places and times

◊  Avoid consuming when you are not healthy enough to do so (except, of course, if you're treating medically with cannabis under a health professional's care)

◊  Avoid overusing cannabis, either in one session or over a period of time

◊  Don't use cannabis to cope with your problems or escape emotionally

◊  Don't mix cannabis with other drugs or alcohol

◊  Respect other adults' choices to use or not use cannabis

◊  Pay particular attention to how your use of cannabis affects the children in your life (see Chapter 6)

If you're new to cannabis, the very best advice is also very simple: *start low and go slow*. Microdosing and moderate dosing are your friends. Let's talk details.

# SO HOW TF DO YOU ACTUALLY CONSUME THIS DELIGHTFUL SUBSTANCE?

There are so many ways! First, there's inhalation, with its suite of sub-categories, including 1) smoking dried cannabis flower, 2) "vaping" cannabis extracts as electronic liquids, or "e-liquids," and 3) vaporizing flower. Next, you have oral consumption. You can eat or drink cannabis-infused products, swallow capsules, or use sublingual tinctures, sprays, and oils. And, last, you have topicals, which include creams, gels, patches, and lubes. There are also some highly concentrated forms of cannabis that I'll address briefly at the end of this section.

Whichever way you choose to consume, my best rec is to seek out full-spectrum products, be it from the flower itself or a product labeled "full-spectrum" or "broad-spectrum." The entourage effect says you'll get the most out of cannabis that way.

# PRESS ONE FOR SMOKING FLOWER

You can use pipes ranging from tiny one-hitters made of glass, wood, or metal to the kind of elaborate blown-glass pieces that have populated head shops for years. I prefer simple pipes because I'm a low-fuss kind of person; mine is a forest green number that's reminiscent of Sherlock Holmes—not the most stylish thing around, but it gets the job done.

You've also got water pipe varieties, from bongs to bubblers to hookahs. The advantage of using a water pipe comes down to comfort: it's smoother (and will make you cough less) to inhale smoke that's passed through water and cooled down. Some people will tell you that bong "rips" produce stronger effects than inhaling from a pipe. Others will tell you that water helps filter the undesirable compounds out, leaving you with cleaner cannabinoids and terpenes. None of this is proven. Still, some people adore (and name!) their bongs.

A bubbler is essentially a small, more portable bong, and a hookah is a Middle Eastern water pipe with which people have traditionally shared hashish or tobacco in smoke circles. It's also possible to smoke dried cannabis flower with a hookah but I'm told it takes a lot of weed.

Next, we have joints, blunts, and spliffs. Joints, or "jays," carry only ground cannabis flower and are rolled in rice, bamboo, or hemp papers. They're tricky to roll right, but in legal states you can buy "pre-rolls"—which are exactly as they sound: joints of named strains that are pre-rolled for your convenience. Personally, I love the juicy sacrilege of buying a joint while paying sales tax—but I hate all the plastic that comes with it.

Blunts are a DIY deal made with ground cannabis that's rolled with cigar or cigarillo paper (and possibly a filter)—lending them a cigar-like taste and smell. Hip-hop pays a ton of homage to this homemade smoke method, and blunts hold a venerated place in weed culture.

You may recognize spliffs, or tobacco mixed with cannabis and rolled in tobacco papers, from Bob Marley and the Wailers' "Easy Skanking." Cool song, bad choice for the lungs.

But wait—is smoking cannabis from a pipe, a water pipe, or a joint *actually* better for your lungs than smoking tobacco or tobacco-laced cannabis? Well, yes. Tobacco is a neurotoxic carcinogen. Weed isn't. (More in Chapter 9.)

Regardless of the tool you choose, smoking weed comes down to the simple practice of setting bud aflame, inhaling smoke, keeping it in your lungs for a moment, and then exhaling. It's the classic mode of consumption, an oldie but goodie, the method still preferred by the majority of Americans who use cannabis,[60] and my favorite way to consume, hands-fucking down.

## PROS OF SMOKING FLOWER

If you want direct experience with the plant, flower is the way to go. (But you don't necessarily have to smoke it—see the sections on vaping and vaporizing flower, pages 93–96.) It's also the most tactile, most natural, most—*ahem*—grassroots way of consuming cannabis. The effects are almost immediate, and the peak euphoria lasts only one to three hours.

You get the full-spectrum of the plant when you smoke flower, including cannabinoids, terpenes, and a bunch of the other stuff in weed that we haven't even identified yet. Get this: a 2019 study of over 3,000 medical marijuana patients showed that, compared to all other products, patients got the greatest medicinal benefit from flower itself.[61]

Plus, flower doesn't break the bank—even top-quality stuff is reasonably priced compared to manufactured products. Smoking flower supports farmers, not a corporate bottom line.[62] It's old school, it's gangsta—and it's definitely *one way* to be a weed mom.

## CONS OF SMOKING FLOWER

You may cough. You will produce smoke. Less risky than smoking tobacco,[63] smoking flower still isn't without risks to your lungs, nor is it discreet. Your breath and your clothes will smell of weed while your eyes might get a bit red, even glassy. (Cue eye drops, mouthwash, and a new shirt.) Smoking weed is neither convenient nor particularly portable. (So, yeah, I one hundred percent get why flower is not everyone's cuppa.) And even though it's positively magical to me now, I admit that I started my cannabis journey *somewhere else...*

# PRESS TWO FOR VAPING

Disposable vaporizers come all-in-one and ready to rock. These are your starter kits, your training wheels, your junior leagues. I dipped my toe in the canna-stream here, and I'm not ashamed to say it.

Some disposable vapes are strain-specific while others consist of proprietary blends of THC, CBD, and terpenes for specific effects like focus, calm, or sleep. Some vapes even feature a way to help you calibrate your dose by buzzing, vibrating, or lighting up after you've inhaled a specific amount (like 2.25 mg).

The second vape option is a reusable pen. Here, you have to buy the hardware itself (including a rechargeable battery) as well as vape cartridges (or "carts") containing either cannabis e-liquid or a more potent product called live resin. (If you've ever seen a tobacco vape, it's pretty similar.) With reusable vapes, you can switch out the carts as you like, and cannabis carts come in dozens, if not hundreds, of varieties.

## PROS OF VAPING

Easy peasy to use. Discreet AF. No lingering smell means you can easily take a puff or two while your in-laws are in the next room.

## CONS OF VAPING

The "vape crisis" that resulted in 2,807 illnesses and 68 deaths seemed *not* to have implicated vaping materials bought on the legal market.[64] Instead, the problems stemmed from illegal vapes with thickening additives like vitamin E acetate, which, it turns out, is really bad to inhale.

But even if you're vaping legal stuff, the whole thing is still pretty new. Up until 2019, vaping was thought to be cleaner and safer for the lungs, but we're learning that that may not actually be true. It's not *not* true, necessarily. We just don't know yet.

Since it's so easy to vape, you can easily overdo it if you're not paying attention. And another thing: terpenes get lost in the manufacturing process. That means, any terpenes in your vapes will have been added back in from another source, which isn't necessarily bad, just not the most natural.

Last, reusable vapes require charging. They come encased in a shit ton of packaging and aren't easily recycled. Maybe this will change soon, but the fact is, vapes aren't environmentally friendly...yet.

# PRESS THREE FOR VAPORIZING FLOWER

In the wide space on the inhalation spectrum between smoking flower and vaping, we have...vaporizing flower. Confusing, right? We just covered all that vape stuff. But this is something entirely different, where you place actual, ground-up flower in a handheld device called a dry-herb vaporizer. Within its chambers, the vaporizer heats the flower material to about 350 degrees Fahrenheit, until the cannabinoids and terpenes in your flower—poof!— well, they vaporize. Seal your lips to the device and inhale the vapor, which is like smoke but not smoke. The Buddha's Middle Way, if you will.

## PROS OF VAPORIZING FLOWER

Vaporizing flower is probably the healthiest inhalation method, and the one that marijuana doctors most often recommend. You'll revel in the smells and tastes! You get a wonderful sense of your weed's flavor, be it fruity, floral, peppery, lemony, woodsy, or even skunky. That's because terpenes tend to burn up a little more quickly than cannabinoids and so, because of the lower temperatures involved, you just *get* more of them when you vaporize.

Shannon Chiarenza tells me that she prefers vaporizing flower to any other method because "you can play around with vaporizing so much more—it feels like you're having a better relationship with the plant."

Another plus is that vaporizing flower is discreet—no smoke! The room in which you've vaporized might emanate a faint weedy afterglow, but nothing like when you smoke. Many people say that their stash lasts longer with a vaporizer, too; and, of course, you get the privilege of handling mother nature's own plant material.

# CONS OF VAPORIZING FLOWER

Vaporizers are dang expensive. Expect to drop about $150 for a decent one, or $500 if you feel like splurging. Still, it's a durable device that should last years if you take care of it. For me, vaporizing flower feels a bit different from smoking; that calm, present, elevated feeling I love is just two degrees lighter in a way I don't enjoy quite as much. Emma Chasen also describes the high from vaporizing as "thinner," though it's rather subjective, she tells me, due to differences in the array of compounds you get from smoking versus vaporizing.

Shannon admits that smoking has a longer and more profound effect than vaporizing. But she appreciates that fact because vaporizing allows her to easily monitor her level of elevation—a real plus for moms. She tells me that newbies might get a little light headed and "confuse that with the feeling of the cannabis," therefore assuming that vaporizing gets them higher. But, overall, she says, smoking cannabis is the more potent of the two. Shannon's pro tip: combine low-dose edibles with vaporizing flower for that mellow body high accompanied by a mental boost.

Flower vaporizers are more environmentally friendly than vape carts and vape pens, but still require electricity and a battery.

# PRESS FOUR FOR TINCTURES AND OILS

You can tote these handy-dandy bottles around in your bag and, with a few drops under the tongue, feel the effects within fifteen to thirty minutes. Cannabis oils come in another oil carrier—like olive or coconut oil—while tinctures can be oil-based *or* alcohol-based solutions of cannabis extracts. Chasen prefers quality alcohol-based tinctures if you're looking for a full-spectrum product because alcohol is a "nonselective solvent," meaning that it helps extract all the good stuff from plant material.

Quality brands, and crappy ones, abound in both categories. Shop around, ask for recs, and read lab results. The most important thing to know about this category is that holding the liquid under your tongue for a minute or more before swallowing will help start absorption via your mouth's mucosal lining and therefore get to work more efficiently. Oils can absorb this way, to a degree, but they will have to be processed by your liver, too.

## PROS OF TINCTURES AND OILS

It's discreet, easy, convenient, no weedy smell, no smoke.

Chasen likes how tinctures give the user an easy way to titrate doses to the milligram and to play with the THC to CBD relationship. "You have more mixed ratio availability," she says. "You can get products with a lower concentration of THC and higher CBD, or a combination of the two, in whatever potency you're most comfortable with."

Indeed, a quick look around most dispensaries will show tinctures in ratios of 1:1, 3:1, 15:1, 30:1, and everything in between. If you don't want to get high, choose a high-CBD, low-THC tincture.

## CONS OF TINCTURES AND OILS

Because it takes fifteen to thirty minutes (and sometimes longer) to feel the effects of oils and tinctures, it can be hard at first to calibrate your optimum dose. As with edibles, people sometimes overdo it by adding more a bit too soon. On the other hand, you can "underdose" with tinctures before figuring it all out. It's not rocket science, but, relates cannabis writer and mom Diana-Ashley Krach, dosing in general "takes trial and error and a lot of experimenting."

Also, good tinctures or oils are pricey.

# PRESS FIVE FOR EDIBLES

Edibles have come a long way from your classic homemade pot brownies. We've got a dizzying assortment of "baked" goods now (cannabis cake balls, anyone?) alongside the super-hot-ATM gummy, chocolate, mint, and hard candy areas. Infused drinks are gaining popularity, as are cannabis teas and honeys. Yep, edibles are big business.

But know this: with edibles, a little bit goes a looooong way. That's because when you eat THC (which is technically Δ-9 THC) the molecule travels to your liver via your digestive tract. In your liver, it's changed into another form, 11-hydroxy THC, which acts more potently in most people. That's why an edible with a low to moderate dose of 2.5 to 5 mg (1 mg if you're uber microdosing) might be enough. It takes a while for your body to complete this molecule-morphing magic trick, so don't go nibbling on your edible again for at least two hours.

A little secret about edibles, however, is they don't seem to work on everyone. This could be because of a group of enzymes that determine how quickly you metabolize cannabinoids, or whether you even metabolize them at all. Some people apparently just can't get high from eating THC unless using the kind of dose that would overwhelm most people whose enzymes fall in the more usual range.

Next, let's take a quick look at quality. Edibles are typically made with one of two types of cannabis oil: distillate or full-spectrum. Eek—more terminology! *I know.* But this is fairly quick and boils down to the fact that many edible companies use a THC extraction process involving chemical solvents. That results in distillate—essentially pure THC oil that's then measured out into edibles recipes. The other method involves heating (aka decarboxylating) raw cannabis flower at about 245 degrees Fahrenheit and infusing the lightly toasted weed into butter or oil. Then, you strain out the flower material and you're left with "canna-butter"—your edible THC delivery system.

So what does this mean for you? Maybe nothing, actually. Most THC edibles are made with distillate, and most people don't know—or care. But since weed momming is all about elevating awareness, I'll add that there are those who swear by the majesty of a full-spectrum edible. Wayne Schwind, owner of Periodic Edibles in Oregon, told me when I interviewed him for *High Times* that full-spectrum edibles yield a smoother on-ramp and off-ramp to the experience and a longer, mellower high than edibles made with distillate.

Why? Because of our friend the entourage effect, the one that says anything with *all* the cannabinoids, *all* the terpenes—and whatever other delights reside in our humble bud—is probably better for you. You know, like whole versus processed foods or home cooking versus the drive-through.

You can also DIY it and whip up a batch of homemade canna-butter. Just make sure you understand the dosing, don't consume too much, and keep those edibles out of little hands.

Oh, and ditto everything I just said for capsules—the way the body digests cannabinoids applies to them as well!

## PROS OF EDIBLES

Elevating with edibles feels really nice. Usually described as providing a "body high" more than a "head high," edibles tend to soften life's edges in pleasant, and at times, vital, ways. (Useful during a global pandemic, for instance.)

Back in the day, home canna-bakers made treats without a reliable way to measure potency; you could eat one or more of those old-school brownies and get high AF, or not at all. But precisely dosed edibles eliminate a good deal of the guesswork. Of course, you'll still want to play around to find your personal sweet spot, but at least you won't be guessing about whether you're eating one or one hundred milligrams of THC with that goodie.

Edibles tend to last. Expect to feel elevated for about four hours with your optimum edibles dose—but note it could be quite a bit longer or slightly shorter, depending on your metabolism, what you've eaten that day, and a bunch of other factors.

## CONS OF EDIBLES

It's way easy to overdo edibles if you're not careful (but don't worry, I'll soon teach you what you need to know).

Also, edibles tend to last. Wait, didn't I just say that was a pro?

Well, it's *both*, depending ultimately on what you want. Unlike inhalation, which is more like a quick hit of chill, edibles are a deep dive into the cannabis sea. That's great if you've got all day, or are dosing for good sleep—not so great if you have to drive carpool at 3.

Personally, edibles relaaaax me, which is exactly what I'm looking for when Saturday night rolls around and I'm up on the couch with a bowl of popcorn and my family's rewatching the *Lord of the Rings* trilogy. But if I've still got work to finish and kids to feed and bathe and homework to sign off on and a pile of laundry collecting dust on my coffee table, I. Just. Can't. Do. Edibles. But maybe that's just me.

# PRESS SIX FOR SUBLINGUAL TABLETS, STRIPS, AND SPRAYS

The only reason I separate these from the other sublingual products out there (tinctures and oils) is that these designer cannabinoid formulas are growing up into their market space and differentiating themselves from the more established stuff. From what I've seen, this category tends to be aggressively branded and marketed toward a specific quality or experience: stuff like socializing, sleeping, sex, focus, and creativity. Tablets and strips may feature interesting blends of cannabinoids, like CBN for sedation, or

THCV for focus, as well as trendy nootropics like vitamin B6, L-theanine, and ginkgo biloba.

## PROS OF TABLETS, STRIPS, AND SPRAYS

These babies can give you the thrill of a good body-mind hack. Wanna hone in a project? Pop a "focus" sublingual strip. Have some pain to kill, but don't want to get high? Try a 5-mg tab of nonpsychoactive THCA. Going to a party? Give a "sativa" tab a whirl. There are cool possibilities here, no doubt, even if the notion of "tailor-made highs" is a little commercial.

Products in this category are also discreet, not at all weedy, and perfect for microdosing.

## CONS OF TABLETS, STRIPS, AND SPRAYS

I'm not a weed snob or anything but I am a little skeptical. Yes, chasing a tailored high is fun, and I agree that this class of product has its place in the ever-expanding cannabis landscape. But do they work? Maybe. The cannabis science field is new enough that we just can't say for sure, and because of natural differences in endocannabinoid systems, the same formulation is probably going to hit different people differently.

In addition to the ECS issue, Chasen tells me that our variable responses to cannabis depend on what we've eaten, our stress level, how hydrated and rested we are, and a bunch of other things. "Our bodies in general are constantly in flux," she says. "Why is it that sometimes we don't have a good night's sleep, and other times we have a great night's sleep? Or we feel a little more anxious one day and not the next? We are ever-changing humans, so it makes sense that medicinal plant intervention would modulate off of this really 'fluxy' aspect of ourselves."

All in all, this category, to me, is a bit like those exquisitely decorated petit-fours in bakery windows; they're so pretty I can't wait to buy them, but when I get home, I'm kinda *meh*. They're also expensive.

# PRESS SEVEN FOR TOPICALS

Salves, ointments, creams, lotions, bath bombs, and skincare live in this category, as do transdermal patches and lubes. Generally speaking, people use THC or CBD topicals (or combos) to help with local pain, inflammation, minor injury, or soreness. Some people rub topicals into their temples or neck to help with headaches, and others reach for cannabis-infused salves after a workout or to soothe pain in their muscles, tendons, or joints.

Infused bath bombs are a sweet way to occasionally add to your self-care ritual, while infused skincare products—marketed for all kinds of things, from acne to eczema to psoriasis—vary quite a bit in quality and price range. There's definitely an argument that cannabinoids, as well as the antioxidants and amino acids found in the plant, could be helpful for skin health. But there's a lot we still don't know.

Topicals as a general rule don't get you high—not really—and that's because cannabinoids don't easily reach your bloodstream when applied to the skin. The first exception here is transdermal patches: if they contain THC, they will likely get you at least a little high (depending on the strength of the patch) because these products are designed to penetrate the skin and enter the bloodstream.

The second exception is a fun one: infused lubes! If you have a vagina, you might try CBD-based lubes to help relax vaginal muscles and ease pain. THC-based lubes may not give you the mind-soothing euphoria of a good smoke but *may* do a funny little thing I've heard described as "getting your vagina high." (More in Chapter 10.)

# HIGHLY CONCENTRATED STUFF

There are even more ways to consume cannabis, like "dabbing," smoking hash, or eating super-potent cannabis concentrates. People who utilize these methods tend to fall into the heavy-duty medical-use bucket or the intense high–seeking bucket—and since I'm neither of those, I haven't gone deep here.

Believe the hype. This shit is *highly* concentrated. Eat or inhale just a little too much of any of these and your limbs get heavy, your brain goes all swimmy, and you're just too damn high. And beyond just getting too high and feeling crappy for a bit, consuming too much THC isn't healthy or necessary for *most* people *most* of the time. Guess I'm kinda old school, but I really can't suggest such concentrated stuff to anyone who's not thoroughly experienced with weed. Sorry, not sorry.

# TOP SIX WELLNESS USES

Great! So what can I take for my anxiety, pain, crappy mood, and all the other stuff, you ask? The top six wellness uses of cannabis for women today are anxiety, cramps, mood, occasional pain, stress, and low libido. Any of those sound familiar?

Look, I don't know you yet, but I'd still venture a guess that at least one of those issues presents a small problem from time to time. Maybe a big problem, and perhaps more often than occasionally. You're a human and a mom—and we're living in stressful days. I get it. Same.

What follows are some notes and tips about what seems to work for a lot of weed moms. (Remember, I'm not a healthcare provider, and this isn't medical advice.)

But first, a quick starter guide on dosing:

**Inhalation:** This includes smoking, vaping, and flower vaporizing.

◊ If you're brand-new/sensitive/know your tolerance is low, choose a flower strain with 15 percent THC or less.

◊ Choose high-CBD, low-THC flower if you don't want to get high.

◊ If you have some experience/aren't sensitive, choose a strain with up to 22 percent THC.

◊ If you're using a vape pen, be aware that vape concentrates are higher in THC than plain flower.

◊ In any case, start with one puff. Wait five minutes.

◊ Add more as needed. Don't exceed three puffs in your first session.

**Ingestion:** This includes consuming edibles, drinkables, tinctures, teas, sprays, tabs, and sublinguals.

◊ If you're brand-new/sensitive/know your tolerance is low, take 1 to 2.5 mg of THC max the first time.

◊ If you have some experience/aren't sensitive, choose 5 mg THC max the first time.

◊ Add an additional 2.5 mg each time you consume until you reach an effective and pleasant dose.

◊ Ten mg is a comfortable "full dose" for many adults (don't start there, work up to it!), though your individual needs may vary.

◊ Edibles take thirty minutes to two hours to take peak effect; never add more edibles before the two-hour mark.

THC in particular is highly dose-dependent. That means a small to moderate amount can have one effect (say, anxiety relief and appetite stimulation). But a high dose of the exact same thing won't necessarily make you *more* relaxed, or hungrier. Instead, it could flip itself around and make you feel anxious and nauseous. *That's* why I'm cautious. I don't want to freak you out—I just want to be honest.

And that's why my dosing guidelines are all about starting so low and going so slow. The first time you consume following these guidelines, you may not get high, and it could end up seeming like a bit of a time waste. But, believe me, it's better *not* to get high at all the first time than to get way too freaking high and have a "bad trip." Moms definitely don't have time for that.

With a bit of practice, you'll learn how to calibrate your dose and wait the right amount of time before adding more. If all goes well, you'll have the rest of your life to smoke (or eat or vape) some really great shit. But, for now, keep it mellow. You can slide up a bit on your per-sesh consumption, if that appeals to you, but only once you've acclimated.

## MODES OF THC CONSUMPTION

| Mode | Common Effects | Onset | Duration |
|------|----------------|-------|----------|
| Smoking Flower | Potential mind and body high—depends on THC and CBD content, terpenes, and other factors | a few minutes | 1–3 hours |
| Vaping | Potential mind and body high—depends on THC and CBD content, terpenes, and other factors | a few minutes | 1–3 hours |
| Vaporizing Flower | Potential mind and body high—depends on THC and CBD content, terpenes, and other factors; usually not as intense as smoking or vaping | a few minutes | 1–3 hours |
| Tinctures and Oils | Potential mind and body high—depends on THC and CBD content, terpenes, and other factors | 15–45 minutes (up to 2 hours possible) | 3–5 hours |
| Edibles (including Capsules) | Body high is often stronger than the mind high with edibles; usually more intense overall than smoking or vaping | 30 minutes–2 hours | 4–6 hours (up to 10 hours possible) |
| Sublinguals, Tablets, Strips, and Sprays | Potential mind and body high; usually not as intense as the above intake methods | 15–30 minutes | 2–4 hours |
| Topicals | Potential pain relief and help for skin issues with little to no high (except for transdermal patches and, possibly, vaginal products) | 15–20 minutes | 2–5 hours |

# USING CANNABIS FOR ANXIETY

First, try CBD. Ten milligrams of oil or tincture is a good starting dose, and you can titrate up from there until you feel an effect. Most studies involving CBD feature a really high dose, but, practically speaking, many people find 25 to 75 mg a day a sweet spot.

If you're looking to add THC to the mix, remember, less is more. Try a strain like Granddaddy Purple or Purple Urkle if you're looking for end-of-day relief that will help ease you into deep sleep. For higher CBD content with a low-to-nonexistent high, reach for Remedy or Canna-Tsu.

And if you're most comfortable with a vape pen, a tea, a tincture, or an edible, look for one marketed as "calming" or "indica" (even though you and I know this isn't an entirely accurate classification). There are many products out there formulated with cannabinoids, terpenes, and even blends of other herbs with a de-stressing effect in mind.

# USING CANNABIS FOR CRAMPS

Tidbit for the history buffs: Queen Victoria, the nineteenth-century British monarch, was reportedly treated with cannabis by her royal physician for menstrual pain. Almost two hundred years later, we still don't have clinical trials on cannabis and menstrual cramps—but there's enough anecdotal evidence showing that it's worth exploring options if you deal with pain on a monthly basis.

While smoking, vaping, taking a tincture, or consuming an edible can provide some pain and mood relief, you'll want to try to get as close to the source of pain as possible to maximize your chances of benefit, because— guess what? You have endocannabinoid receptors in your reproductive tract, too!

Here's where suppositories come in. A handful of companies have developed "weed tampons" (the term's a bit misleading because we're talking about suppositories, not actual tampons). Essentially, they consist of CBD and/or THC in a vagina-safe delivery system like cocoa butter. The whole thing comes in a small, tapered cylindrical shape that's easy enough to insert while it's a solid; then, your body heat melts the product and the liquid absorbs through your vaginal walls.

As we've seen, THC and CBD can both relieve pain—though better together. They're anti-inflammatory and, when used vaginally, may help soothe and relax uterine muscles and promote circulation. Since science tells us that inflammatory prostaglandins peak during periods, it makes sense that taming inflammation (essentially what NSAIDs like ibuprofen do) could help. But, again, we don't know for sure. There are no FDA-approved cannabis treatments for sucky periods, just optimistic entrepreneurship and some women who are now much happier for a few days a month.

## USING CANNABIS FOR STRESS

If you manage momming today *without* exerting gobs of your mental energy stressing TF out, I'm happy for you. Really. But if you're human, as I am, maybe you haven't totally managed to kick stress's ass to the curb yet.

Cannabis helps—it really, really does. Among connoisseurs, Sour Diesel and Super Silver Haze are two strains renowned for helping shift perspective. For moms, that end-of-the-day shift from a goal-oriented "work brain" to a more process-oriented "family brain" is crucial.

I really can't overstate exactly how *fundamental* cannabis is to my stress management as a mom. Here's a little secret about me: I was once a pretty carefree person, but becoming a mother brought out my hidden control freak–perfectionist boss lady. Which is cool, because I can manage a lot: kids, work, dog, meals, social calendars, cleaning, gardening, doctor's appointments, and all the rest. You know, *making lists, keeping people on task*. The downside is that I can be rigid, critical, and relentless in my drive to get things done, and done well. But fortunately, like I said, *cannabis helps*.

For daytime stress relief, I like Cannatonic or Critical Cure—two CBD-rich strains that won't get you very high, if at all. Lemon Kush is a favorite of mine for transitioning from work brain to family brain. With its light, lemony flavor and uplifting energy, it's a great after-work choice that helps soften the edges without putting me to sleep. It's higher in THC, so make sure that's a safe choice for you. If it's bedtime and stress is still weighing you down, try the winner of multiple Cannabis Cups, Gorilla Glue #4. Its deep, heavy chill will help you, like Elsa from *Frozen*, to *let it go*.

## USING CANNABIS FOR MOOD

If you're living in a female body, you're probably acquainted with hormonal mood swings. Hormones—you know, those lovely chemicals that make us deeply *want* partners and babies, but at certain times of the month also make us want to run away screaming from all of them?

Whether you suffer from run-of-the-mill mood fluctuations or from the more serious premenstrual dysphoric disorder, hormonal mood swings are tough. For a long time, I didn't realize how irritable and unbalanced I felt for about a week every month until *after* my period would begin and then I'd be like, *ohhh, right*. But once I started marking premenstrual days on my calendar and treating myself a little kinder when I wasn't feeling my best, things improved. Awareness is half the battle, right?

And the other half? It's the Jack Herer strain for an uplifting and creative break. It's Harlequin for a mostly nonpsychoactive (i.e., CBD-dominant) dose of mood stabilization. Or it's God's Gift, a strain that takes me to such a deeply relaxed (and sleepy) place that being pissy straight-up slips my mind.

## USING CANNABIS FOR PAIN

Whether it's acute, chronic, or neuropathic—and no matter where it lives in your body—it's one hundred percent true that pain really sucks. Fortunately, this is one of the things cannabis does *really* well. If you're dealing with chronic or severe pain, see a cannabis healthcare provider. But if you're dealing with run-of-the-mill pain that you'd normally treat with OTC stuff, you might consider giving a 1:1 ratio of THC to CBD a try. Edibles are a great choice here if you know your dose. Just pop a CBD and a THC edible of equal amounts. If you don't know your dose yet, you're going to have to play with it a bit, but make sure to start low (remember, start at 1–5 mg THC for edibles) and go slow (don't add more your first time; wait two hours before adding more any other time).

As long as you pay attention to your dosing, you can DIY it by mixing any kind of THC product with CBD. For instance, if you have a THC vape and a CBD vape, take alternating puffs. Or combine a low-dose THC edible with a few milligrams of CBD tincture. Or take a pinch of THC-rich flower mixed with a pinch of CBD-rich flower; then, as they say, put that in your pipe and smoke it. Alternatively, you can find all kinds of products in premixed 1:1 ratios.

But what about when you want to take a nine-pound hammer to your pain *and* get high at the same time? Well, there's Nine Pound Hammer, the heavy-hitting strain that can obliterate both your pain and your desire to get up from the couch. Because it's a powerhouse, go with Nine Pound Hammer—or related strains like Grape Ape and Romulan—only when you've got a backup parent or other caregiver to help with the littles.

On the other hand, if you just need to give pain a little nip in the bud so you can comfortably move your body, try something like Jack Herer, Blue Dream, or Sour Diesel. They're all energizing strains that might provide the little bit of relief that can make the difference between being active and sinking further into the (c)ouch.

## USING CANNABIS FOR LOW LIBIDO, PAINFUL SEX

Many women find cannabis incredibly helpful for relieving pain associated with sex, getting and staying in the mood, and for those deep-in-your-core orgasms. *Yes, please.* Chapter 10 covers this in juicy detail. See you there.

# CALIBRATING YOUR EXPERIENCE FOR WELLNESS AND FUN

Remember, cannabis is a complex matrix containing at least five hundred different compounds that appear to work best as team players, not soloists. And, as plant medicine, its effects will vary from person to person. So let my suggestions inform you—but serve merely as a springboard for your own canna-journey.

I'll leave you with a thought from cannabis writer and mom, Diana-Ashley Krach, who tells me, "The thing about cannabis that's *so great*, and also *so challenging*, is that it gives you autonomy over your body—but there's a lot of trial and error." With some patience, you can discover the right mode of consumption, dose, and product to meet your unique needs and wants. Don't give up.

# BEFORE YOU GO SHOPPING

Ready to hit the dispensary? Great! Just a few more tips...

I know you've shopped before, and you're a mom, so you're probably really good at finding the last jar of creamy peanut butter while holding a baby and opening a juice box for a toddler. I may have passed you in the aisle doing the exact same thing. But, believe me, this is a *different* kind of shopping experience; the legal market offers a dizzying number of choices, and if you don't want to be overwhelmed, I recommend asking yourself a few questions before you go:

1. Which modes of consumption am I comfortable using?

2. What's my goal for this purchase?

3. How do I want to feel after consuming?

4. What will I be doing while under the influence of cannabis?

5. How long do I want my supply to last?

6. What am I willing to spend?

# DISPENSARY CHECKLIST

Bring...

◊ ID (*everyone* gets carded at a legit dispensary)

◊ Cash (until banking regulations change, most transactions involving THC are cash-only)

◊ A clear sense of what you're looking for

*Don't* bring...

◊ Your kids, your dog, or anyone under age 21

Now, hit the dispensary (or call for delivery), and have yourself a blast!

# CHAPTER 6

# BEING THE MOM YOU WANT TO BE... WITH CANNABIS

## BEDTIME, aka THE WITCHING HOUR

Remember *Mary Poppins?* Near the beginning, Mr. Banks, father to Jane and Michael and employer of the titular character, cheerfully marches home from his job at the bank while singing about his domestic life and parenting duties, or lack thereof. To refresh your memory:

"It's 6:03 and the heirs to my dominion are scrubbed and tubbed and adequately fed! And, so, I'll pat them on the head and send them off to bed! Ah! Lordly is the life I lead!"

Sound familiar?

I thought not. (As you probably remember, it's not exactly true in *Mary Poppins*, either, because—as Mr. Banks is about to discover, the nanny has quit and the children are missing.)

And, now, for a bracing dose of reality, aka game time—errrr, bedtime. This is how it goes in our home (and possibly yours?): After an hour of pregame ritual, including a session with whichever Harry Potter we're currently reading and the painfully slow supervision of teeth-brushing and pajama-donning, I'll hug and kiss my son, hand him a couple of stuffies (cats, always cats), and walk out. After that, he may call me back once or twice to fetch water or find his sleep shades, but nothing too taxing. Bedtime with my son is like a lightning round of UNO.

My daughter's bedtime, on the other hand, is a baseball game with extra innings. We must kiss and hug somewhere between fifty and five hundred times. It's sweet, yes, but long. Then we must pray—her idea—and God forbid that I am not sincere and passionate in my devotion. I squeeze her hands. I screw up my face. *Dear God*, I silently pray. *Please let this be over soon.*

At seven years old—imaginative and bright—my daughter's nighttime fears include the usual suspects of bad dreams and closet monsters, so she bids me to spin a "good dreams story," full of unicorns farting magic fairy dust. And to triple check the closet, which I'd be happy to do if I had an ounce of stamina left. We're at the bottom of the ninth inning and I spent most of my energy on the hundred-and-one kisses.

"Goodnight!" I sing, inching optimistically toward the door.

My heart soars with the prospect of *me* time as I tiptoe to the staircase, when a shriek emanates from the untidy pile of quilts under which my dear daughter is lying.

"Open the door wider!" she commands. Or, "Close it an inch more!"

*We're going for extra innings tonight*, I sigh to myself like a burnt-out pitcher, only with a bit more rage. There will be another round of closet-checking, another round of adjusting the pillows, and fresh water to fetch—followed, of course, by ten or two hundred more kisses and hugs. Look, I'm lucky to have such a warm and loving person as a daughter. And, yet, night after night, game after game, extra inning after extra inning, it's enough to make a mom really hate baseball.

There are dishes piled up in the sink. Work emails to return. Netflix shows to watch for ten minutes before falling asleep. A husband to—errr, snuggle. I haven't even showered today. I'm a good mom, but a human one. My patience has limits, and those were officially breached a while back.

But...if I've had the foresight to take a few puffs of one of my favorite chill strains, like Kosher Kush or Blue Zkittlez, game time looks and feels different. It may start similarly: I'll lean over, one hand on my daughter's headboard and one on the bed, angling for a hug and kiss.

"I love you to the moon and back," she says, pulling my head to her face.

"I love *you* to the moon and every single star in the entire universe. Including Alpha Centauri and Sirius A and Sirius B."

"And back?" asks my daughter, still clutching my head.

"And back. *Of course.*"

My neck is starting to ache in this awkward position, so I climb into bed and snuggle up. We talk about school and that annoying kid Ryan. We marvel at the shapeshifting dance of candlelight in the hallway and wonder if there's a universe where a girl just like my daughter is receiving her letter of acceptance to Hogwarts. We fervently hope that this is true.

We still pray. I still check the closets and adjust the door. There may be lingering calls for water or any number of other things, but the big difference is I'm okay with all of it. Not gritting my teeth, not watching the clock, not wishing I were someplace else. I'm definitely still me—just more attuned to my kids' emotional needs. More generous with myself and my time.

With extra innings in the bag and the kids tucked in, I'll go downstairs to tackle the dishes and fold the laundry with my husband, but I probably won't erupt into fits of anger because he *totally blanked* and let his driver's license expire or forgot to mail an important check. We'll still talk about it—I just won't lose my shit. Later on, I may even be amenable to a bit more than snuggling; cannabis is good for that, too. (See Chapter 10.)

Look, I'm not saying I need cannabis to parent. I'm not saying I or you—or anyone—should habitually light up to deal with life, even if your life also features insanely long bedtime rituals. But I also know I'm not alone in feeling that cannabis, in the right circumstances, actually makes me a better parent.

I asked Sara Ouimette, a cannabis-friendly licensed marriage and family therapist in California (where cannabis is both medically and recreationally legal) about parenting while partaking. "If a parent is quite high around their kid, I can see how the child might notice mommy or daddy feels different, or 'far away' right now," she tells me. "But if it's in a subtle way that makes the parent feel more connected and more present with the child, then that's going to be a positive experience for the child."

She elaborates on the dose-dependent aspects of weed-momming: "If a microdose or a small dose of cannabis is going to open you up and give you more oomph, or joy, when playing with your kids, or bring out that younger part of you...then by all means, it might just enhance your time with your kids."

# TABOOS

When I first started noticing how profoundly cannabis shifts my parenting, I kept mum to my friends and community. It felt wrong somehow, like admitting to only having sex with my husband while shit-faced (nope) or swallowing a cocktail of pharmaceuticals to deal with my editor (nope again). I was afraid that parenting even mildly under the influence of cannabis would be seen as a cop-out at best—or neglect and abuse at worst. It's sad, but true, that stigmas and taboos around cannabis use remain. And when it comes to perceived failure in the category of moral uprightness, few in our society are judged more harshly than moms.

Ironically, the one person I felt comfortable telling about my newfound delight around parenting was my husband. I had once been judgmental of his pot use, both before and after children, but now, on some level at least, I got it. When consuming responsibly, I'm not a different person or a chemically forged supermom. What I *am* is a less harried version of me. A more chill, more appreciative, and, quite honestly, more nurturing version—like the me from a universe just one click away, a me who doesn't stress nearly as much about things that don't *actually* require stressing.

Now that version of me, I admit, doesn't mix with writing on deadline, or operating a motor vehicle, or doing anything that requires my sharpest intellect and hand-eye coordination—you get the picture. But it mixes incredibly well with building fairy houses, playing (but not winning) at board games, and running around the park with my kids and our dog. I don't use or recommend weed in every parenting situation—that's certain. But for some of the mundane tasks and in the most leisurely moments, cannabis is a win-win for our family. I get a break from my mental habits of worrying and scheduling and directing, and they get the most fun version of me for the occasion. And, this, my husband understands perfectly. When I told him, he didn't even judge *me* for judging *him* about pot and parenting those many moons ago. (Thanks, baby!)

It took a while for me to ponder my newfound realization and eventually find some kind of peace before I could share it with most other moms in my life. But once I came out of the weed closet and admitted to those nearest and dearest that I love to smoke weed and hang out with my kids, all kinds of other weed moms started coming out of that closet, too. The first time I found myself watching kids on the playground after school and getting an earful from another mom about how she prefers indicas for anxiety, I knew things were about to get interesting.

I listened to some OG moms who started smoking cannabis in college and still enjoy it from time to time. I also listened to moms without much previous experience who'd heard about CBD or low-dose THC products and were trying it for pain relief, to sleep better, or to rekindle their sex drive. Even moms who weren't quite ready to dive into the new world of cannabis were eager to hear about it. Some of the moms I spoke to were stay-at-home parents, and some were lawyers or teachers or business owners or restaurateurs. Their common thread? Curiosity about the new world of legal cannabis and what it means for all of us.

# HOW CANNABIS UPS WEED MOMS' PARENTING GAME

The first time I talked to Arlene, I felt like I'd known her a long time. She has a way of making me feel like we're coconspirators in something marvelous. And we kind of are. She's worked in public relations for many years—and since discovering cannabis—has chosen to represent cannabis brands on the cutting edge of wellness and plant medicine. When I want to know what's new and kick-ass in the cannabis space, I talk to her.

"I think," Arlene says on the phone, "the issue for me boils down to anxiety." Her two kids, ages five and seven, are active and social—and so is Arlene. It's just that the chaos of playdates and parties at Chuck E. Cheese, what she describes as "one of my five least favorite places in the world," are not really her thing.

"And it got to the point," Arlene confides, "where even the thought of a playdate was overwhelming. It was a chore for me." But Arlene lives in a suburb of LA where kid-centered activities are the backbone of the social scene. As her children grew, she realized how important play opportunities for kids and what she calls "those mommy friendships" really are. Before discovering cannabis, Arlene was leaning on wine and margaritas to cope with some of the social overwhelm of parenting.

"It helped me take the edge off and it was great....But on those days when I was coming home from work and maybe didn't have a substantial lunch—it wasn't the best thing to do, you know. I'd get—not drunk, but maybe a little more buzzed than I should—as I was trying to figure out how much to drink to make the environment tolerable.... But I started feeling a little self-conscious.... I didn't want people to think I'm *that* drunk mom."

Wine also came with some unpleasant next-day effects. "As I get older," Arlene tells me, "it's like every glass matters. I just *cannot* hang in the same way." So when she'd drink to unwind on a Friday or Saturday night, she says the morning after, "I'd just be worthless."

The funny thing about alcohol, as I learned in a conversation with cannabis nurse Jessie Gill, is that, "while a lot of people will reach for a glass of wine at the end of the day to relieve stress, it actually *contributes* to stress and creates a cortisol reaction." Researchers have indeed found up to a 3 percent cortisol increase for every unit of alcohol consumed.[65] An excess of cortisol in the body is associated with irritability, anxiety, and insomnia, among other things.

For Arlene, feeling like she wasted hours trying to recover from the very thing that was supposed to make her feel better in the first place just wasn't adding up. So a couple of years ago, she pivoted toward edibles for events like birthday parties or park playdates. "I have them in my purse, and if during the process I need to mellow or get more centered, I just pop another one." She found that she was no longer uncomfortable in the midst of those chaotic scenes. "I wasn't overwhelmed, I wasn't anxious," she shares. "I was right where I needed to be."

Of course, it's all about balance. A tiny bit of sedation while parenting can be a good thing. (Chuck E. Cheese, anyone?) But a lot of sedation? Not a winner.

Besides, overdoing it with THC can actually contribute to anxiety, as we learned in Chapter 4—another great reason to stick with microdosing and moderate dosing.

Arlene finds her happy place for socializing with low-dose THC-infused gummies or mints. While she likes to smoke cannabis, too, she prefers edibles when on the go because of how discreet they are—particularly when compared to her old habit, alcohol. "You know," she says, laughing, "I couldn't exactly refill my wine at parent-teacher night."

Arlene grew up in California with conservative Mexican-American parents who, in part because of the harsh impact of the War on Drugs in their community, felt negatively about cannabis. "Drugs of any sort, especially cannabis, were taboo and not part of the 'American Dream' idea that my parents had set out for me: learn English, go to school, get good grades, go to college, have a better life than we did, rinse and repeat," she tells me, chuckling. On top of that, Arlene's husband is an active-duty service member for whom cannabis is off limits. She says some people in her community believe that cannabis is something that only the "fringes of society partake in." As such, she's felt the sting of social disapproval at times. "People talk," she tells me. Her parents were initially disappointed when she, as a mother in her mid-thirties, came clean about her use.

But, more and more, Arlene's noticed shifting attitudes. That's likely in part because legalization in California did not bring any of the doomsday scenarios that anti-cannabis groups feared, but also because Arlene habitually and proactively addresses potential concerns from her community—including from members of her church and the parents of her kids' friends. After a while, even her own parents have grown more comfortable. "My dad," she enthuses, "now enjoys edibles from time to time, and my mom is going all out with CBD rubs. She *loves* telling her friends about it."

Jennifer, a New Hampshire mom I interviewed about what cannabis means in her life, has a lot to say. As a mom to a six-year-old boy with autism and a genetic disorder called fragile X syndrome, Jennifer says that the years since his diagnosis have been hard on her. To make the thirty to forty hours a week of therapy and doctor's appointments possible for her son, Jennifer stopped working as a nutritionist and began focusing all her energy on helping him thrive to the best of his ability. But a part of her was lost in the process.

"Becoming a mother," she tells me, "—it rocks your personal world. You're floundering around trying to find out your new identity, and who you are in your new body, and with this little person now attached to you."

Meanwhile, Jennifer was dealing with fibromyalgia, anxiety, and PTSD. She rediscovered cannabis about a year ago after not having indulged for decades. "I smoked pot in the 1990s, like a lot of Gen-Xers," she tells me. Because fibromyalgia and intensive parenting were leaving her in the kind of debilitating pain where getting out of bed was sometimes more than she could handle, she applied for a medical card through her state program and found relief.

During the week, Jennifer only uses cannabis after her son and husband are asleep. "I call it my 'magic hour,'" she tells me, "where I explore whatever it is that nourishes me that day." That might look like coloring, or listening to The Cure, or playing clarinet, or working with the Tarot. It's helped create space in a life that's, by necessity, focused on her son's needs.

For Jennifer, cannabis has been a means to self-discovery. "I realized that by silencing my right brain and silencing my creativity, I silenced the magic in my life. It's important," she says, "to believe in impossible things."

Tinctures are now Jennifer's favorite way to consume because they're discreet, and because she can easily find the kind of ratios she needs for the best effect. The pain-relieving effects of cannabis last well beyond her magic hour.

"It's given me a life back," she says. "I still have days where I'm very fatigued and in pain. Today is that kind of day, actually," she tells me over the phone. "But I have pants on and I'm sitting in my car—not in bed." And that's huge.

What's more, Jennifer and her husband own a small share in a new, legal pot farm in neighboring Maine. She's optimistic about the future of the industry, and of plant medicine. "It's so interesting," Jennifer muses, "how this one little plant has transformed almost every aspect of my life."

✹ ✹ ✹

Genevieve is a mom in her late forties who owns a brand development firm, has a busy social life, and is the mother of a first grader with a flair for the dramatic. I sat down with her in a bright kitchen just a mile from the beach in Carlsbad, California. Well, *I* sat while she bustled around the kitchen, wiping counters and making tea.

Not long ago, Genevieve went through a rough patch and was prescribed anti-anxiety meds that didn't seem to help much. Her doctor doubled the dose, but those, too, failed. She, like Arlene, was in the habit of enjoying wine—sometimes even leaning on it in those difficult moments at home—but was also becoming aware that drinking regularly could affect relationships with her wife and daughter. She also noticed certain perimenopausal changes in metabolism and decided to cut down on those alcohol sugars. So she tried cannabis. Like a lot of women new to the world of legal weed, she started with a vape pen that delivers THC in small, measured doses.

"I don't get stoned," Genevieve tells me, pouring hot water into our mugs. "I just microdose." And when she does, she finds that her energetic and argumentative daughter doesn't trigger her like usual. After a full day at work, her daughter's defiance used to get under Genevieve's skin. "There are some parents who can just laugh it off, but I'm not one of them," she tells me. Cannabis helps Genevieve manage her mood while staying on top of her parenting game. "I can see my daughter for the young child she is," she tells me, smiling, "instead of a little monster trying to make my life miserable."

The reason cannabis tends to have that kind of soothing effect on people has to do with the endocannabinoid system. "Cannabis compounds engage our ECS to facilitate homeostasis," cannabis educator Emma Chasen tells me. "And that typically manifests as less stress and more chill for most people."

But, just like with anxiety, there's a dose-dependent effect here, too. Cannabis, in small doses, increases attentiveness and helps you just *be*—present, content, and peaceful. But, in the wrong dose, cannabis can absolutely make you check out and lose track of all kinds of things, from the fact that your kid asked for dinner about an hour back to what you *literally just said* three seconds ago. That, my friends, is way too high to parent. My advice? Don't ever go there when you're around your kids, or anyone else's kids.

If you start low and go slow, you needn't worry about spacing out. Gradually you'll settle into a sweet spot as a weed mom who's nailed how to chill TF out *while not compromising* your executive functions. For those of you digging that alcohol comparison, getting a wee bit high is akin to having a glass of wine—not like drinking an entire bottle.

Genevieve's found her sweet spot. When microdosing from her pen, she can get lost in a craft project or a puzzle with her daughter. They toss the balloon back and forth, play airplane, or have pillow fights. You know, the kinds of things that kids love and parents *don't*. Best part is, Genevieve feels her daughter's behavior has turned a corner. They're getting along better, and it seems to Genevieve that a slight reorientation on her part has perceptibly changed their dynamic.

Genevieve's wife chooses not to partake, but it hasn't been an issue between them. And while they haven't yet talked to their daughter about cannabis, "I think," she tells me, sitting down across the table, "she knows something is different. I'm just more present. And she can feel it."

Jenn Lauder is the mother of a twelve-year-old girl and the director of marketing and advocacy at an herbal product company in Portland, Oregon. She and I met in an online group, and when we talk on the phone, my distinct impression is of an energetic, smart, and articulate woman who's also extraordinarily thoughtful in her parenting choices. Cannabis is part of her life—"an extremely valuable tool"—but Jenn's careful to say that it's only one item in a wide swath of self-care practices like yoga and meditation that help her as a person and a parent.

Speaking to the "checked-out" stoner stereotype, Jenn makes clear that conscious cannabis use is one way she checks *in* with herself instead of zoning out or escaping. Because of the way cannabis works with the ECS, in the right doses it makes most people feel more relaxed, euphoric, and emotionally warm. As such, it can be a game changer in the parent-child dynamic.

I asked Carl Hart, PhD, professor of psychology at Columbia University, about the stereotype of the "checked-out stoner" and how it relates to parenting. A psychologist, neuroscientist, and drug policy expert, he's authored or coauthored over sixty peer-reviewed articles on drug use, drug addiction, and drug treatment. He's conducted lab experiments and written the textbook on the cognitive functioning of cannabis users, called *Drugs, Society, and Human Behavior* (McGraw-Hill Education, 2014, coauthored with Charles Ksir).

In an affidavit presented in New York's Family Court, Hart asserts his opinion that responsible, recreational marijuana use does not compromise one's parenting ability:

> "Based upon my thirteen years of experience testing individuals during and post drug-induced intoxication under carefully controlled conditions, it is my opinion that casual, recreational marijuana use does not interfere with one's ability to provide

effective and responsible parental care. As is the case with alcohol, during marijuana intoxication some cognitive operations (e.g., response time) may be temporarily slowed (as measured in seconds), but the intoxicated individual is able to respond to environmental stimuli in an appropriate manner. Marijuana intoxication lasts no more than two to four hours, depending upon the individual's level of experience with the drug. It is important to understand that even during the period of intoxication, the user is able to carry out her/his usual behavioral repertoire; e.g., engage in appropriate social behaviors, including responding to emergencies."

What's more, Hart's clinical research shows that once the effects of cannabis have worn off, there are no lingering or long-term brain or behavioral changes that can be found in the recreational user. Even the most reliable physical symptom of cannabis use, elevated pulse, peaks at about the ten-minute mark and subsides within about two hours. In other words, just like with alcohol, you can be intoxicated by cannabis in the evening without feeling any aftereffects the next morning. However, the metabolites for cannabinoids can remain in the urine for weeks; since most drug tests rely on urine samples, they are notoriously imprecise when it comes to detecting intoxication.

Even while under the influence of cannabis, Hart's study subjects were able to respond appropriately to social situations and emergencies. His research shows that long-term cognitive effects are not measurable in cannabis users, who—in this study—came from all walks of life, including from a variety of professional fields. In short, his research indicates that "recreational use of marijuana does not undermine responsible parenting."

Jenn and her husband, with whom she cofounded a digital magazine on pot and parenting called *Splimm*, embrace the idea of responsible cannabis use. "We're open with our daughter about what this is, and that it's not for kids," she tells me. They've had many iterations of "the talk" that we'll cover in Chapter 8. Jenn, like me, keeps cannabis safely padlocked and has taught her daughter how to recognize it in case she's ever to come across it—like at a friend's house.

Jenn is comfortable vaping or eating low-dose, homemade edibles while parenting, but she and her husband—who also uses medical marijuana for pain associated with a digestive disorder—rarely smoke cannabis at home. When they do, they ensure they're in separate and enclosed quarters. "It's not that we're ashamed or embarrassed," Jenn tells me, "but we don't want our daughter exposed to smoke."

Jenn's quick to talk about what responsible use around her daughter means. She doesn't get crazy high, or catatonic, or forget to pick her daughter up from school. "There are many experiences besides intoxication that cannabis can provide," she tells me. Once in a while, she does enjoy smoking a joint and getting high—it's just not something she's comfortable doing around her kid.

While Jenn recognizes that cannabis use, like that of alcohol and other substances, can cross the line into problematic use, "the negative effects," she tells me, "are mitigated because it's a pretty benign substance generally." Ultimately, it boils down to intention. "If your intention is to enhance your wellness or be more present throughout the day—those are pieces of responsible use." But if you're consuming cannabis out of compulsion or habit or boredom, that's a sign that you probably need to reexamine your relationship to the plant. (See Chapter 9 for more.) "I don't want to be one of those people who says, 'no worries, it's cannabis, it's all good.' We lose credibility when we say that."

In part because her family lives in Portland—one of the most progressive cities in the country when it comes to cannabis—Jenn has embraced the synergy of pot and parenting and is more than happy to share what works. The best dose for Jenn, for myself, and for a lot of other moms, is just enough to shift our energy from an outward-focused, work-and-responsibilities perspective to one that's emotionally attuned.

# RACE, PRIVILEGE, AND WEED MOMMING

Professor Hart, who's studied drug use and drug users for his entire professional career, is also the first African American tenured professor in the sciences at Columbia. When we spoke, he reminded me that though Black and white people reported using cannabis in roughly equal numbers, Black people in this country suffer disproportionately at the hands of law enforcement and family courts. Black men are incarcerated for cannabis-related offenses at much higher rates than white men, and Black mothers are significantly more likely to have their children taken away by Child Protective Services than white mothers are.

Jenn, who is white, is also quick to point out the privileges of her skin color when it comes to being a mom who publicly admits—and celebrates—her cannabis use. But even for someone like Jenn, it's been a slow progression toward her current level of openness. Her family lived in Baltimore before moving to Portland, and she says that because Maryland was then a prohibition state (now it's medical-only), she had her speech ready in case CPS ever showed up at her house.

In legal states today, fewer and fewer parents are penalized for weed, but legal issues remain a dilemma for many mothers living in nonrecreational states and for women of color all over the country; sadly, consuming this plant at the wrong place/wrong time or using cannabis if you're living in non-white skin could lead to a loss of freedom or child custody. The awful truth is that in the US today, people of color—particularly Black people—still face greater risks to their freedom and safety simply *by living their lives normally*.

I spoke with Natasha Best, who works to dispel stigmas online as the Stoned at Home Mom, about skin color and weed as a mom. Natasha's the daughter of a Black man and a white woman, and she tells me that getting in trouble for weed is "definitely more of a thing that people of color worry about." She recounted a recent driving experience when, though she'd done nothing wrong on the road, a police officer drove right next to her for far too long while staring intently into her car. Natasha had cannabis she'd recently purchased in the car, and though she has a medical card and wasn't high, she still worried. "It was so bizarre and scary," she says. "I was thinking, if he pulls me over, I don't know what's going to happen."

Shali, a mom of two in Oakland, California, tells me that she notices increasing numbers of neighbors, friends, and coworkers who are open about their cannabis use. But as a mixed-race woman who presents as Black, she still gets occasional side-eye when patronizing dispensaries in more affluent neighborhoods. "I do feel like there's a stigma when you're a person of color and have weed rather than say, a white college student would be," says Shali. And even after adult-use legalization in California, a white neighbor called the police on her for using cannabis at home. She says one of the officers seemed to be looking for something to give her a hard time about— asking question after question about her home life and habits. "I smoked a blunt in my backyard—which is *legal*," Shali recalls telling them. "I'm not driving. I'm not bothering anybody."

Because I believe that it's every woman's right to use this plant in a safe and health-promoting way, I need to speak up in any forum available to me about how responsible cannabis use should be normalized for women of every color. I need to speak up when women of color are penalized or questioned for the very same things I enjoy; I'm confident in my ability to make responsible choices around cannabis and parenting, and I know other weed moms of every background and skin color can do the same.

## Weed Moms Speak on Being a Weed Mom of Color

"Being a biracial woman of color and a mother comes with a multitude of challenges. I feel like adding cannabis to the mix both adds to these challenges and helps with these challenges... Unfortunately, Black mothers are stereotyped as more troubled or unfit to parent compared to white mothers... Just because some of us use cannabis, it doesn't make us bad mothers. I believe cannabis actually makes me a more patient and understanding mother. It helps me to let go of my daily stressors. It helps me to be more imaginative and playful with my child. Overall, I wish it was more readily available to mothers and less stigmatized for the mothers who do use it. —*Kania, mom of 1, Michigan*

"...Cannabis helps me be a better mom. From PMS pains and anxiety to temper tantrums and potty training, cannabis gives me the same experiences that it gives my other mom friends. It heals... We already face the stigma that moms who use cannabis aren't good moms. Moms of color want the same benefits from cannabis—just the same as white women." —*Shabria, mom of 2, Illinois*

"There are so many people, mostly Black individuals, who are incarcerated for something that I am able to do legally. It's insane to think that all these people are still sitting in jail, while many are profiting off the same thing that put them there. Especially when it's considered 'essential.' It just blows my mind."
—*Natasha Best, the "Stoned at Home Mom"*

"I know that because I am a woman of color, I have to be extra careful on when I pick it [cannabis] up so I don't get pulled over. I have to be careful when I do use it so I don't alert the neighbors nearby. My kids come number one, so I don't want them to be in danger or have someone call the cops on me or CPS because they put this stigma on me... Because of the history of racism in this country, we are automatically put in this box that we are worse. We are bad mothers, we are drug addicts, we're not responsible, we deserve to have our kids taken away. Black people are more likely to get higher sentences for weed possession or usage than a white person. Our lives will always be different because of the color of our skin." —*Kandice, mom of 2, Arizona*

# PREGNANCY AND CANNABIS

I spoke with Marissa Fratoni, RN, a cannabis nurse and maternal health specialist in Massachusetts, about the difficult questions surrounding use during pregnancy and breastfeeding. "We don't have a full understanding of what all the risks are," she tells me, adding that we do know that cannabinoids cross the placenta and also pass into breastmilk.

Ethically, it's impossible to do clinical research measuring the effects of cannabis on a fetus or a baby, so we have to rely on observational studies, surveys, and self-reports. That kind of data is important, but incomplete, Fratoni points out. "The research we do have hasn't been able to show that cannabis is harmful," she says, "but neither is it able to show that it's *not* harmful."

A 1994 study in Jamaica found no differences at the one-month mark between babies who'd been exposed to cannabis in the womb, and those who hadn't.[66] But other studies have found lower birth weights, motor skill delays, and cognitive issues in children who had been exposed to cannabis prenatally. Because these are naturalistic rather than controlled studies, a number of potentially confounding factors—like use of alcohol or other drugs—can complicate findings. There's also new research in California pointing to higher rates of prenatal cannabis use, but no statistically significant outcome for newborn babies.[67]

And then there's researcher bias. "We do have a lot of studies seeking harm," says Fratoni. On top of that, many studies only look at data from women who smoke THC-rich varieties of cannabis and do not compare results to other forms of consumption, like edibles, tinctures, or even CBD.

Still, there are reasons, like help with nausea and vomiting, why some pregnant women would like to use cannabis. (I get it: my nausea with both pregnancies was basically a disability!) And women who are already medical marijuana patients for MS or autoimmune diseases may prefer to continue managing their symptoms with cannabis instead of turning to pharmaceuticals—some of which also carry unknown risks for a developing baby.

"We can't look at it as black and white," Jessilyn Dolan, RN, a cannabis nurse, researcher, doula, and legal cannabis grower in Vermont tells me. "If a pregnant woman has to go on six pharmaceuticals to take care of her rheumatoid arthritis, and that increases the risk of miscarriage, but she can use a moderate amount of cannabis and get the same symptom relief—that makes a lot of sense." But Dolan's quick to add that no one can make that decision for a pregnant woman. "You have to know your laws and weigh the pros and cons for yourself," she says.

Some OBGYNs and midwives do test prenatally for drugs, including THC, while others don't, and, depending on your state, testing positive for THC while pregnant can trigger an automatic call to Child Protective Services. For recreational and wellness uses, pregnancy *isn't* a good time to try cannabis. Get to know your laws and talk to a cannabis nurse or doc if you're considering using cannabis for a medical condition while pregnant.

# BREASTFEEDING AND CANNABIS

Breastfeeding moms may be interested in cannabis for help with postpartum depression, anxiety, and insomnia. But, like in pregnancy, the risks aren't entirely clear.

"We don't have enough information to rally around to say 'yes, this is safe, go ahead,'" Fratoni tells me. "But we *also* don't know about a lot of other medications that pregnant and breastfeeding women are taking." She believes that, with time, a clearer picture of the risks and benefits will emerge, and that—instead of making decisions *for* women—practitioners need to empower them to make informed choices.

In the meantime, keep in mind that the official recommendation of the American College of Obstetrics and Gynecology is to avoid cannabis during pregnancy and breastfeeding, and that in your state you could face legal risks for using—including mandatory drug rehabilitation, jail time, or termination of your parental rights. It varies a lot by state, so I recommend doing your research and talking to a cannabis healthcare provider knowledgeable in maternal and child health for more information.

# JUST ADD CANNABIS: TIPS FOR MIXING CANNABIS AND PARENTING

Cannabis and parenting can be a fantastic pairing when you're engaged in low-risk activities with children, such as:

◊ Making purple and green polka-dot spiders out of play dough

◊ Coloring, drawing, painting, or crafting

◊ Any kind of pretend play (*seriously!*)

◊ Gardening (you may want to do a quick coordination test first—in any case, avoid operating a lawn mower or chainsaw)

◊ Reading to your children, or listening to them read

◊ Watching a movie or TV show together (take it from me, *My Little Pony*'s super-trippy)

◊ Playing a board game (though not necessarily if you want to win)

◊ Co-parenting with a sober spouse

◊ Socializing responsibly with other weed moms (see Chapter 11)

◊ Saying goodnight to your children, especially if it involves lots of praying

Don't risk using cannabis when:

◊ Caring for a baby or toddler alone

◊ Driving

◊ Using machinery

◊ Swimming, watching your kids swim, or spending time around *any* body of water unless you are with a non-stoned adult

◊ Trying a new product or dose

◊ Parenting in a stressful or anxiety-producing situation (unless it's a purely social setting, where cannabis actually helps you relax and chat with strangers)

◊ Parenting in any situation where safety requires your quick reflexes, like if you decide to take your five-year-old rock climbing or skydiving

◊ Parenting in the midst of divorce or separation, especially if your soon-to-be ex may try to hold it against you

◊ You are pregnant or breastfeeding, unless you are treating for a medical condition and are under the care of a cannabis-knowledgeable health professional

◊ Any situation where your gut tells you to abstain. You will have many years ahead of you to enjoy cannabis. One day you can even be a cool, stoned grandma—just not while caring for littles.

Be that conscious consumer—I have faith in you. Know your stuff. Respect your personal tolerance. Though there's a bit of a learning curve to finding the right modes and doses of consumption while combining motherhood and cannabis, my experience—and many other moms' experiences—reflect that responsible use and momming are one hundred percent compatible. Laws and social norms are changing rapidly, and they're all moving in one direction: toward more access, more openness, and more elevated uses of cannabis. Being a weed mom isn't a passing fad. We're here for the long haul.

# Weed Moms Speak on How Cannabis Affects Parenting

"It 1,000 percent makes me more patient." —*Natasha Best, the "Stoned at Home Mom," Oklahoma*

"Mama doesn't need to get high to cope with life. It's not about getting out of my head, but tuning into it." —*Rachel, mom of two, Massachusetts*

"I strongly believe it makes me a better mom.... Cannabis slows down my thoughts. It helps me be more patient and more present. I'm not thinking of the million things I have to do. I'm focusing on *them*, on *their* life." —*Jessie Gill, cannabis nurse and founder of MarijuanaMommy.com, speaking on the* Your Highness *cannabis podcast*

"It's absolutely helped get through some of the drudgeries of parenthood and to be more fun and creative and silly.... in a moderate way, cannabis can be wonderful for parents." —*Reya, mom of one, Idaho*

"I have high-functioning anxiety and depression, and my ten-year-old daughter is severely ADHD. Cannabis allows me to get out of my own head and be wild and crazy with her. We've had so many adventures that I never would have imagined, so many memories that would have never been made if I was still hiding out in my house. Cannabis gave me a relationship with my daughter that I never would have had, and I am so, so thankful for that." —*Stephanie, mom of one, Illinois*

"I don't have much hands-on support, as an older mom to two little ones, and I have [generalized anxiety disorder] GAD. I find cannabis, in small doses, helps immensely." —*Anonymous mom*

"After having my children, two boys, my anxiety was at an all-time high due to hormones, moving, and my new role as caretaker of these tiny beings bent on self-harm... Using cannabis allows me to relax, really savor and be present in the moment with my children, have more patience and overall, be a fun mom unplagued by exhaustion, mental strain, and anxiety. It also alleviates my aches and pains so I can keep up with them. And then at night, I can pop an edible and sleep like my husband, blissfully happy and soundly, throughout the night. It's helped my motherhood journey be that much more positive." —*Anonymous mom*

## CHAPTER 7

# KIDS, TEENS, AND CANNABIS USE

As a general rule, kids and cannabis don't mix. But there *are* exceptions. In this chapter, we'll take a brief tour of pediatric medical uses for CBD, and even THC. We'll also talk about the risks involved in accidental—or intentional—cannabis use by kids and teens; the cliff notes version, in case you're wondering, is that even in very large amounts, THC isn't fatal. However, it's our absolute responsibility as parents to keep cannabis out of the hands of little ones and to provide age-appropriate education at every stage.

## KIDS AND CBD

Even if you've never heard of Charlotte Figi, she's partially responsible for the fact that you've heard of CBD. The epileptic girl from Colorado became the nation's poster child of medical marijuana because her remarkable journey with CBD-rich cannabis oil was as extraordinary as her mother's dedication to procuring it and educating the world about why.

In 2006, Charlotte Figi was born with a severe form of epilepsy called Dravet syndrome. As a baby, Charlotte suffered from up to four seizures a day—some of which lasted hours. By the age of two, her development had slowed, and she began to show autistic-like behaviors that only worsened. She stopped talking, was confined to a wheelchair, and relied on a feeding tube for nourishment. By five years old, Charlotte experienced up to fifty seizures a day.

Her family tried every cocktail of pharmaceuticals prescribed by Charlotte's doctors—none of which stopped her seizures. In 2011, out of options, Charlotte's mother Paige researched CBD and gained permission from their home state of Colorado to try a dose of high-CBD, low-THC extract in a desperate attempt to mitigate her daughter's life-threatening seizures.

The results were nothing short of incredible; with CBD, Charlotte experienced her first seizure-free week since she was a baby. She began making eye contact and communicating with her family; eventually, she walked again, fed herself, and played with her twin sister—things her family thought she'd never do again. People who met her said that Charlotte was warm and genuine—an observer of people, a lover of nature.

But for the Figis, sourcing CBD was a problem. At the time, Colorado had established its medical marijuana program—and voters were poised to okay recreational weed—but few growers were working with CBD-rich strains; there wasn't demand. Searching for a regular source of quality CBD, Paige Figi reached out to a family of seven brothers in Colorado Springs, who had been experimenting with a variety of low-THC hemp known as "Hippie's Disappointment" because it didn't have enough THC to get high on. The Stanley brothers agreed to grow more of that CBD-rich strain, which they renamed Charlotte's Web—now one of the most well-known and respected CBD brands around.

Over the next several years, Charlotte's story sparked a movement. She was featured on CNN's multipart documentary, *Weed*, hosted by Dr. Sanjay Gupta, whose public reversal on cannabis in 2013 paved the way for more favorable mainstream media coverage of the topic. These events coincided with, and bolstered, the public's changing perceptions of cannabis and helped spur legalization efforts in other states. And from states without legal access, "medical refugees," or families with sick kids seeking legal cannabis therapy, flooded to Colorado. Paige Figi, who fought hard for access—and against stigma—cofounded a nonprofit, Realm of Caring, to provide education and advocacy around the therapeutic use of CBD. And weed rapper MC Flow wrote and performed her moving song, "Oh, Charlotte," at Red Rocks with Grammy-winner Jason Mraz.

Eventually, the CBD-based antiepileptic pharmaceutical Epidiolex was approved, though the Figis and many others still preferred CBD oil in its more natural form. It's no exaggeration to say that Charlotte, and the CBD named after her, were two of the most important forces behind the CBD-based health and wellness juggernaut we know today. Sadly, Charlotte's own story ended in April 2020, when she passed away of a COVID-19 infection at the age of thirteen. Her legacy lives on, as does the public's new and growing acceptance of CBD as medicine.

# CBD AND EPILEPSY

CBD-based Epidiolex is approved by the FDA to treat kids over two years old with Dravet syndrome, which Charlotte suffered from, or another seizure disorder called Lennox-Gastaut syndrome. The efficacy of this highly concentrated form of CBD has been shown using three separate double-blind, randomized clinical trials. It's given orally, isn't without side effects, and must be overseen by a doctor.

When I spoke with David Berger, MD, a board-certified pediatrician in Tampa, Florida, and founder of Wholistic ReLeaf, he told me he prefers a good-quality CBD supplement to Epidiolex. He's even had success treating other seizure disorders in children besides the two that Epidiolex is approved for, and he's done so with much smaller overall doses of CBD.

# CBD AND AUTISM

Autism is another area where CBD for kids shows promise. Dr. Berger recommends CBD for pediatric patients with autism and finds that symptoms of anxiety, aggression, and self-harm can be reduced or alleviated—either with CBD alone, or when combined with a carefully titrated quantity of THC.

A 2019 study of 188 children with autism found that 30 percent experienced significant improvement in symptoms such as restlessness, agitation, and rage attacks when given a solution of 20:1 CBD to THC.[68] An additional 53.7 percent of children in the study showed moderate relief with the treatment, which was given in addition to—not in place of—the patients' existing regimen of meds. The results are encouraging, but it's important to note that it's only an initial look at the intersections of autism and cannabis and that the study didn't include a control group.

# OTHER POTENTIAL PEDIATRIC USES OF CBD

Some parents give their children CBD for help with anxiety, insomnia, PTSD, and hyperactivity, and you can find online parent groups like "CBD Moms Support" and "CBD Oil for Kids," dedicated to sharing information on the topic. Research hasn't yet validated these uses for kids; unfortunately, we may not have better answers any time soon because studies on cannabis are notoriously difficult to get approved and funded—more so if those studies involve kids.

Dr. Berger, who's been working with plant medicines in many forms—not just cannabis—for his entire medical career says, "I don't see CBD as risky unless there is a negative reaction to it," adding that he's seen that only twice. Generally speaking, he says, as long as you have a "verified product that's tested for all of the various toxins, including molds, mycotoxins, solvents, metals, and pesticides, it should be safe when following a good dosing protocol." If you think CBD may help your child, I suggest speaking with a cannabis-knowledgeable healthcare professional who can point you in the direction of quality products and appropriate dosing.

# KIDS AND THC

Marinol is the pharmaceutical name for a synthetic version of THC that's prescribed to both adults and children who suffer from nausea and vomiting associated with chemotherapy. Aside from that particular use, there's no general consensus about whether kids should be using any amount of THC.

Those under twenty-one with a qualifying condition like cancer, pain, PTSD, anxiety, depression, Tourette syndrome, and others, can apply for a medical marijuana card in some states, and there's no doubt that some of those young patients have experienced real improvements. As I mentioned a moment ago, the "medical refugee" influx to states with legal THC access for underage patients continues. Let me be clear: no one is looking to get kids high, but in cases where other approaches have failed, some parents and pediatricians are open to therapeutic doses of THC.

"I'm very cautious with THC," Dr. Berger tells me, "especially for pediatric patients." Therefore, he starts with small doses of THC alongside CBD and titrates up gradually to find the therapeutic dose. Parents tell him that "it's very uncommon for their kid to look high or stoned—that's not at all what we're going for." Many doctors are afraid to touch the subject of cannabis in pediatrics, but because Dr. Berger had been a holistically oriented MD for twenty years before medical cannabis even became an option, he considers it just another tool in his box.

# "RECREATIONAL" CANNABIS AND YOUTH: QUICK FACTS

### ...on prevalence of use

◊ In 2019, 43.7 percent of high school seniors self-report ever having tried cannabis, 22.3 percent report last month use, and 6.4 percent report daily use.[69]

### ...on health and safety

◊ Cannabis is a low-toxicity substance, and there's no scientifically validated literature documenting fatality in humans; the DEA's own resource guide states that "no deaths from overdose of marijuana have been reported."[70]

  » However, overconsumption can cause unsafe behavior and poor decision-making, which can, in turn, lead to accidental death.

  » If children ingest a very large quantity of THC, they can require hospitalization and intubation.

  » In extremely high doses, THC can also affect cardiovascular function.

◊ Edible cannabis is processed differently from inhaled cannabis, and the effects of edibles tend to be much stronger.

  » Edibles pose the biggest potential harm for kids because infused gummies, chocolates, or cookies can be mistaken for treats.

  » Some ERs and Poison Control Centers have seen an uptick in pediatric patients with accidental cannabis exposure—primarily caused by edibles.

### ...on mental health

◊ Human brains are still under construction until about the age of twenty-five; adding psychoactive substances during this time may impede healthy development.

» Frequent adolescent cannabis use has been associated with greater risk of developing schizophrenia.[71]

» Critics of the above-mentioned study point out that those at increased risk of schizophrenia are more likely to self-medicate with cannabis, and that it's not cannabis necessarily that causes these conditions to develop.

» A 2019 study found a small but significant relationship between adolescent cannabis use and depression, anxiety, and suicidal ideation later in life.[72]

» As above, critics point out the higher rates of self-medication among those prone to mental health conditions.

### ...on cognitive development

◊ Contrary to what was once thought, adolescent cannabis use does not appear to cause lower IQ.[73]

◊ A 2018 study showed that teens who use cannabis regularly showed deficits in impulse control, memory, and perceptual reasoning.[74]

» Another 2018 study showed that memory capacity returned to full function in adolescents following one month of cannabis abstinence.[75]

### ...on substance abuse

◊ Some research shows that starting regular cannabis use before the age of eighteen is correlated with cannabis use disorder later in life.[76]

» Certain environmental and genetic factors may contribute to *both* early-onset use *and* developing cannabis use disorder; in other words, it's possible the relationship isn't a causal one.

### ...on comparisons to alcohol

◊ Underage alcohol use is strongly associated with fatal car crashes, unsafe sex, sexual assault, unplanned pregnancy, and increased risk of nonautomobile-related injury.[77]

### ...on legal and social considerations

◊ Some US middle and high schools permit random drug testing of students.

  » Middle and high school students can lose their ability to participate in sports or other activities for cannabis use.

  » Minors also risk criminal prosecution for possession and distribution.

◊ You can lose custody of your children and be prosecuted for child endangerment or child abuse if they ingest or use cannabis found in your home.

The research, combined with the legal landscape, is indeed complex. For every group of studies finding harm from adolescent cannabis use, you can track down at least one rebuttal. It's true that research funded by NIDA (the National Institute on Drug Abuse) and NIH (the National Institutes of Health) is more likely to seek harmful effects, and independent research is harder to establish and fund.

A 2019 largescale review of human and animal studies on age-related differences in how cannabis affects the brain found some interesting results.[78] For instance, executive functioning appears to be more impaired in adolescent cannabis users than adults, and overall effects are much worse in "heavy and dependent users." The review found that adolescents may have greater susceptibility to dependence, but difficulties in learning and memory observed in adolescent cannabis users tends to decline once they are no longer using it.

Dr. Rav Ivker, the cannabis-friendly osteopath in Boulder, tells me that small amounts of THC are unlikely to harm anyone—child, adolescent, or adult.

He supports limited medical marijuana access for youth but warns against high-potency and frequent THC use in young people, regardless of whether it's for medical or recreational purposes. "These adverse consequences," he tells me, referencing the studies on schizophrenia and other mental and cognitive changes observed in studies, "result usually from daily use—kids that are getting high every day and smoke several times a day."

In my view, we can cautiously surmise from the data that there are definite risks to adolescent cannabis use but that those risks are perhaps not as pronounced or long term as we once thought. Far from advocating a weed free-for-all, what I'm saying is this: some degree of underage substance use is inevitable. Instead of exaggerating the dangers, responsible adults should state them clearly—without fear-mongering and misinformation—while providing sane approaches to teen substance education. In other words, encourage adolescents to delay experimenting with cannabis and understand the risks without unduly demonizing the plant or those who benefit from it.

# CHAPTER 8

# THE TALK: MOMS ON THE FRONTLINE OF THE CULTURAL SHIFT

"No drug, including marijuana, is completely safe, especially for teenagers. Yet the mischaracterization of drugs such as marijuana...may be the Achilles' heel of current drug prevention approaches because such messages too often contain exaggerations and misinformation that contradict young people's own observations and experiences. As a result, many teens have become cynical and lose confidence in what we, as teachers, parents, and other caregivers tell them."

—*Marsha Rosenbaum, sociologist, former director of the Drug Policy Alliance's San Francisco chapter, and author of Safety First: A Reality-Based Approach to Teens and Drugs*

Jessie Gill was a hospice nurse when an on-the-job accident left her with a spinal injury and debilitating pain. The New Jersey native tried at least a dozen different pain medications, including Valium and numerous opioids—all of which either didn't work the way she needed them to or caused intolerable side effects. She was on disability, unable to work, play, or be fully present for her kids. So, finally, having little to lose, she gave medical cannabis a try.

At the time, Gill's eighteen-year-old daughter couldn't believe that, after all she had learned about marijuana's harms in her school's DARE program, her mom was becoming a pothead. "*What* are you doing?" Gill recalls her daughter questioning incredulously.

But Gill's daughter, who was studying science, was savvy enough to have understood her mom's health struggles—and the immediate results got her attention. Very soon after starting her medical cannabis regimen, Gill got off all her other pain meds and regained her former sense of self. She could play boardgames at the kitchen table and go to her kids' events. Soon, she got back to work—this time as a cannabis nurse on a mission to educate patients about the healing potential of the herb, and as a founder of MarijuanaMommy.com.

Speaking of her daughter, Gill tells me, "She had to unlearn DARE—and that was at first a bit tough. But when she saw the results, she was a believer."

Gill's son was in the third grade when she became a medical cannabis user, and she knew she'd have to prepare him for the stigma he might face from friends or family members. Eventually, Gill tells me, knowing that he was going to start the DARE program in school, she decided to take a closer look at the curriculum and find out what kids were learning about the plant she had found so helpful—a medicine that literally gave her back her life.

What she found wasn't encouraging. DARE programs vary somewhat, but as a rule they take a "prohibitionist" approach and tend neither to acknowledge the plant's medical potential nor appreciate that cannabis and other drugs are fundamentally different. "We're teaching kids that cannabis is akin to heroin. When they find out it's not true, they won't trust us," says Gill.

So she did something about it. Gill writes and speaks frequently on the topic of moms and cannabis and developed a fact sheet she calls a DARE alternative.

**The Talk: Moms on the Frontline of the Cultural Shift**

# WEED MOM Q&A

**Q: Should I tell my children about my own cannabis use?**

**A:** Short answer is that there's no definitive one. It depends on where you live, the ages of your children, your relationship with them, your spousal or co-parenting situation, your job, and, of course, the unique needs and capacities of your children. If it's possible to discuss your relationship to cannabis without causing undue risks to any of the abovementioned, I'd say to err on the side of truthfulness. As legalization efforts march along and an increasing number of Americans are tuning in to the healing and pleasurable uses of the plant, I stand up for the idea that cannabis can and should be normalized in American families.

Normalizing cannabis, of course, doesn't mean we give kids and teens access, nor does it mean we condone early or heavy consumption. It *does* mean we stop demonizing it and be truthful about the good and the bad. We own our choices—on both the personal and the familial levels—because we're smart and conscious and strong as hell. Educate, uplift, empower—*that's* how weed moms roll.

**Q: What factors should I consider when choosing to talk to my kids about cannabis?**

**A:** Regardless of what you choose to tell them about your own use, I strongly recommend educating tweens and teens about cannabis. For younger kids, honesty and openness are the weed mom way, but be cautious about disclosing your personal use under the following circumstances:

◊ *Cannabis is currently illegal in your state, or you are using it illegally...*

It's risky to use cannabis illegally, and your comfort level vis-à-vis that risk is entirely personal. Here are five examples of illegal use: 1) buying on the illicit market, 2) growing at home when you're not authorized to, 3) buying cannabis in a nearby legal state and bringing it home to a prohibition state, 4) deliberately misleading a health professional about a medical issue in order to obtain medical marijuana, 5) when your job specifically prohibits cannabis use.

Today I live in a prohibition state, and yet, here I am, writing a book all about weed and moms while admitting to #3 above—there's risk in it for me. But I know which way the wind is blowing—toward legalization, or decriminalization at a minimum, all across the US. And, so, I'm willing to take the small-enough risk because I believe in ending the stigma and normalizing responsible use. And I'm white.

Since the beginnings of prohibition, the risks of using cannabis have always been much greater for people of color. If you're a Black or brown mother, no matter where you live, deciding whether or not to incorporate this wonderfully healing plant into your self-care repertoire is a tough choice that I have no business weighing in on. We all have the same rights to conscious cannabis elevation; yet, the racist underpinnings of the drug war and the enduringly unequal way drug laws are enforced mean that your risks are greater. Racism fucking sucks.

All weed moms need to speak up for equity and justice on this issue because there's no reason Black and brown women should be treated differently on this, or any other question of health and parenting. Consider supporting the Last Prisoner Project (seeking to free those in prison for marijuana distribution, who are disproportionately Black and brown); the Equity First Alliance (promoting equity in cannabis business and in cannabis-related law enforcement); Root & Rebound (helping people who were previously incarcerated find work in legal cannabis); Success Centers (dedicated to helping marginalized communities with entrepreneurship and economic growth, including in the cannabis space); or National Bail Out (not cannabis-specific, but still an important piece of social justice to help provide bail money for those who can't afford it—on Mother's Day they even have a #FreeBlackMamas drive). Educational resources about social justice and cannabis are also archived on the Family Law & Cannabis Alliance site.

No matter who you are, I encourage you to get to know the laws and the precedents where you live. If you're in a prohibition state, look up the arrest stats for cannabis and find out what happens after arrest. For instance, do those arrested for cannabis have to attend twelve-step meetings, or drug education, and do they lose custody of their kids?

You can, of course, minimize your risk for legal trouble if you're discreet, but, sadly, there's no truly risk-free version of illegal cannabis use. With all my heart and soul, I hope it changes—and stat.

◊ *You're in an abusive or unstable spousal relationship...*

If you're in an abusive relationship—whether the abuse is physical, emotional, sexual, or financial, seek help. The National Coalition Against Domestic Violence (NCADV) lists hotlines, like 1-800-799-SAFE. Find this one, and a lot more, at https://ncadv.org/get-help. You can also find a state-by-state list of resources at the Department of Health and Human Services site for women and relationship safety (www.womenshealth.gov).

Your safety, and that of your kids, is priority number one.

An unstable partnership is a little harder to define, but I'm confident you'll know if you're in one. When my husband and I went through our rough year, we separated and reunited so many times we literally lost count, and he sometimes says that he actually lived out of his car during that time because that's where most of his stuff lived.

And even though it may have smoothed out some of the worst of the heartache, shame, anger, fear, and confusion I felt then, I'm glad I didn't use cannabis at that moment. Chaos + weed + parenting don't mix well, so please, weed moms, partake when you're settled in your home life.

◊ *You're co-parenting with an ex who might try to use cannabis against you in custody proceedings...*

Even good people do shitty things when hurt and angry. Don't make the mistake of assuming your ex will be reasonable about your responsible weed use. Splits, even kinda amicable ones, can bring out the worst in people.

I asked Thomas M. Huguenor, JD, of the San Diego-based law firm, Huguenor Mattis, A.P.C., about the question of custody. Huguenor, a board-certified specialist in family law, let me know that even in a legal state like California, federal law still applies. Therefore, cannabis use can potentially cause a problem for a mother when the other parent chooses to make it one.

Ultimately, he writes, courts are meant to look to "the best interest of the child" in custody decisions, and the whole picture—including each parent's relationship with and ability to care for the child—is taken into consideration. Of course, if the child is seen to be at risk because of a parent's cannabis use, that would be a factor. Examples of putting a child at risk include driving under the influence, exposing a child to secondhand smoke, keeping cannabis in an accessible place, or allowing a child to accidentally consume cannabis.

Huguenor writes that the relative novelty of cannabis as a recreationally legal drug affects the courts, too. Judges, who have probably had personal experience with alcohol, are more likely to be "knowledgeable as to the type of alcohol use that poses a risk in child custody situations, but less likely to know the type of cannabis use that poses little or no threat in child custody situations."

All this is to say, use a heavy dose of caution if child custody at stake. If you're living in a prohibition state, quadruple it. (I'm not condoning illegal use here, just providing information.)

◊ *You have a pending legal situation, or any interaction with Child Protective Services...*

I hope this goes without saying, but just in case: don't give well-meaning (or not-well-meaning) but clueless representatives of the drug war any reason to give you shit, make your life hard, or take your kids. This goes for cops, prosecutors, judges, CPS workers, immigration authorities, and parole officers. Even though responsible cannabis use may be a great stress-reliever for your legal troubles, in this situation, it's just not worth the risk.

◊ *Your kids aren't ready to talk about cannabis...*

Kids (like adults!) vary in maturity, vocabulary, and grasp of subtleties. You know your family and your situation—I trust you to figure out how and when to start the conversation about this important subject.

For instance, if your children aren't old enough or mature enough to limit their conversations about cannabis with the public (including their peers), then work on those public/private distinctions first. They need to understand that you believe cannabis is safe *for adults, in the right quantities, at the right times*. But because this belief isn't shared by everyone, it's important that they know what to talk about out in the world and what to leave at home.

If you do choose to delay your conversations about cannabis, remember that you probably don't want your kids learning about the subject, or about your use, from others first. So don't delay forever, weed moms!

**Q: Does cannabis legalization lead to more teen use?**

**A:** You might think it would, but the data says otherwise. Multiple states have run the numbers on youth and weed and found that adult-use legalization impacts underage use very little. In some cases, underage cannabis use even declines post-legalization. For instance, the Colorado Department of Public Health and Environment reports that cannabis use in high school students declined slightly between 2011 and 2017[79] (legal retail sales took effect in 2014). And in Oregon, cannabis use among eleventh graders fell in the year legal sales started.[80]

**Q: I'm ready to talk with my kids about cannabis! Now how TF should I do this?**

**A:** The yoga teacher in me wants us all to take a big breath together. Innnhale. Exxxhale. It's going to be okay. You're their parent. You love them. You can do this.

First, I want to acknowledge the fact that talking to kids about cannabis may feel quite different for mothers of color in this country than for white mothers. Shali, a Black mom in California whom you met in Chapter 6, has two sons, ages 13 and 23. Her older son occasionally uses cannabis, and Shali worries about him getting pulled over with weed in the car or flagged for holding a joint in public. "Your white counterpart might be able to get away with that," she tells him, "but you have to be more careful." Unfortunately, the discussion with your kids will indeed vary—not just depending on their ages—but on your family's skin color, where you live, and what policing is like in your area.

Jessilyn Dolan, a mom of two, a cannabis nurse, and a legal grower in Vermont, reminded me that it's okay for us moms to acknowledge how uncomfortable all the conversations around kids and cannabis can be— while simultaneously remembering that we *really need* to have them.

I wish I could provide you with a perfect script for talking to your kid about cannabis at any age, but I can't. "There are no simple, ready-made answers, just thoughtful conversations," Marsha Rosenbaum, author of *Safety First: A Reality-Based Approach to Teens and Drugs*, tells me. Drawing from the experience and insight of dozens of weed moms, along with my own research into drug education programs, the next section covers a set of ideas, signposts, and important safety practices to share with your kids by age and stage.

### ◊ *Ages 0–2*

Unless your kids are verbal super-geniuses, there's not much in the way of cannabis education that will find fertile ground yet. My recs are simply: 1) to consume in healthful doses at the appropriate and safe moments, 2) to keep your cannabis locked and out of reach, and 3) to love and care for them. Done.

Well, *almost* done. I want to talk about padlocking your cannabis, and I mean NOW—even if your dear little is not yet making eye contact or rolling over. Why? One, it will establish a good habit that will serve you well from the day your baby learns to crawl until they're old enough to (maybe) enjoy a legal toke. Two, the extra step of opening up a locked box to access your stash will encourage mindful, deliberate use, which, as you know by now, is key to weed momming! And three, in the event CPS or police ever visit your home, you'll be on more solid ground if your cannabis is safely out of reach.

My plea to padlock cannabis in your home applies to *all* products— but particularly to edibles. No matter how little your little ones are, no matter your circumstance or living situation or the fact that they're not even walking yet, cannabis edibles that aren't locked are a danger to kids' safety. Fortunately, there are lots of cool storage options out there. See the appendix for recs.

◊ *Ages 3–5*

This age group might feel a bit young for broaching the topic—and I'd never presume to make the decision of when's the perfect moment for your littles to know about cannabis. But weed momming is about conscious use and integrity, so I encourage you to consider opening up.

Age-appropriate conversations here can be very simple. Karissa, a medical cannabis user who's a mom to twin four-year-olds in Montana, tells her twins, "this is Mommy's medicine and it makes me feel better." Erica, another medical user and mother to a five-year-old in Massachusetts, relates that her daughter doesn't know the word *cannabis*, "but she knows it's my medicine and that medicine is private." Erica takes pharmaceuticals in addition to cannabis to help her manage fibromyalgia and PTSD—and she talks about her medications similarly. "In that way, it's just become normal for my daughter," she says.

My daughter was four and my son seven when we started talking about cannabis—it was becoming a big part of my working life and, slowly, my personal life, too. Plus, their dad had a history with which, by then, they were also aware. Even though we lived in California at the time and recreational cannabis was legal, I encouraged them to talk or ask questions about the subject *at home*—emphasizing that while I wasn't ashamed of it, I wasn't yet comfortable having conversations about it in public, either.

My spiel went something like this: "This is something Mama uses sometimes. You can call it cannabis, but people also call it by a bunch of other names, too. For me, it's a little like medicine because it helps when I have a headache or am worried. I also enjoy how it makes me feel. For most adults, it's okay to use cannabis sometimes; but some adults want to use it more than is healthy for them (like Daddy!). Some kids with cancer and other diseases use it, too, and it helps them, but only when a doctor tells them it's okay. But for most kids, it's not okay to try because your brains and bodies are still growing, and using cannabis would make you feel sick."

And that's more or less it—simple, repeatable, and informative enough for this age set. Remember, kids need a lot of repetition, so don't be surprised if you find yourself having some version of this conversation again and again. Count on it, in fact. Provide the same simple and reassuring message each time: cannabis is good for a lot of things, just not for kids.

If you enjoy edibles, this is the right time to start education around safety. Show them edibles packaging and make it clear that THC gummies, candies, cookies, and the like may *look* like treats but *aren't*. You may choose to show kids the tin of mints or the blister-packs of gummies and point out that the packages are hard to get into for a good reason: because eating them will make kids sick. Most states require the pot leaf or THC symbol on the packaging: show them these indicators and point out that if they ever come across these (like at a friend's home) they should let them be, and let you know. Just as we inform our kids that alcohol, pharmaceuticals, and household cleaning products aren't safe for kids—we *must* take this step, too.

A quick note on packaging: some states require resealable child-resistant packaging for all cannabis products, but generally I'm not a fan. First of all, all the extra packaging is plastic—not the good kind of hemp-derived bioplastic, either (come on, cannabis industry!). Second, child-resistant packaging isn't always as child-resistant as you'd think. Can your child use a pair of scissors? Then he or she can hack at least some of the "child-resistant packaging" I've seen out there. So please don't rely on whatever plastic your canna-goodies come in. Padlock your stash, weed mom style.

I'm going to push the envelope a bit here and say that choosing to consume, or not, in front of your children is up to you as long as you don't expose them to secondhand smoke. I've spoken to weed moms on both sides of this question, and I haven't quite figured it all out for myself yet. I feel uncomfortable at the thought of consuming cannabis in front of my kids— but why? I drink wine occasionally in front of them—or coffee—and those also aren't for kids.

Prohibition, past and present, *that's* why. Growing up with DARE, Just Say No, and the War on Drugs distorted our view of what's normal, what's responsible, and what's okay. With this book, I'm standing up to say that responsible use of plant medicine *is* perfectly okay. And yet, the question of consuming in front of kids remains.

Marissa Fratoni, cannabis nurse and maternal health specialist, tells me that "the whole comparison with alcohol has given me pause. I've been at parties with small children, and no one thinks anything about filling up a glass of wine or chugging down a bottle of beer, but cannabis is still taboo." She goes on to say, "I don't condone lighting up in front of a child. But, for parents, I think we need to find these points of normalization."

Rachel, a mother of two in Massachusetts who uses cannabis for hormonal mood issues and other conditions, has a thoughtful contribution to the consumption convo. "My daughter," she says of the older of her two children, "doesn't physically see me smoke, as I don't want her to mimic that behavior, nor do I want her to be around smoke—so I keep it 'hidden' in that regard. She will see me dip outside and she's occasionally seen me through the window, which I don't love. But, ultimately, I don't want to HIDE it like I'm being naughty. I don't sneak around because I don't want THEM to sneak around."

Far from presuming to tell you what's right for you and your kids, I offer these perspectives as food for thought, with a few additional questions: What are the norms you want in your family? How transparent can you comfortably be with your kids? Did you grow up in an open and honest family environment? What kind of family environment do *you* want to create?

Another way into the cannabis conversation for littles is through story. *It's Just a Plant* by Ricardo Cortés is a charming picture book geared toward little ones that portrays a parent's use of medical marijuana in a way that normalizes responsible use and reassures the younger set. You can easily adapt the message to fit whatever ways you make use of cannabis (e.g., to relax, to sleep better, etc.).

◊ *Ages 6–10*

With this age group, you can introduce the broad strokes of humans' long and—with the exception of the last century—*peaceful* coexistence with cannabis; tell them that hemp and marijuana can be used for all kinds of things, from fiber to bioplastics to food to medicine to something fun that changes your mood or your outlook. Tell them it does good things for the environment by absorbing heavy metals and carbon from the soil and that it's a new and growing field that creates jobs and is good for local economies.

Sarah Danielle Rossignol, mom to an eight-year-old boy in Massachusetts, works as a grower and processor of medical cannabis. Her partner is also on the board of directors for a regional growers' group, so they visit local farms and greenhouses and bring their son along when possible, she tells me. Choosing to share parts of her working life with her son means that he knows about cannabis for arthritis, cancer, anxiety, and more. "I hope," she tells me, "that he grows up seeing that we are helping so many people."

I suggest telling your kids about why *you* use it. For headaches? For getting deep into the groove on your yoga mat or out and about in nature? To subtly take the edge off in a way that won't leave you feeling queasy or lackluster the next day? If you drink alcohol you may want to compare and contrast the two, pointing out that one is legal everywhere in the US while the other isn't—yet.

Six- to ten-year-olds aren't too young for a little lesson in critical thinking about the inconsistencies between alcohol and cannabis policy. Why is the substance that's associated with more harm (car accidents, assault, alcohol poisoning) legal, while the other *isn't*? Talk about how racism contributed to the drug laws as we know them, and how a disproportionate number of people of color are in jail for nonviolent drug-related crimes. Use words they can understand, of course. But tell them.

The same basic message you imparted to the littler ones applies at this age: cannabis is medicine for some adults and relaxation for other adults—sometimes it's both. But it's also something that kids' bodies and brains can't yet handle, and it would make them feel sick if they ate an edible or inhaled from a vape. Keep them updated on identifying edibles, and normalize cannabis as you would other things that touch your shared lives. Padlock your stash. And rock on with your responsible, weed momming self.

◊ *Ages 11–13*

I've said this before, and I'll say it again: there are (much) worse things than weed out there, but otherwise-healthy tweens and teens don't need an ECS-altering addition to their fast-morphing, hormone-flooded brains, either. Adolescents are mercurial enough as it is.

Jessie Gill, the cannabis nurse in New Jersey we met earlier, tells me, "I teach my twelve-year-old about cannabis in a similar way to alcohol and sex. There are responsible ways for adults to consume alcohol and engage in sexual contact—but there are also many potential risks and dangers that are difficult for kids to understand and manage."

While it's true that most kids won't smoke weed at this age, some will be exposed by peers—and a portion of those will indeed try it before high school. According to NIDA, 11.8 percent of eighth graders (thirteen to fourteen years of age) have used cannabis in the last year. And, again, though smoking weed isn't a sure route to ruin, early and frequent cannabis use *is* associated with negative outcomes that none of us want for our kids. Gill talks about brain development with her son—particularly the fact that tweens and teens have a prefrontal cortex in a period of flux and growth. And that means there are greater risks of addiction and misuse for younger people.

Your messaging for this age group can grow more complex, subtle, and wide-ranging—just like the plant herself. You can toss out fun facts—Shakespeare may have smoked cannabis!—and add a history lesson by comparing it to alcohol prohibition of the 1920s. (During alcohol prohibition, alcohol was still plentiful, but untaxed. Nonregulated moonshine was also more dangerous to make and drink than its once and future legal counterpart. Parallels to the cannabis industry abound here!)

Educate your tween on why some people use it for medicine or fun or wellness, as well as the ways it can be consumed, its multitudinous slang aliases, and the fact that it's totes possible to abuse weed. (OK, probably *don't* say totes.) If you or someone biologically related to your child has a family history of addiction and mental health diagnoses, it's a good idea to start talking about those, too.

Tweens may be curious about what flower, vapes, topicals, or tinctures actually look like, and you may or may not choose to show them your stash (and then lock it up again!). Remember, the goal here is to be someone they'll trust not to spin the truth: be genuine and up front, to the extent that they, and the relationship, are ready for. And answer their questions. I can't say it enough, but I'll try. *Answer their questions. Answer their questions. Answer their questions.*

And last, love the crap out of those wonderful, changing humans you get to share your life with. You might need a little emotional reframe here and there if you're dealing with one of them, so…rock on with your weed mom self.

## ◊ Ages 14+

Here's where shit gets real. According to a 2019 NIDA survey, 28.8 percent of tenth graders and 35.7 percent of twelfth graders had used cannabis in the past year, though much fewer said they use it regularly.[81] In both legal and illegal states, there's plenty of weed floating around, and the majority of high school students say they know someone they can buy it from. If you haven't talked about cannabis with your teen yet, time's a wastin'.

The approach I endorse here is called harm reduction, and it's all about teaching people strategies for prioritizing their own safety and well-being. It's based on the notion that expecting total abstinence from every drug for all people at all times is, well, it's impossible. Reality, and at least ten thousand years of human history, reflect that people like to change moods and alter perceptions. It's part of our deep genetic and cultural heritage. Harm reduction advocates tell us that abstinence-only approaches to drugs like Just Say No and DARE *don't* lead to less drug use by kids. Instead, they lead to riskier, less informed drug use.[82]

I was definitely part of the Just Say No generation; in elementary school my teachers played TV clips of Nancy Reagan, who confidently assured us all that drugs were a scourge that would most certainly lead to death, poverty, and insanity. Her message echoed, of course, the ridiculous "this is your brain on drugs" eighties commercial featuring an egg sizzling in a frying pan (remember?) and generally reflects the abstinence-only, light-on-information model of drug education.

After watching those clips in elementary school, we got T-shirts and, I think, some pizza. And voila: my generation's drug education. Whatever drugs I went on to try or decline had little to do with that message, or the T-shirt.

Research shows that abstinence-only drug education (just like abstinence-only sex ed) doesn't work, as evidenced by the fact that nearly half of high school seniors admit to having tried illegal drugs or misused prescriptions,[83] and accidental overdose is the leading cause of death in people under fifty. But despite its failures, abstinence-only drug education is still the dominant approach taken by educators and parents. It's often accompanied by threats of dire consequences for a single infraction; but punitive policies like "zero-tolerance" can stigmatize and alienate teens—perhaps making them feel like a bad person if they do try drugs. (It's worth remembering here that alcohol and nicotine are *also* drugs—and they cause far more health problems and death than some illegal drugs.)

Punishment resulting from a shame-based abstinence model also discourages teens from talking. As anyone who's dealt with teens knows, this is the opposite of what we're looking for. Parents want teens to call if they're too messed up to drive. Parents want teens to confide what's going on with them. And parents want teens to ask a trusted adult for help when they need it. But if parents only communicate about drugs by lying and threatening, teens won't trust us. Plain and simple.

Now, my two aren't quite teens yet, but I've picked a side in the abstinence-only versus harm-reduction debate, and it all boils down to a few essentials:

1. I want my kids to be safe and healthy.

2. I realize that, as they age, some degree of experimentation is both human nature and developmentally expected.

3. I want my kids to trust me and the information I provide.

So, that means...

4. I choose honesty about cannabis and other drugs in the degree of detail they're ready for.

5. I choose to teach my kids how to keep themselves safe and informed. I don't rely on fear-mongering or threats of punishment, but I do tell them what science says about young brains and cannabis.

Other features of harm reduction include the belief that everyone, even young people, can learn how to own their health and well-being in order to make good decisions. Harm reduction says that people make choices based on their own set of circumstances, some of which we can't understand—even as a parent. The approach acknowledges that, even though we discourage it in teens, it's a human impulse to seek out mind-altering substances from time to time. It also distinguishes between use and abuse.

And the whole approach makes so much sense. The Netherlands has long taken the enlightened path to drug policy; even though cannabis isn't wholly legal in the Netherlands (despite those ah-mazing coffee shops in Amsterdam where you can indeed smoke a jay in public), it's decriminalized and destigmatized. That doesn't mean youth use is encouraged—far from it. Indeed, analyses of Dutch drug policy and outcomes from the 1980s onward have consistently found that harm reduction doesn't encourage drug use, but it does help people stay safer if they choose to engage in it.[84]

A quick US example might drive home the point even more. Youth who receive a comprehensive sex ed curriculum are more likely to wait for sex, use condoms, and show lower rates of teenage pregnancies,[85] abortions, and STIs than youth who receive abstinence-only sex education. Knowledge is power, people.

# SAFETY FIRST

The Drug Policy Alliance's Safety First program for ninth and tenth graders in participating schools is insanely helpful for parents, too. Along with drug education, they teach critical thinking skills that come in handy when teens are faced with conflicting information about anything from drugs to sex to politics.

Sasha Simon, manager of the Safety First program, offers a sobering perspective that teens, on average, spend upwards of eight hours a day in some form of online entertainment (and this was pre-COVID!), including chatting, gaming, texting, and video messaging. In other words, teens aren't only learning about drugs from school and parents, said Simon in a virtual seminar, "they get information from each other and online." [86]

One critical thinking strategy taught in the Safety First curriculum is the CRAAP test, which guides teens to check a source of information for:

**Currency:** Is it up to date?

**Relevance:** Is the article or website intended to provide the information you seek?

**Authority:** Is the author qualified to write on the topic?

**Accuracy:** Is the information verifiable through other credible sources?

**Purpose:** What are the author and publisher aiming to accomplish with this work? To educate? To sell? To entertain? To accomplish a personal or political goal?

To become more critical thinkers, young people should be encouraged to question and cross-reference information, particularly if a source doesn't give both pros and cons. If young people have the skills to inform themselves and the trust to ask an adult for help when they can't tell fact from fiction, they're on much firmer footing in relation to their own health and well-being.

In the Safety First curriculum, educators lead students through fact-check exercises, where they use real-world internet research to evaluate statements like, "Cannabis is safe because it is natural" (only partially true), and "Edible cannabis is safer than smoked cannabis" (only true for the lungs). Students learn to apply the CRAAP test to web articles addressing these questions and assign each source a rating from 0 to 3 for reliability based on how they meet the criteria. (I know more than a few adults who could learn a thing or two from the CRAAP test, too. Just sayin'.)

Another page from the Safety First playbook parents can lean on includes ten points of drug safety. They are:

1. Understand that abstinence is still the safest choice.

If, however, a young person understands this fact and still chooses to engage in experimental drug behavior, they should:

2. Develop drug knowledge, including skills to evaluate the credibility of sources.

3. Understand dosing; how much is a small, a medium, and a large dose?

4. Start low and go slow.

5. Practice moderation and reduce heavy use.

6. Be conscious of set and setting—where you are, who you're with, and how you're feeling beforehand.

7. Check the substance, aka "drug checking," a service offered at raves and music festivals. It helps rule out potentially fatal stuff like fentanyl that can be present in (non-cannabis) party drugs. When it comes to cannabis, it's important to determine that the substance isn't what's known as K2 or "spice," a synthetic, potentially lethal drug that looks a bit like potpourri and is sometimes sold on the street as cannabis (legal cannabis dispensaries will never sell K2).

8. Refrain from mixing substances.

9. Know how to respond to an emergency. Seek help; don't isolate. Call 911 in an emergency.

10. Understand drug policy in your school and state. Zero-tolerance policies can cause a teen to lose opportunities.

What really strikes me here is that this kind of drug education gives young people credit for their intelligence and trusts that, with guidance, they can learn how to pilot their own well-being. It discourages early drug use and provides real information about risks. But, should teens experiment, they'll have the information that will help them make healthier and safer choices—and possibly save their life, or a friend's. This approach tells teens, "I believe in you *and* I'm here for you." Isn't *that* the message we should be sending our kids?

The entire Safety First curriculum is available via a free download from the Drug Policy Alliance's website, and I strongly recommend acquainting yourself with it if you've got a teen.

And last, a quick tip: if you're finding it difficult to communicate with your teen, you might suggest they speak with another adult that they like and you trust (like a cool aunt). This person could sometimes be their go-to person for tough topics.

# HARM REDUCTION AND CANNABIS

When it comes to cannabis, harm reduction rejects the bogus claim that it's a "gateway drug."[87] Most people who try or use cannabis don't go on to use other, more dangerous stuff like cocaine or meth or illicit opioids.[88] As a quick example, of the 124 million Americans who've tried cannabis, less than 2 percent have tried heroin.[89] In reality, and in direct contradiction to the gateway theory, cannabis is increasingly considered an "exit drug" that helps people taper or quit opioids and alcohol. While cannabis use disorder (weed addiction) is absolutely real (see Chapter 9), the majority of teens who use cannabis don't use it daily.[90] Preexisting mental health problems have been found to be the greatest risk factor of cannabis abuse by teens.[91]

So, while I'd never claim it's a *great* idea for teens to use cannabis, I believe in realistic, pragmatic parenting that's, of course, informed by values. There are worse things for teens than smoking weed, and that's a fact. I will never try to impose my beliefs or parenting style on your family, but if you agree that kids need education, guidance, and empathy to navigate this weird-ass world and all the conflicting messages in it, then I also hope this discussion gets you thinking and talking to your partner or co-parent, and, ultimately, your kids, too.

## Weed Moms Speak on Educating Kids about Cannabis

"I'm going to set the bar at, 'this is a grown-up activity. And it affects grown-ups differently than kids.' But if I *had* to choose, I'd rather have my child experiment with cannabis than with alcohol. There's a number of reasons around that. I can go into toxicity, or the types of behaviors that tend to happen with each one. I just think alcohol is way riskier." —*Jenn Lauder, mom of a 12-year-old, Oregon*

"Ideally, I'd like her to wait on *everything* until her brain is developed, but I don't think that's realistic. I also don't want her to ever feel like she has to hide it from me. In fact, I want to be there when she experiences intoxication so that I know she's safe, and we can talk about limits. And she likes that idea—for now. Obviously, I'm not going to be punitive but I'm going to try to help her make the best decisions." —*Reya, mom of a teen, Idaho*

"Cannabis isn't something [my kids] see or smell. I'm responsible. But there *is* going to be conversation about it once they're old enough—and I don't want it to be like what was given to me. You know, that drugs are all bad and they're all going to kill you. After I smoked weed for the first time as a teenager, I was like *lies! I was told all lies!*" —*Kristin, mom of 1, stepmom of 1, Connecticut*

# CHAPTER 9

# IF THINGS GO WRONG: DOWNSIDES AND RISKS TO USING CANNABIS

> "Any source that's all positive or all negative—just forget it."
> —*Marsha Rosenbaum, sociologist and author of* Safety First

It's only fair to admit that there are potential downsides to weed. Evidenced by the fact that I indulged you in some of them right off the bat, you know that I'm not afraid to explore the topic. Weed momming is all about conscious and informed use, so let's dive in.

## SO WHAT COULD GO WRONG?

◊ You could have a **bad trip**, aka "green out," and hate everything about the way you feel for the duration of that super-shitty experience.

◊ You could experience **deficits to your short-term memory** with long-term, heavy use.

◊ You're at increased risk of cannabis-induced **psychosis** if you have a history of mental illness. And even if you don't, months or years of overconsumption could lead to developing psychological problems like **anxiety and depression**. Heavy usage early in life may be associated with greater risks of **schizophrenia**.

◊ There may be **risks to your heart** from using a lot of cannabis, particularly if you have a preexisting heart condition.

◊ Though no clear link between smoking weed and lung cancer has been proven, you'll likely **cough and experience diminished lung health** if you smoke anything in large quantities.

◊ With excessive consumption, some people develop **cannabis hyperemesis syndrome** (CHS)—frequent and uncontrollable vomiting.

We'll get into each of these in more detail in this chapter, but the elephant in the room is, of course, substance abuse:

◊ Known as **cannabis use disorder** (CUD), it can wreak havoc on your life in many of the ways that substance abuse usually does. You'll find a discussion of this important subject here, too.

## BAD TRIPS

Experiencing a bad trip, aka "greening out" or "freaking out," may have already happened to you at some point. In case you don't know what it feels like, I'll tell you: it royally sucks. While cannabis usually works on your ECS to help bring you into balance, too much can do the opposite, forcing you out of homeostasis and into a really uncomfortable place.

The common side effects of using weed include dry mouth, aka "cotton mouth," and temporary lapses in short-term memory, like, "Dude, what was I just saying?" You could get really tired, too.

Moderately uncomfortable symptoms of greening out include:

◊ Dizziness

◊ Nervousness or mild paranoia

◊ Shortness of breath

◊ Heart palpitations

◊ Agitation

◊ Disorientation, confusion

◊ Nausea

◊ Sweating

Next-level symptoms of a bad high might look like:

◊ Chills

◊ Full-blown paranoia and panic attacks

◊ Profuse sweating

◊ Fear that you're having a heart attack, or dying, as a result of a rapid pulse

◊ Vomiting

**Fact:** In heavy doses, and for certain people, cannabis can act a bit like a psychedelic. In other words, some people—when *really* high—will get light visual or audial distortions with weed, similar to what they might experience on psilocybin (magic mushrooms) or LSD. Michelle Janikian, a cannabis journalist and author of *Your Psilocybin Mushroom Companion* (2019) tells me, "Psychedelics are more powerful substances than cannabis, but cannabis is also a psychedelic in some ways because it can shift your perspective—it *does* alter your consciousness."

Here are some tips to avoid greening out:

**Start low and go slow!** It's always your best bet for avoiding unpleasant highs. Pay attention to product, timing, and dose while experimenting with differing quantities of THC and CBD. If you're worried about overconsuming THC, reach for lower-potency strains when smoking, vaporizing flower, or vaping e-liquids, and wait five minutes between each puff. As we discussed in Chapter 5, start with a low-THC edible or tincture dose if you're new (1 to 5 mg) and increase by only 2.5 mg each subsequent time you consume until you've reached your ideal threshold. Don't do dabs or concentrates.

Use caution when trying a new-to-you product—whatever the form of consumption—and remember, microdosing is your friend.

**Buy your weed on the legal market.** Pesticides, molds, solvents, and fungi, frequently found in lab tests of stuff bought on the illicit market, can contribute to unpleasant symptoms like allergic reactions.

**Pay attention to your set and setting.** "Honestly," says Janikian, "your mindset and your environment impact your emotional experience no matter what you're doing, but in an altered state of consciousness, you're more sensitive. So things like your surroundings and the people you're with will impact your experience in general...and they can really affect how you process the experience." For instance, being in a loud or unfamiliar, or not entirely safe place (even a fun one, like a concert) is likely to feel uncomfortable if you're not used to being "elevated." To minimize the risk of bad trips, stick to comforting and familiar places and people.

**Care for your body.** Make sure you're sleeping enough, that you've eaten well and are hydrated before your sesh, and that you've done what you can to nurture your well-being. Though cannabis helps you relax and shake off emotional baggage, you don't want to reach for weed (particularly in high doses) if you're super-stressed, undernourished, or emotionally out of whack.

**Don't mix cannabis with other substances!** Bringing alcohol into the mix significantly increases your chances of greening out because alcohol boosts the absorption of THC. What may feel like a moderate amount of alcohol and weed, when combined, can quickly push you into green-out territory.

## What to Do If You Ever Get Too Damn High

First, try to relax. Remind yourself that this, too, will pass. If you're caring for children—and please don't designate yourself the responsible party if you're ever trying a big dose or a new-to-you product—call in for reinforcements from a partner, friend, or family member. You don't even need to explain—

tell them you're not feeling well and leave it at that. Make sure your kids are being looked after by someone you trust, then take care of your own needs.

If at all possible, get yourself to a familiar or favorite spot—preferably one that's chill, quiet, and private. Take frequent sips of water to hydrate, but don't guzzle it because that could worsen nausea. Speaking of nausea, a few nibbles of a cookie, cracker, or dry cake can help quell those queasy sensations. Just don't go overboard. I hate to be the bearer of bad news, but you may vomit. It's unlikely if you've stuck to the guidelines, but stomachs vary.

Speaking of kindnesses, call in support if you have someone who'll help you process feelings and sensations. A good friend or partner (who also knows the deal) will not judge or shame you for getting fucked up. Instead, he or she will pat your back, get you a glass of water, and wait it out.

No matter how crappy you feel, remember that *it's temporary.* If you've smoked, the peak of the bad trip should only last about an hour. If you've scarfed too many edibles, you could be in for an uncomfortable stretch, but even potent edibles should start to wear off between three and six hours after you start feeling the effects.

Try to be curious about any negative thoughts or feelings that arise. What are you telling yourself, and is it both true and kind? Janikian recommends treating an unpleasant trip "a bit like a meditation practice— with compassion or curiosity—instead of wishing the experience were over, or resisting it."

Keep in mind that you may feel like you're going to die from too much THC, but no one ever has from THC intake alone. Of course, accidental death or injury is possible if you're so high you lose some of your motor control, so don't drive while high, ever, and avoid any kind of risky situation. You'll be okay—sooner rather than later.

Here are a few more ideas for dealing with a bad trip:

◊ Take an easy walk.

◊ Sit outside in a pretty spot and observe nature (but don't go wandering into the wilderness); natural rhythms tend to be calming—as do natural light and fresh air.

◊ Watch a comedy or listen to music.

◊ Go to sleep.

◊ Take a shower.

◊ Try adding CBD. It's generally thought, but not proven, to moderate THC's high because it partially blocks the brain receptors that respond to THC.[92] Many people find relief from greening out with a few puffs from a CBD vape or a dropper of sublingual CBD tincture; at the very least, CBD may help quell your anxiety—one of the most uncomfortable side effects of being too high.

◊ Chew on peppercorns or sniff their aroma. B-caryophyllene, found in cannabis and peppercorns, is an antagonist for CB2 receptors (a part of your endocannabinoid system) and may help increase the sedative effects of THC, thereby helping to chill you out while you're waiting to come down.[93]

◊ Drink some lemon water. Limonene, the terpene found in citrus that's also a component of certain cannabis strains, may help soothe and refresh you.

◊ Try aromatherapy. Linalool, the aromatic terpene in lavender, interacts directly with the limbic system for a calming and restorative effect.

If you're seriously greening out, your heart may race and you may feel like you're dying; though you'd have to have consumed ungodly amounts of THC (like in the range of 70,000 mg, or 7,000 to 14,000 edible serving sizes) to suppress your central nervous system enough for THC to be fatal (and remember there's no documented case of that ever happening), it's okay to have someone drive you to the ER or to call an ambulance if you feel you need it.

There are reports that ERs and poison control centers saw an increase in overconsuming patients due to recreational legalization, which has led to greater numbers of cannabis-naïve people (including canna-tourists) trying weed. Docs and EMTs tend to treat acute cannabis overconsumption with a recommendation to sit in a quiet room, hydrate, and wait it out. If a person is severely agitated or paranoid, they might administer an antianxiety drug, like a benzodiazepine, or fluids for dehydration. In a rough moment, some folks need reassurance from proximity to medical professionals and life-saving equipment. Remember, it's perfectly okay to seek medical help if you're scared.

Most people who use cannabis responsibly won't experience the dreaded green out, but there's a small chance that even a moderate dose of THC won't agree with you. Unpleasant reactions to moderate doses of cannabis are very uncommon, but they're also not impossible. The more you know, weed moms!

## MEMORY

An interesting study spanning twenty-five years found that adults who used cannabis heavily over the course of their lives had poorer short-term memory recall for a list of fifteen words[94] than those who—wait, what was I saying?

Just kidding. The memories of chronic weed users were worse than those who didn't partake.

After adjusting for a bunch of other factors, like alcohol use, activity level, and mental health, they found that every five years of heavy cannabis use produced greater declines. However, the total differences are pretty small: on average, cannabis consumers could recall eight-and-a-half words of the fifteen, while nonusers recalled nine. The researchers also found that executive functioning and processing speed, two other indicators of cognitive function, were not affected by pot. Other evidence points to CBD in particular as a neuroprotectant that may offset the memory impairment of THC.[95]

# MENTAL HEALTH ISSUES FROM OVERUSE

Mental health is a big ol' bucket, but an important one. Boulder osteopath Dr. Rav Ivker tells me that he's seen people suffer from "depression, fatigue, a sense of distortion of time and space, irritability, and higher levels of anxiety" with long-term and heavy use.

Because the positive potential for cannabis—and particularly THC—for mental health is dose-dependent (a little can help, a lot can make things worse), it stands to reason that many of the negatives come from heavy use. Let's take a look at what those might be.

## Anxiety

◊ In the short-term, THC's effect on anxiety is dose-dependent. "All other things being equal, THC appears to decrease anxiety at lower doses and increase anxiety at higher doses," a researcher from the University of Washington's Alcohol and Drug Abuse Institute concludes, adding that, "CBD appears to decrease anxiety at all doses that have been tested."[96]

◊ Long-term studies are lacking, but mental health professionals point out that any pharmacological anxiety intervention, including cannabis, can't work all on its own; over time, you have to address the underlying reasons for your anxiety and adjust your mental habits in order to gain benefit. Without accompanying therapy, meditation, or a sustained practice of self-reflection and emotional growth, it's likely that anxiety symptoms will continue, or even worsen—with or without cannabis.

## Depression

◊ Some data shows that while a majority of medical users' depressive symptoms are relieved immediately after using cannabis, long-term dependence on cannabis for coping may result in higher levels of depression over time.[97]

## Bipolar Disorder

◊ A 2015 study found that using cannabis resulted in improved mood for people with BD.[98]

◊ Another from the same year found cannabis use in BD populations was associated with positive mood, but *also* found that users experienced more manic and depressive symptoms after smoking weed.[99]

◊ A British review of six previously published studies on cannabis and BD found that smoking weed might worsen, or even bring on, bipolar symptoms.[100]

◊ Other researchers found that those with BD who smoke marijuana are about seven times more likely to develop cannabis use disorder than the general population.[101]

◊ CBD, *sans* THC, shows promise for helping those with bipolar: an ongoing Brazilian study is tracking the effects of CBD alone for bipolar patients; results are expected in 2022.

## Schizophrenia

◊ A widely cited study from the 1980s found a link between cannabis use and schizophrenia.[102]

◊ Since then, there's been plenty of debate. Some research has backed up that evidence linking cannabis use to schizophrenia, and other research has pointed to the flaws in equating association with causation; for instance, those with, or at risk for, schizophrenia may be more likely to self-medicate with cannabis.

◊ Another study found that "cannabis use precipitates schizophrenia in persons who are vulnerable because of a personal or family history of schizophrenia."[103]

◊ CBD reduced psychotic symptoms associated with schizophrenia as effectively as a common antipsychotic med called amisulpride—and did so with fewer side effects than the pharmaceutical.[104]

# Psychosis

◊ Described by the National Institute of Mental Health as a "loss of contact with reality," psychosis can manifest as hallucinations or simply believing thoughts that are inconsistent with reality (such as feeling like the target of a conspiracy). Remember how cannabis, in heavy doses and with some users, can act a bit like a psychedelic? A psychedelic cannabis experience could register as "psychosis," but its effects are only temporary. If, however, psychosis persists—as can be the case with heavy users who are also genetically predisposed—it could lead to a diagnosis of schizophrenia.

◊ In a European study, 30 percent of new cases of psychosis were found to occur among daily, high-potency pot users, prompting the researchers to conclude that there is a relationship between the two, though not necessarily a causal one.[105]

So, what does all this mean for us weed moms and potential weed moms? It's challenging to parse it all out, to be sure. But here's a quick rundown of the most salient factors when it comes to mental health and cannabis:

1. In most of the data, it's hard to determine which came first—mental health issues or cannabis use.

2. Where negative effects from cannabis use are found, studies have looked at THC, not CBD.

3. Heavy use of THC over the long term comes with the greatest risks.

4. Cannabis users who are also predisposed to psychiatric disorders are most at risk for adverse mental health events.

We're deep in the realm of botanical medicine here, and it just doesn't translate to simple answers. To add to the confusion, studies done at different historical moments and by different researchers often come to wildly divergent conclusions; much of the research we have on cannabis is funded by government agencies that aren't particularly warm to the plant in the first place.

Jessilyn Dolan, a cannabis nurse we met in the last chapter, tells me that since beginning her job in research at the University of Vermont, she's become more skeptical of, well, research. "I want to know who's funding it," she tells me, "along with what their initial hypothesis was, and how they've come to their conclusions." In other words, agendas—both pro-cannabis and anti-cannabis—can absolutely influence the outcome of a study.

By all means, pay attention to research. But at the same time, advises Dolan, "You are the expert of your own body. This is plant medicine, not a lab-derived pharmaceutical. As long as you are safe and go slow with clean cannabis, you're not going to hurt yourself." And in the process, she says, "You're doing your *own* experiment, your *own* research."

## POSSIBLE CARDIOVASCULAR RISKS

There isn't a ton of reliable research yet, but we do know that cannabis raises your heart rate. While this effect isn't really noticeable for most people after a moderate intake of THC, high doses, like I mentioned earlier, can cause noticeable heart palpitations and discomfort.

Researchers haven't been able to provide a causal link to atherosclerosis (narrowing and hardening of the arteries) resulting from cannabis use, but there's some evidence that THC can contribute to platelet aggregation. Some say there may be a link between weed and increased risk of heart attacks.[106]

Others point to research showing lower overall levels for blood sugar, insulin resistance, and obesity, among cannabis consumers—markers that may contradict the idea that cannabis is bad for your heart.[107] To confuse matters even further, a large-scale review found a lack of sufficient data to determine the cardiovascular effects of cannabis use for good or bad.[108]

Bottom line: if you're living with a heart condition, investigate and talk to a doctor who's well-versed in cannabis's potential effects on your heart health before consuming.

## LUNG ISSUES

I'm guessing that if you've ever hung out with serious stoners, you've heard the chronic cough that tends to accompany them. Research has found cilia damage, some degree of airway inflammation, increased phlegm, and wheezing—none of which sound like a recipe for optimum lung health—among long-term and heavy marijuana smokers.[109]

However, researchers haven't found a link between smoking cannabis and lung cancer. What's more, a comprehensive study comparing tobacco and cannabis smoking found that *moderate* cannabis use isn't associated with adverse effects on lung function.[110] But even without a proven link to lung cancer, it stands to reason that long-term, heavy exposure to cannabis smoke will affect your lungs; I mean, the whole process involves inhaling hot, foreign matter that also contains particulates.

In my experience, moderate cannabis smoking has neither given me a chronic cough nor reduced my lung capacity; I'm actually a better, more dedicated runner since becoming a weed mom. If I were part of the "wake and bake" crowd, or used cannabis all day, every day to cope with symptoms, I'm sure the outcome would be different; in other words, quantity of exposure matters. But even if you're a low to moderate consumer, it's important to know that the act of smoking cannabis isn't risk-free.

Fortunately, there are many ways to consume this wonderful plant, and while smoking flower is hands down my favorite mode (for effect, taste, and ritual), you can—and should—avail yourself of other methods if you want to fully protect your lungs.

If you, like me, prefer smoking flower, you can reduce your risk of lung injury in the following ways: 1) Don't smoke heavily, 2) Mix it up with a flower vaporizer or edibles from time to time, 3) Avoid tobacco and tobacco-laced cannabis products, and 4) Smoke from a pipe or bubbler instead of a joint so that you inhale only cannabis smoke, not the smoke of the rolling paper, too.

## CANNABIS HYPEREMESIS SYNDROME

CHS brings on gnarly GI symptoms and occurs in a very small subset of longtime, daily cannabis users. When large amounts of THC are repeatedly dumped onto brain receptors, those receptors may end up flipping the script on the ways they respond to cannabinoids. Essentially, we're talking about an overload and a dysregulation of the endocannabinoid system, resulting in:

◊ Nausea

◊ Vomiting, often severe

◊ Abdominal pain

◊ Weakness

◊ Sweats

◊ Weight loss

◊ Dehydration

For most people with CHS, the nausea and vomiting last only a few days but tend to recur if cannabis is used again; if it persists longer and isn't treated, someone with CHS could die of dehydration—so take it seriously if this ever happens to you or someone you know. People with CHS often find that hot showers ease their symptoms temporarily, but the only real, known treatment for CHS is quitting cannabis altogether.

In my experience, many cannabis lovers accept that CHS is super-rare, but real, while some are threatened by the notion that cannabis could ever cause any harm. Obviously, I disagree.

# WEED MOM Q&A

**Q: Should I ditch alcohol for weed?**

**A:** A great question, but a purely personal choice. My thoughts about alcohol vs. weed echo those of cannabis nurse and CEO of GreenNurse Group, Sherri Tutkus, who tells me that, "While cannabinoids support all of our body systems, alcohol is toxic."

As legalization progresses, greater numbers of people are coming out of the "weed closet" and admitting they've been living alcohol-free with the use of the good herb for years—a category sometimes called "green sober," or "Cali-sober." Even if it's not fully legal everywhere (yet), the fact that it's available for adult use in several big states means that the whole subject is getting easier and easier to talk about.

Quick stats: In 2020, 47 percent of US cannabis consumers said they preferred the effects of cannabis to alcohol, and one in three survey respondents said they either drink less or have quit drinking entirely since cannabis became legal in their state.[111] Independent data backs that claim up, showing that per-person spending on alcohol declines an average of 12.4 percent in counties with legal access to cannabis.[112]

I spoke with Adi Jaffe, PhD, psychologist, author of *The Abstinence Myth*, and founder of a multipronged lifestyle program called IGNTD. Jaffe, who has his own story of past substance abuse, specializes in shame-free approaches to help clients develop healthier relationships to substances and live their purpose. He tells me he's had clients in AA who'd completely given up alcohol for cannabis but felt compelled to lie about it because of cannabis's legal status, and because of the emphasis on total abstinence that stems from perennially popular twelve-step programs. Now, with increasing legalization, reduced stigma of cannabis use, and alternatives to the twelve-step approach, more "green-sober" folks are willing to share their experiences.

Since legal weed came into my life, I've shifted mostly from alcohol to cannabis and am seriously loving it. While I wouldn't describe myself as "sober" and will still have a glass of wine or a cocktail from time to time, the hormonal migraines that plagued me for several years after my pregnancies are less frequent and intense when I mostly skip alcohol. And at forty, I was diagnosed with an autoimmune disease that suddenly explained symptoms like joint pain and achiness I'd had for years despite being a flexible yogini and a yoga teacher. Autoimmune diseases are linked to that murky internal process of chronic inflammation, whereby—in super simple terms—the immune system overreacts to create pain and a host of other problems. Alcohol promotes inflammation; cannabis is a known anti-inflammatory. So pivoting away from alcohol toward weed—well, for me, it adds up.

Now, when I do drink alcohol, I notice the achiness, fatigue, and headaches ramping up—often before I've even emptied the first glass. Sometimes I'll still choose to partake (I mean, what's a Seder without wine?) but the pleasant taste of alcohol and the social, buzzy feeling aren't really worth feeling like crap.

But that's just me.

Your health and your life are your very own business and I hereby give you permission—that is, if you haven't already—to take full-frontal responsibility for all of it. If not you, who?

You may not change your drinking habits at all when you add cannabis to your repertoire (though, again, please no mixing of the two). You may reduce or moderate your drinking, or you may quit it altogether. No judgment. Stay open, stay curious, stay awake and aware. That's all I ask.

**Q: I have, or have had, a problematic relationship with alcohol (or pills, or whatever). Is cannabis a good idea for me?**

**A:** If you have a problematic relationship with alcohol or any other substance, Jaffe tells me it's extremely likely that trading one for the other is going to lead you down the same road. Though the potential harms of cannabis are fewer and less serious than those of alcohol or opioids, substance abuse is substance abuse—and even weed can mess up your life. Short answer? Don't swap out one thing for another thing unless you've gone deep into why you were misusing substances in the first place. Even with a new and improved suite of neurochemical effects that will flow to you from cannabis (compared to alcohol or opioids), your underlying problems will catch up quickly.

If substance misuse is part of your life story, you're absolutely not alone. The struggle is real—and it can devastate. And, yet, always remember that you're allowed to grow and to write yourself a new story. With therapy, yoga, meditation, forest-bathing, commitment to a spiritual tradition—or whatever it is that spurs you on your evolutionary path—you're allowed to flip the script on substances.

If you've examined your history and behaviors, if you've learned to love and accept yourself and are committed to staying conscious in whatever you do, then I have no authority to tell you whether adding cannabis to your life is a good idea or a bad one. In truth, I have no authority on anything that relates to you. YOU get to decide.

## UNHEALTHY PATTERNS

Some longtime weed moms I've spoken with talk about how they've learned to modify their use of cannabis over time—in large part by recognizing habits that weren't working. Reya, a mom in Idaho (whose name has been changed at her request), tells me, "I've been in patterns where I've been smoking too much. For me that looked like lethargy—and I was kind of apathetic about life, like I lacked enjoyment." Shifting away from daytime use toward evenings-only helped her become more mindful about consuming, as did letting go of the idea that she had to smoke first if she wanted to clean the house, or practice yoga, or do some creative writing.

"When I first started writing seriously," she tells me, "I would be getting high first. It helped create so many ideas and I really enjoyed it, but eventually it started to backfire." Reya tells me that, over time, her stoned writing sessions became decreasingly fruitful, so she'd get increasingly higher in pursuit of that creative mojo. Eventually, she tells me, she needed to stop using cannabis to try to get things done and pivot toward more occasional use that was all about enjoyment. She once took a six-month break, and that served as a helpful reset to make her more mindful of what she missed about cannabis, and what she didn't. "If you start to depend on it for creating a certain feeling," Reya shares, "that's when it turns."

# CANNABIS USE DISORDER

Increasingly, cannabis is being researched and utilized as an "exit drug" that helps ease cravings and rewards for a number of substances like alcohol,[113] nicotine,[114] opioids,[115,116] methamphetamines,[117] and cocaine[118]. In some cases, it's CBD alone that's being investigated as addiction therapy; in other cases, the focus is on THC, or a combination.

But cannabis use in itself can also become a problem. Cannabis use disorder (CUD) appears in the *Diagnostic and Statistical Manual of Mental Disorders (DSM-V)*, published by the American Psychiatric Association and, according to NIDA, about four million people in the United States met the criteria for a cannabis use disorder in 2015.[119] Compare that to the prevalence of alcohol use disorder, at 14.4 million,[120] and the deadliness of opioid use disorder, which accounted for nearly 47,000 deaths in 2018.[121] CUD isn't nearly the public health threat that those two problems are.

On top of that, the data on CUD may not accurately reflect numbers of people who actually have a substance abuse problem with cannabis. For instance, the diagnostic test, called CUDIT-R, considers daily use problematic; however, at least three million Americans are registered medical marijuana patients who use cannabis as medicine, in many cases, for *frequent*—but not necessarily *disordered*—cannabis use. The test also doesn't ask about dosage or total THC intake, or a bunch of other information that would provide clues to disentangle problematic use from helpful use.

I think it's still worth checking out an online version of the CUDIT-R if you're interested; information is a good thing, as long as you know how to interpret it. But bear in mind that the results are potentially misleading. Let's say you microdose twice a day, four days a week, and feel pleasantly elevated for a few hours each on those days—that counts the same as someone who wakes and bakes every day and gets high as the proverbial F when they do. Clearly, those are different kinds of use.

Some of the questions, on the other hand, are helpful for evaluating weed's place in your life, like *how often during the past six months did you find that you were unable to stop using cannabis once you had started?* And *how often during the past six months did you fail to do what was normally expected from you because of using cannabis?* Personally, I can say that this doesn't happen to me—ever. Cannabis helps me accomplish what I need to, and then relax when the time's right.

Don't get me wrong. CUD is absolutely real. Even though some canna-folks still believe that cannabis mainly supplies compounds similar to what our bodies already make (true) and that therefore you can't become addicted or dependent (false), all you need to do is listen to a few real-life CUD stories to get it.

For instance, in a podcast from Colorado Public Radio called *On Something* (recommended!), the author Neal Pollack discusses the worst of his CUD:

> "I wasn't just getting a little high. I was smoking huge amounts of weed all day, every day.… I started having public meltdowns. Personality-transforming public meltdowns. I would lose my temper, yell at waiters. I was a drug addict."

I've seen CUD up close. I've been married for seventeen years and counting to a really good man who, nonetheless, for a period of time, prioritized getting high over almost everything else. And though I wasn't even aware of the depth of his problem until my terrible mistake blew every secret in our relationship wide open, I absolutely knew *something* was wrong. And it was devastating to both of us.

My husband has changed his ways around weed since then, and I've forgiven him for hiding his cannabis abuse from me—just like he's forgiven me for betraying him. And while I'm not proud of my husband's past abuse of weed or of my affair (I mean, *duh*), I promised to be real with you. So I think now's the time to bring in my husband's CUD story—in his own words.

**Can you describe your history with weed?**

When I was smoking a lot, it would greatly affect my cognitive ability, my memory, my social abilities. And I'd have really bad trips that were dissociative, like psychotic episodes. I felt like I was splintered into multiple pieces, all of which were screaming at me for attention. All the negative feelings I had about myself—they would just come out all at once.

I also had delusions of grandeur. For instance, I trained like a maniac to compete in the 1996 Olympics—only, I forgot to pick a sport.

One time I drove up to Santa Ana for a work thing—this was about seven years ago. I parked in the parking structure, smoked a bowl, and threw away the lighter and the weed because I was "quitting."

Then I walked across a plaza area with a fountain. About halfway through the plaza, I realized I had *no idea* what city I was in. It could have been Chicago, or LA, or New York, or Venice, Italy. I just had *no idea* where I was. And that kind of thing happened to me more than once. It was the cumulative effect on my brain of smoking so much, for so long.

**How did your relationship with weed change over time?**

For years, I would quit—I'd be smoke-free for a few months. Then I'd smoke once. Then again a little while later. And, gradually, the intervals would decrease, and I'd be smoking all the time.

After starting to smoke again, there was always a sweet spot where things would be good. Then I'd come down on the other side of the bell curve and I'd become a decrepit antisocial hermit who could barely function.

To really change that, I had to quit entirely for a long while. I went to NA and therapy and all that, and, eventually, I just realized that getting high all the time wasn't worth it—that I could focus on my relationships, my career, my life, or on weed.

**Can you talk a bit about what NA (Narcotics Anonymous) was like for you?**

I think generally you're going to find some shit in an NA meeting that, if you're someone who just abuses marijuana, you can't relate to. In twelve-step programs, they put so much emphasis on "clean time" that if you fuck up or make a different decision, it affects your whole identity. Some people probably need to do abstinence-only. But twelve-step programs don't really recognize that it's not the same for everyone.

**Where are you with cannabis now?**

I quit entirely for a while—maybe it was about a year and a half. In the last eight months I've done it, I think, six times. For me, not smoking at all might be worse than smoking once in a while. I still like getting high, but I don't do it that often anymore.

**What do you think about me becoming a weed enthusiast, a weed mom?**

Honestly, it *has* bothered me at times, but, overall, I actually really like it when you get high. You're more pleasant to be around—and more malleable (he says with an evil grin).

**Any advice for potential weed moms?**

It's just about moderation for yourself, your individual makeup. Getting high can help you with insight and self-reflection. If you don't get too high and you don't use it too much, you're able to carry that reflection forward.

# CANNABIS DEPENDENCE AND WITHDRAWALS

When my husband quit weed cold turkey, he was no fun at all to be around for a couple of weeks. He had trouble falling asleep, and when he did get to sleep, nightmares hit hard. He'd wake up thrashing, fighting off an unseen threat. He was irritable and moody and unpredictable, and though the fact that he was still really pissed at me played into the moment, the weed withdrawal made everything so much worse.

CBD helped.

But did he really need to go to rehab for weed addiction? Not exactly. What he needed was five weeks away from his responsibilities. Five weeks of therapy, medication management, and strategizing in order to recalibrate—well, everything.

With heavy and longtime use, symptoms of cannabis withdrawal can include:

◊ Anxiety

◊ Brain fog

◊ Cold sweats

◊ Depression

◊ GI issues

◊ Headaches

◊ Insomnia

◊ Irritability and mood swings

◊ Nightmares

Withdrawal symptoms from cannabis are not considered life-threatening the way withdrawal from alcohol or opiates can be; with cannabis, they tend to appear within a day or so of abstinence and to peak around day ten, gradually subsiding over the next two to three weeks. Helpful practices during this time (and always!) include rest, hydration, nutrition, exercise, and mind-body disciplines to both relieve stress and cultivate mindful attention.

If you or someone you love is struggling with CUD, you can start exploring more formal options by calling the Substance Abuse and Mental Health Services Administration national helpline at 1-800-662-4357. Depending on your needs, you may also want to check out SMART Recovery (smartrecovery. org), Marijuana Anonymous (marijuana-anonymous.org), an app like I Am Sober, or the IGNTD program.

# RECOGNIZING A PROBLEM WITH CANNABIS

Most adults, says Jaffe, have some intuition that their use is becoming problematic before it veers dramatically off course. Still, he says, "you may not know *exactly* when you've crossed that line." So he offers a few signposts to help identify the territory.

## SNEAKING AROUND

"The moment," says Jaffe, "you start hiding your use from others, it's time to do a little self-check-in." For instance, if you're slipping away to consume while covering your tracks from a partner, or if you don't want others to know how frequently or heavily you're using cannabis, that's something to look at. Sneaking and lying, Jaffe tells me, "create shame, struggle, and a disconnect from the relationship—which will cause problems downstream."

An exception, of course, is with kids; while I never recommend lying, there are legitimate reasons we may consume privately or refrain from full transparency with the little ones in our lives.

Another exception concerns the legal status of THC in your state and the biases, stemming from a century of prohibition, that some people still have toward weed. Legalization makes it easier for many of Jaffe's clients to talk about cannabis with the people in their lives, he tells me, but stigmas remain. If your partner, mom, or best friend looks down on the herb or disapproves of you using it, that's a relationship and education issue more than an indicator of substance misuse—we'll discuss relationships in the following chapters.

## DEFENSIVENESS

If you're feeling defensive with people in your life around your use, Jaffe tells me it's something to be curious about. "It's important to be able to self-reflect," he says. "And sometimes, other people are a better reflection of us than our own perceptions."

"We are social animals," he tells me, which means, among other things, that our loved ones' perceptions matter to us. If you're using cannabis in secret because you know your partner wouldn't approve and wind up feeling angry or attacked when he or she calls you out, that's defensiveness.

## SUBSTITUTING WEED FOR ALL SELF-CARE

According to Jaffe, another sign that you've gotten off track with cannabis is if you pivot away from self-care activities like exercise, massage, yoga, meditation, and hanging out with friends in favor of getting high. "If you notice that you feel stressed," he says, "and every time you feel stressed you jump on cannabis because it's easy and it's there—then start paying attention to the other ways of getting relief." Just like no single human being can meet all your needs for love and connection, cannabis isn't the answer to all of your self-care needs.

## NOT ENGAGING WITH YOUR KIDS

Jessilyn Dolan, who worked in the field of substance abuse before becoming a cannabis nurse, acknowledges that overuse can decrease a parent's willingness and capacity to meaningfully interact with kids. "If it makes you a wonderful parent and you're out on the playground—awesome," she tells me. "But if you're using cannabis all day long and just sticking your kid in front of a screen and watching TV with them," she says, then cannabis probably isn't serving you and your kids' highest good. If you ever *do* find that cannabis detracts from your ability to parent the way you want to, then, please, take a step back and rethink.

But I want to add a subtle reframe here, or maybe just a question for you to hold. Moms today are—almost universally—overcommitted, overtaxed, overstretched, and tapped out at least some of the time. No matter how many children you parent, whatever your job or financial situation, or how much support you have, I'd bet you can identify. And yeah, *at least some of the time*, that's me, too.

If you let it, cannabis can help you reflect and mindfully step back from what's not working in your life. Say you have a client who's draining your time and energy, or you're struggling to meet a goal of home-cooked meals for your family every night. Or say you hate running the PTA. Stepping back from what *isn't* joyful in your life is a super-bad-ass weed mom move because it frees your energy up for the things that do matter to you. You *don't* have to be a supermom, you just have to love your kids, love yourself, and keep growing.

A few other signs that you may be getting off track with cannabis include:

◊ Getting cranky when you can't use cannabis

◊ Consuming with increasing frequency

◊ Using increasingly potent products to produce the same effect

◊ Overconsuming in a way that compromises safety

◊ Wanting to stop, but not feeling up to it

## CHANGING THE PATTERNS

So far, there's no clinical protocol that's specific to cannabis use disorder, though cognitive behavioral therapy and other kinds of talk therapy are usually recommended. No medication has been approved by the FDA, either, though doctors do sometimes prescribe sleep aids or anti-anxiety meds to lessen the discomfort.[122] Interestingly, helping with anxiety and sleep are two of the things CBD may do best; many people, including my husband, have found that CBD does indeed ease the discomfort of tapering off THC—all without the high.

Some people who overuse weed can self-correct, while others may need a more robust intervention like therapy or a short-term treatment program. A cannabis-friendly therapist can also help you renegotiate your relationship to the plant.

Jaffe's approach is all about examining the underlying issues—the *why* behind the overuse. "Odds are," he tells me, "if you understand that, you can change your relationship to it. Then maybe you don't have to quit forever. Maybe you can change the pattern instead." Overusing anything—from sugar to caffeine to weed to alcohol to pills—is about *coping*, so Jaffe encourages his clients to understand their stressors and to develop a range of strategies to meet those needs.

We all have shit to deal with in life, and for us moms, stresses are amplified by the complicated realities of balancing family, work, and self—compounded, of course, by cultural expectations about being a mother and a wife or partner. For instance, says Jaffe, if you feel trapped in your job, or your marriage, or your financial situation, *those* are your problems—the substance abuse is just a symptom.

Without mincing words, Jaffe tells me, "*If your life sucks*, there's no substance, no amount of porn, no behavior, no intervention of an outside source that's going to make that better without fixing the problems you have with your life." Jaffe's approach—in stark contrast to much of the addictions field—isn't all about quitting and staying quit:

"I don't care if someone gives up using, or moderates it. I'm agnostic as to the outcome...the idea that it's an all-or-nothing game is absurd. It doesn't play out in other fields—not in medicine, not in psychology, not in construction.

There is no other field where 100 percent success is the *only* measure of success. The world is full of gray, and the blacks and whites are pretty rare."

✹ ✹ ✹

So, to bring our conversation full circle, even though our beloved Mary Jane is helpful, healthful, and healing in so many different capacities, there *are* risks to loving her too much. Inform yourself. Be moderate and mindful; reflect on why you're consuming, how it affects you, and what you can do if overuse ever becomes an issue. Be informed, conscious, and uplifted—the weed mom way.

# CHAPTER 10

# THE BIG O: SEX, RELATIONSHIPS, AND CANNABIS

I've had plenty of wonderful orgasms in my life, but never the G-spot kind until, well, until I smoked a bowl of Sour Diesel, generously applied THC serum to my lady parts, and got down to playtime with my husband.

Inhaling the fragrant smoke, my endocannabinoid receptors were massaged and my sense of touch ignited. And the serum's effects were like a sprinkling of fairy dust on my most sensitive parts. You know the medieval paintings of the saints, or the Virgin Mary, with those glowing, golden orbs encircling cherubic heads upturned in prayer? That was me—only the glowy orb emanated from deep in my center and pulsed itself in unrelenting waves of *hell yeahs* through my entire body. Afterward, I felt positively weak with pleasure—like a pool of molasses or well-kneaded dough. Virgin, indeed.

Turns out, sex and cannabis have a long history, and people from many walks of life and many different historical moments have sung its praises in the boudoir; tantric texts from hundreds of years ago allude to cannabis as an aid to ritualized lovemaking, and nineteenth-century French artists enjoyed hash-inspired sexual liberties. Today, many weed enthusiasts agree: sex and weed are a great combo.

Historically, cannabis's medicinal properties have been put to use for women's sexual and reproductive health, according to Michelle Weiner, DO, who practices in Florida. There's evidence, she says, that cannabis flowers, seeds, and stems were used in midwives' medicinal preparations to help with childbirth, menstrual cramps, heavy bleeding, menopause, and low libido.

When a 2017 Stanford study of 51,000 Americans showed that cannabis users of all races and demographics have on average 20 percent more sex than nonusers,[123] weed lovers the world over nodded their heads knowingly. In another study, 68.5 percent of women who get down while high describe sex as more pleasurable, 60.6 percent say weed improves their sex drive, and 52.8 percent find their orgasms more powerful.[124]

Research has found that the endocannabinoids anandamide and 2-AG play a role in sexual arousal for women,[125] and from that we might hypothesize that a plant-derived cannabinoid such as THC could also contribute to that sexy feeling.

But cannabis does more than enhance sex. It promotes bonding and feelings of compassion while opening up a pathway to intimacy and communication with a partner—all of which is vital inside *and* outside those sexy moments. What's more, partnered moms and single moms alike tell me that intentional cannabis use helps them cultivate self-acceptance and self-love.

# WHY CANNABIS IS AH-MAZING FOR SEX

Good sex is *really* good for you. It lowers stress and anxiety, boosts immunity, lowers blood pressure, and enhances connection; for some, sex is also an elemental part of spirituality.

Cannabis, too, helps lower stress and anxiety. It's a known vasodilator, meaning that it widens blood vessels and increases blood flow—*très* helpful when it comes to arousal and orgasm. Cannabis relaxes your muscles, heightens sensitivity and sensation, and helps you get deeply present. And if you have PTSD-like symptoms around sex, cannabis can help deprioritize those thoughts.

Sex and intimacy educator Ashley Manta tells me that, when it comes to women and sex, cannabis is such a helpful tool because "it helps address the things that are getting in the way of pleasure." Pain, stress, worry, self-consciousness, feeling disconnected from your body—these are all common things that hang us up. "By intentionally choosing cannabis products that address those factors, you can enhance your sexual experience," says Manta, who coined the term CannaSexual® to mean someone who consciously chooses cannabis for elevating pleasure and intimacy.

For moms, a bit of herbal relaxation can also help us shift from our parenting-and-getting-shit-done brain, where we live a lot of the time, to our pleasure-focused brain. But, like all things cannabis, it's a dose-dependent kind of deal. Get too high and you may just wanna cuddle up with your partner (or a bag of chips) and binge on Netflix. Or, you could go so far down a mental rabbit hole wondering about whether the island of Crete really *is* the long-lost city of Atlantis that you forget what your body is up to. Let's be honest: being too deep in your own head isn't a good thing when it comes to sex. Fully in your body, responsive to your partner, and consciously elevated: *that's* where cannabis and sex come alive.

Let's explore some of the many areas where cannabis in the bedroom (or wherever you wanna do it) can lend a hand.

## DESIRE

Your sex drive is an important part of you and may have even contributed to the fact that someone now calls you Mom. (Hey there, adoptive moms, mamas who didn't carry or breastfeed, mamas without vaginas—I see you, too! Kindly disregard whatever doesn't apply to you here.) But, for some of us at least, becoming a mother did a number on the ol' sex drive. From pregnancy to breastfeeding to diaper slinging to carpooling to the endless list of tasks that moms tend to take on—often in addition to our day jobs—sex can absolutely get harder to feel psyched about once you're a parent and a female in a culture that expects so much physical and emotional labor from us. Add to that the sheer physical exhaustion of it all, the lack of time and privacy, new financial stressors, and the feeling of being "touched out" by babies and toddlers who use your body as a twenty-four-hour gym—sometimes sex is the last thing on your mind.

Cannabis can help. Remember the studies I mentioned a minute ago? People who enjoy weed regularly have 20 percent more sex on average, and a majority of women who consume find themselves more aroused and better satisfied with their sex lives. It makes a lot of sense: if sex and connection *actually feel great* for mind and body, you're likely to be in the mood more often. "Wheels that are in motion stay in motion," LA-based sensuality coach Carli Jo Cabrera tells me. "The more sex you're having, the more sex you want. It's a flow, just like everything else."

It's a total stereotype and—if you ask any sex therapist—an unfair claim that men in hetero relationships want more sex while their female partners want less. That happens, sure. But sometimes there's a libido mismatch the other way around—more than one weed mom I've talked to wishes her male partner were up for more play time. In fact, about 30 percent of men experience diminishing sex drive as they age. Either way, cannabis, can help even out an unbalanced libido on the sexy see-saw for two, says Jordan Tishler, MD.

If you're a mom in a relationship with another woman or any human adult, for that matter, there's no guarantee that you and your partner will always want sex at the same time; it's the reality of real-life relationships. But if you or your partner *want* to want sex, then infusing your sex life with the good herb is definitely worth a go. I'll talk soon about what to use, and how.

# AROUSAL

Desire and arousal are not precisely the same. Desire is about *wanting* to have sex, and arousal is about the physical response to foreplay, or to various sexy visual stimuli—such as glimpsing your partner's naked torso or watching him or her fold the laundry. For people with vaginas, cannabis aids in the arousal department via its action as a muscle relaxer. It's those perineal muscles all around the vagina, anus, pelvic floor, and vulva that need to relax enough to promote circulation and make sex both easier and more pleasurable.

Anyone with a vagina can benefit from these effects, I think, but women with endometriosis, pelvic inflammatory disease, or other conditions that tend to cause painful intercourse often need pain relief in addition to relaxation, and cannabis is great for that, too.

With the right product and dose, cannabis can also do good things for your head space when it comes to sex. Carli Jo talks about the challenges— particularly for mothers—of transitioning between different roles and head spaces. "When we're being boss ladies—we're running the family, we're running the job—we are in a different operating system. You can call it masculine, you can call it the hunter, there's different versions of it, but it's very task-oriented, goal-oriented," she says. There are tons of benefits to being in that head space out in the world, but when it comes to sex and sensuality, she says, "it's really helpful for women to be able to switch over to the gathering operating system—the feminine side of us that's softer, more process-oriented, and open to possibilities." (It's not about submissiveness to a male partner, nor is it exclusive to hetero sex—it's simply about opening up. Many men, too, can benefit from cultivating receptivity and the feminine side of their natures.)

Speaking to those difficult transitions, Manta tells me that "women and women-identified people typically need more time to get ready for sex," and cannabis can help us put aside those work and parenting roles. Decreasing stress and anxiety and focusing your awareness on the here and now are incredibly important parts of pleasure.

Some women find that they produce more lubrication while high, and others report little difference in that area. But if you also add THC topicals or weed-infused lubes to the mix, the increased sensitivity may boost your pleasure and your natural lubrication. If both you and your partner have vaginas, it sounds like a double-win to me.

For male partners, Dr. Tishler says that judiciously incorporating inhaled cannabis can help lessen anxiety, increase focus, and boost blood flow and erections. Too much weed for men, however, tends to have the opposite effect, because "some focus is required to maintain an erection and sustain the mechanics of sex," Dr. Tishler said on an appearance of the *GreenNurse* show. Women can enjoy a somewhat higher dose; but for men, less is more.

Just a quick reminder here, that—as in so many things—intention matters; smoking or ingesting any kind of weed product isn't a magic horny button. And while slathering on your THC lubes and serums may or may not spark a warm tingle in your nether bits, combining cannabis and sex in a healthy way requires you to *want* sex, to feel safe with your partner, and to get down willingly. If you are unhappy or unsafe or unattracted, cannabis isn't your Band-Aid, relationship therapy, or no-hassle divorce. However, if you *do* want sex with your partner and just find it kinda difficult at the moment, I predict some good times ahead in your bedroom. (Or in a 420-friendly hotel somewhere far, far away from your home and your spawn.)

## Weed Moms Speak on Cannabis for Pain-Relief before or after Sex

"I call it the 'velvet vagina.' It was like a miracle. I couldn't believe that cannabis fixed so many of my problems and made sex really, really good." —*Shannon of WeedMama.ca, mom of 2, Vancouver, BC*

"I had endometriosis and adenomyosis. I now have pelvic floor dysfunction among other chronic illnesses. For me, [cannabis] is the only way I will engage in any kind of sexual activity. It makes me feel sexier and more confident—not to mention that sex is just better all around. It also helps me with post-sex pain, muscle fatigue, and spasms I tend to experience right after I orgasm. It's godsent for my marriage and overall self-esteem." —*Anonymous mom*

"For me, having endometriosis makes it difficult with pain. So topicals and certain strains act as muscle relaxers in a sense, making it less painful." —*Diana, mom of 1, Massachusetts*

# ORGASM

While there's plenty of good sex to be had without orgasm, let's face it: orgasms are healthy and important and *wonderful*. They flood your brain with endorphins, those feel-good neurotransmitters, and promote healthy circulation and longevity. And since cannabis helps release dopamine while engaging your endocannabinoid system to boost your sense of well-being, it's like a triple scoop of *yes pleases*. Already-pleasurable sensations are deliciously heightened with cannabis—from holding hands to massage to couples yoga to everything else you and your partner might do to and for one another.

# SATISFACTION

Satisfaction is related to intimacy and connection. In other words, once play time is done, how do you feel about the experience, your partner, and yourself?

Manta tells me that cannabis works really well for quieting down the voices in our heads that get in the way of connection. "We have so much shame, we humans—especially those of us who've been socialized female," she tells me. "It's *so hard* to talk about sex, even with our partners. Cannabis can help break the walls down a little bit and reduce some of the inhibitions you have around sharing yourself and being vulnerable in the sexual space so that you and your partner can see more of each other and come from a beautiful, openhearted, nonjudgmental space." A big ol' amen to not letting shame and anxiety run the show!

The satisfaction phase holds a lot of therapeutic benefit for relieving stress and bonding with your partner. A study has found links between anandamide (which, as you recall, THC mimics) and oxytocin—the so-called hug hormone.[126] In other words, it appears that THC boosts pro-social, bonding behavior. But most of us weed moms didn't really need a study to show that, because it's obvious that a little elevation from our friend ganja increases the pleasure of snuggling and feeling close.

> ### Weed Moms Speak on Improving the Sex-Related Symptoms of Menopause
>
> "Menopause made orgasms *meh*. Cannabis brings them back with a vengeance!" —*Jennifer, mom of 1, New Hampshire*

# SOLO SEX IS BETTER, TOO

Yes, cannabis can enhance your sense of connection to a partner, but it also deepens self-awareness. In solo sex, we can learn to slow down, to breathe, and to be present with sensation—all without the emotional and practical complications of a partner in the mix. Indeed, masturbation is a natural and healthy part of sexuality and another area where cannabis adds flair.

Carli Jo, who helps women in relationships awaken to their sensuality, prefers the term "self-pleasure" over masturbation, she tells me, because masturbation tends to be driven by the goal or endpoint of orgasm. "Self-pleasure," she says, "is the whole body, the mind, the spirit, the energetic body.... In self-pleasure we can really have our awakening and learn about the instrument that is our body—to find out what we like and don't like."

Even if women come to her for coaching because they want better sex with a partner, Carli Jo first encourages her clients to explore solo sex. And, sometimes, she says, cannabis can show the way.

She tells me about her own experiences while in training as a sensuality coach a few years ago. While studying tantra and solo sex, she says, "I was having a really hard time getting out of my head and experiencing pleasure." She'd been a cannabis consumer on and off in her life, and she remembers a particular moment when—faced with another self-pleasure assignment from her mentor—she looked over at a California-grown joint sitting on her dresser. "And I had this thought—'what about combining these?'"

So she smoked the joint, tried again, and, to her surprise, found herself out of her own head, fully present in her body. "It was the most amazing experience of my life," Carli Jo tells me. "I was swimming inside of my vulva.... I even drew my orgasm. It was so magical!"

But when she went to her next coaching session and reported what happened, she was quick to disqualify her own experience. "It was cannabis," she recalls telling her coach. "It wasn't *me*, it wasn't *my* body." Instead of agreeing with her, Carli Jo's coach pointed out that it *was* her body—cannabis just showed her how that kind of pleasure was possible. "If you're willing to bring in cannabis in a really mindful, intentional way," Carli Jo tells me, "you're opening yourself up to possibilities that were already there for you. Cannabis just lifts that veil to see that your body *is* capable of such awesome pleasure."

Cannabis has been an integral part of her practice in that it helps some women who have a hard time relaxing and getting out of their heads. But she's quick to point out that the good herb is only one piece of the picture for awakening to sensuality—and not a requisite one.

Speaking of her initial awakening to self-pleasure with the help of cannabis, she says, "I have achieved that much and *more*, with cannabis and without. You just gotta do what you gotta do to connect with that sensual side of you."

If you're new to combining cannabis and sex, both Carli Jo and Ashley Manta suggest that self-pleasure is a perfect vehicle for discovering how your body responds and calibrating your optimum product and dose. Some women even report that self-pleasure yields more powerful orgasms than partnered sex, in addition to better acceptance, and love, for oneself.

# WHAT CANNABIS CAN DO FOR YOUR RELATIONSHIP

## ENHANCING COMMUNICATION AROUND SEX

"We're afraid to give sexual feedback because it sounds like criticism," Manta tells me. But as cannabis helps reduce shame and promotes feelings of connection, it can also help you give and get feedback more openly. Instead of freaking out and going into a shame spiral ("OMG I must be a terrible lover because my partner had to tell me to move my finger three inches to the left," says Manta), we can more easily hear our partners' needs and desires, and express our own.

## INCREASING EMOTIONAL INTIMACY

Good sex is an excellent relationship glue, amirite? But in addition to sex, cannabis can help deepen emotional intimacy. "Cannabis can be a numbing agent, but it can also be an amplifier," Sara Ouimette, Berkeley-based, 420-friendly LMFT tells me. Intimacy requires a depth of feeling in both people, and mindful cannabis use as a couple can actually enhance your feelings of connection in and out of the bedroom.

"It really helps you slow down," Manta says. "And that's where the juice is for connection. We go, go, go all the time—produce, produce, produce, hectic, busy, on full speed constantly....Cannabis helps you slooooow down so you can really enjoy every moment."

## INCREASING KINDNESS AND EMPATHY

Here's where I'll bring back the idea of cannabis as a light psychedelic; don't worry, I'm not talking about crazy light shows or breathing walls— I'm talking about cannabis's ability to shift your perspective. For a lot of people, that perspective shift tends toward the more compassionate, more accepting side of their nature.

Journalist and author Michelle Janikian gives me an example of a two-degree shift that makes all the difference: "This happens to me with my partner," she says. "I'll be mad at him for not doing enough around the house. And then I'll smoke a joint and realize, *oh my god, he does so much*. We *both* do so much, and there's no reason to feel resentful."

## SEEING YOUR PARTNER ANEW

Sometimes we get stuck in our beliefs about our partner, or we're so focused on what the relationship *used* to feel like that we can't see what it is now. No matter how long you've been with someone or how well you know them, there's *always* more to discover. Sometimes we just forget to keep looking. At its best, cannabis gives us the ability to see even the most familiar interactions, the most mundane moments, in a fresh light. And that can do so much for cultivating a sense of appreciation—the kind that sometimes erodes in the midst of all the messes and busyness of a kid-centered life.

## EASIER DATING

I've heard from single and dating moms, too, about how the cannabis-enhanced practices of masturbation, mirror-gazing (a practice of gazing at your own image in the mirror for an extended period of time while using affirming self-talk, like *I love you*),[127] and inner journeying have transformed their self-understanding and ability to own what they want in life and love. Yeah, cannabis can absolutely be part of your emotional, mental, and spiritual growth. (More in Chapter 13.)

# WEED MOM Q&A

**Q: How do I talk to my partner about wanting to bring cannabis into our relationship and our sex life?**

**A:** The short answer is to offer information, destigmatize the subject, and talk with your partner about trust, safety, and good boundaries. You might start by mentioning some of what you've heard (or read in these pages!) about what cannabis can do to enhance your shared sex life.

CBD is an easy first-time product, since it doesn't get you high but—for some people at least—packs many of the same pro-relaxation benefits. You could suggest that the two of you start with a little CBD-enhanced bath, or a few puffs from a high-CBD strain while you're finessing the mood. Or you could mutually microdose with THC to test the waters—because, as I've said about a million times—it's better to *not* get high while learning about your ECS and calibrating your optimal dose than it is to get uncomfortably stoned. Believe me—ain't nobody having good sex that way.

## Weed Moms Speak on Sharing Weed with a Partner

"My husband was a drinker and did not like to smoke at all. Then drinking became less fun and more annoying (as he did when drunk). I slowly eased him into smoking and away from booze. Nine years with no alcohol, and we smoke together every day. We are truly happy with each other 99 percent of the time (can't be always). We are on our twentieth year of marriage, and we are besties. And the people at the dispensary love it when we come in together."
—*Bekki, mom of 2, Massachusetts*

But, before you even reach for that flower, vape, edible, or lube, talk to your partner about what draws you to cannabis-enhanced sex. For instance, do you need pain relief to make it more enjoyable, or are you searching for a way to turn the volume down on anxiety or past sexual trauma? Are you looking for a better way to transition from your mom or work brain to your sexy brain? Chances are, if you let your partner know how you think cannabis can help both of you in the bedroom (whether or not *they* choose to partake), they'll be more understanding.

Trust, safety, and boundaries are hugely important if you want to bring cannabis into your shared sex life—and cannabis won't just make these appear if they're not already alive and well in your relationship. Plus, whenever you bring *any* new element to sex, you'll want to talk about what's okay and what's not okay with each of you. Cannabis doesn't tend to lower inhibitions in the same way alcohol does, but it *can* make you feel more sensitive—so talk about what that might mean. What are you comfortable with sexually, and what's your partner comfortable with? How will you communicate about trying new things when enhancing your sexy time with cannabis?

Another way to gently experiment with altered consciousness in your relationship is simply to get a little high and give one another massages: no strings, no pressure—just a loving give and take.

## Weed Moms Speak on Tension with a Nonconsuming Partner

"My husband is straightedge (no drinking, smoking, or drugs), and I vaporize only in the bathroom. I never used cannabis before it became legal in Massachusetts, and now I grow my own. My husband does not love it, hates the smell, etc., but knows it's the best option for managing a bunch of medical conditions. Out of respect, I keep his involvement with anything cannabis-related to a minimum. Do I wish he'd get high just once? Absolutely! And I think it'd help with some of his medical conditions, but alas here we are." —*Kristen, mom of 2, Massachusetts*

"My boyfriend doesn't partake, and I do. We try and work it out, but he just generally dislikes it due to his job. We live separately still, so I just smoke in my bathroom and air out the place before he comes over....He knows I need it and he's accepted and agreed to that. He just wishes it was federally legal so I didn't run any risk for either of us." —*Danaca, mom of 2, North Dakota*

**Q: My partner can't or doesn't want to partake. How should we handle it?**

**A:** With respect, weediquette, communication, good boundaries, and love.

I asked Sara Ouimette, LMFT, about when cannabis becomes an issue between couples. "If the person who's using cannabis feels checked out or distant when they're high," she tells me, "then I can see how that's problematic." But if the person choosing cannabis uses it as a tool for self-reflection in a way that improves their ability to be present and to connect, then Ouimette sees how it could feel enriching for the relationship.

Arlene, one of the cannabis-loving moms I interviewed back in Chapter 6, is married to a man who can't consume because he serves in the military. Her use, however, isn't a problem in the relationship. Unless there are underlying tensions between partners, she tells me—in which case cannabis could become yet another thing to argue about—people can often accept one another's choices as long as those choices do no harm.

Think of it this way: if one of you enjoyed alcohol responsibly and the other didn't drink, that probably wouldn't be a deal-breaker. Given the fact that millions of Americans abstain from alcohol for reasons of health, religion, or recovery, I assure you that there are many, many couples who successfully negotiate these differences. In other words, it doesn't have to be that hard.

As I mentioned a moment ago, addressing any stigmas your partner may be harboring about weed is a great idea; you can provide helpful information about why you're choosing to consume, what you're consuming, and its benefit to you. And then—so as to avoid coming off like a weed-crazed maniac or simply an annoying partner—back off.

Remember, you don't need your partner's permission to decide to give cannabis a whirl on your own, kid-free time. But courtesy and respect are vital to a happy partnership, and totally weed mom to boot—so figure that into your equation as it makes sense to you. In any case, hiding weed use from your partner is always a bad idea. As discussed in Chapter 9, it'll sow the seeds of shame and mistrust—which are truly the antitheses to love. Believe me on that one.

Another thing you can do is to practice good weediquette. Vapes, sprays, tinctures, and edibles are the more discreet choices because any kind of smoke will emanate that distinctive, lingering aroma. And for your abstaining partner—whether the choice is due to job concerns, recovery, or simply a personal preference—that smell can feel like an intrusive reminder of what they're *not* doing. You'd never smoke in the house with your kids anyway, so keep the courtesy up for all nonconsuming people in your life if you choose to smoke. In addition to smoking or consuming outside, putting on a new shirt afterward, rinsing with mouthwash, and using eye drops can also help to reduce conspicuousness, and quite possibly, your partner's discomfort.

Using cannabis responsibly can help your partner come around. Like we talked about in Chapters 5 and 6, there are a slew of ways to ensure you won't go overboard or put yourself or anyone else at risk. And, as we covered last chapter, it's vital to stay engaged with your roles and responsibilities (or renegotiate them, if needed), because owning up and showing up are both pieces of conscious weed momming.

Remember, as long as you're functioning well in your life and causing no harm, you're entitled to the form of relaxation that works best for you. Still, try to be patient with your abstaining or objecting partner. The cultural tide is turning, and, for most Americans, cannabis is no longer a big, hairy monster lurking in the shadows. "Attitudes," Arlene tells me, "are changing quickly. In many cases, it's only a matter of time."

**Q: Is it possible for cannabis to detract from sex?**

**A:** Yes! Manta tells me that anytime you use cannabis to numb yourself out or escape, it's going to negatively impact sex. "If you can't handle your partner and the only way you can be around them is stoned, that is not going to lead to a positive sexual experience." The point, she says, is to be more present, patient, and open—not to escape.

## Weed Moms Speak on Partners Who Don't Partake but Are Generally Cool with It

"My husband is in law enforcement so until it was recreationally legal, he had a problem with it. It was definitely an enormous source of tension as he knew it was something that helped me, but he didn't want it to affect his career, our kids, etc. Now it's something he's totally fine with—even suggests it at times I don't think I need it." —*Natalie, mom of 3, Massachusetts*

"I'm bipolar and use it to medicate, and my husband 100 percent understands and doesn't give me any grief about it." —*Molly, mom of 3, Colorado*

"My longtime boyfriend does not smoke...but he never minds if I smoke or take oils or tinctures 24/7. It's my only medication—no prescription medications at all. So it's never been a problem for us. He even goes and gets it at the dispensary for me when I cannot make it." —*Celeste, mom of 2 and grandma, Massachusetts*

"My hubby cannot until it's federally legal. He's finally comfortable with me doing it on the regular. It's not easy but we are currently in a good place and agreement about things." —*Amy, mom of 2, Colorado*

"He likes bourbon, and I don't drink. I like my weed, and he doesn't smoke. It works out well—would be too expensive if we both smoked and drank!" —*Tara, mom of 1, Massachusetts*

Along similar lines, she tells me, *anything* you're using to escape—whether that's alcohol, other substances, food, work, or even sex itself—won't serve you well in the bedroom. "Whatever you're using as a vehicle for not dealing with what is actually going on," she tells me, "is going to come back and bite you in the ass later."

The other way that cannabis can detract from good sex is if you're being haphazard about your choices. "If you pick up a mystery joint at a party or you're eating an edible that you made at home and you don't know the dose—you're really rolling the dice as far as whether it's going to be a positive experience for you, or a really uncomfortable one," says Manta. Again, cannabis and sex are a perfect pairing when the two are served up mindfully and with ample consideration of how, when, what, why, and—of course—with whom.

**Q: What's the best stuff for getting down? Deets, please!**

**A:** Take a stroll through your dispensary and you'll find loads of cannabis products formulated to enhance sex—from teas blended with aphrodisiac herbs to topicals for heightening sensation to bath bombs packing both THC and romantic essential oils. The main question here isn't "What works best?" but "What do you like?" and "What are you and your partner comfortable consuming in intimate situations?"

It'll require some experimentation because your ECS will not respond in the same way as mine, or your best friend's, or your sex therapist's, or your partner's. If you choose an intake method involving inhaling or ingesting THC in some capacity—in other words, if you choose to get high for sex— aim for the sweet spot of relaxation before it crosses the line into sleepiness; aim for excitement without the urge to jump out of bed and organize your spice rack.

Manta tells me that, because everyone's ECS varies, there's really no way of predicting with accuracy the strains that will turn you on. But she does recommend following your nose and going with the most appealing terpene profile. Limonene is often experienced as invigorating—so a strain with a fresh, lemony scent may be a good choice if you need a boost. And caryophyllene has a more relaxing effect on many people, which can help you get grounded in your body if you, like so many of us, spend a lot of time in your head. Just like our preferences for different kinds of sex can vary with our menstrual cycles, Manta finds that women's weed preferences can vary at different points in the month, too.

And as far as dosing goes, always start low if you're new to combining weed and sex. A 2.5 mg edible, or a single puff of a vape or a joint, may really be enough. "You can always add more, but you can't subtract," Manta says. "And if you've gone too far, you're kinda fucked—and not in the fun way."

**Flower:** Inhaling is probably the easiest mode of intake for sex because it comes on quickly, doesn't last all day, and has a beneficial effect on both body and mind. Whether you're smoking or vaporizing flower, you can experiment over a period of time with a few or even several different strains to find what brings you to the sweetest spots. Remember that each kind of sex has its own mood, and a single strain probably won't meet all your needs for sex-positive elevation.

I happen to love Sour Diesel, which helps me feel—as our friends from Jersey Shore used to say—DTF. For me, it intensifies *all* the sensations from touch to kissing and well beyond, but your own ECS is a precious snowflake, and there are many strains in the proverbial sea: I encourage you to do some experimenting and find what you (and your partner, if applicable) dig. Believe me, it's worth it.

If, on the other hand, my husband and I are looking for a slow jam lovemaking session, then a more laid-back strain like Gelato is what I'll reach for. To be perfectly honest, I'm going to be so chilled TF out on this strain, especially if it's late in the evening, that my husband will have to do a lot more of the actual work—but he doesn't seem to mind. Like I've said, he hardly uses THC anymore, and from time to time he gets off on being the sober one who (with full consent, of course) does with me as he will.

For a midday quickie, which doesn't happen often because *kids*, I prefer a high-CBD strain to lessen anxiety and help me stay clear-headed enough to get back to work afterward. Harlequin and AC/DC are both nice-tasting

CBD-rich strains. AC/DC won't get you high at all, but if you're sensitive to THC, Harlequin has just enough to provide a little extra tingle.

Other strains frequently mentioned in the sex and weed convo are Black Jack, Zkittlez, Wedding Cake, Jillybean, and Do-Si-Dos. There are so many fun possibilities here, friends, and thankfully you have the rest of your life to experiment with becoming a happy, healthy, sexually awakened weed mom.

**Vape:** If you're vaping e-liquid with a vape pen, you can go strain-specific and find a product made from one of the strains listed above. Just remember that, with e-liquids, some of the materials in the complex cannabis matrix are lost in manufacturing. Terpenes may be extracted from some other plant material and added back into the THC mix later. That's well and good I suppose—just not my preference. A few brands are doing full-spectrum vape liquids or live resins with no fillers or additives; I recommend looking into them if vaping is your choice.

An increasing number of vape brands are moving toward mood-specific formulas, which include sexy ones. They may be worth checking out, too. See the appendix for recs.

**Edibles:** Edibles give you that sweet body high, which typically translates to reeeeelaaxation; touch is also amplified by about a hundred. That's why some weed moms swear by the edibles route for sex. Sharing an infused truffle or two (depending on the total milligrams of THC) can be a lovely segue to getting your groove on together, but remember that edibles take a while to kick in. Thirty minutes is kinda the minimum here, and it could even take up to two hours to reach peak effects, so proper timing is key.

If you're an edibles newbie, stick with 1 to 5 mg of THC the first time and increase by 2.5 mg each subsequent session until you get where you want to be. It takes a bit of trial and error, true, but it's the fun kind. In the appendix, you'll find some chocolaty recs that pair wonderfully with activities of the sensual variety.

Here, as is often the case with cannabis consumables, it's the waiting game that gets a bit annoying. If you know your perfect edibles dose (the one that gets you high but doesn't put you to sleep) and how long it typically takes to kick in, you can plan ahead and pop that truffle anywhere from thirty minutes to two hours in advance of any planned sexy time. But if you're inexperienced with edibles, you may initially find it a bit of an unreliable method for getting in the mood. In that case, I suggest either reserving the experience for a weekend away when you'll have more free time or consuming a low-dose edible about an hour before the kids go to bed.

**Tinctures, Oils, Teas, and Sublingual Sprays:** If you're looking to tone down stress and anxiety, or need pain relief without the high, you may want to start with CBD-centered stuff like a 10:1 tincture or spray, or a CBD-heavy tea. A typical starter dose is between 10 and 25 mg; read the label and titrate up or down to find your minimum effective dose.

If you do want to add THC to the mix, dose your tinctures and oils in the same way you would edibles: start with up to 5 mg of THC if you're brand new, or simply take the dosage you *already* know works to get you elevated, not high AF.

**Suppositories, Lubes, and Serums:** For women with dyspareunia (painful intercourse), Patricia Frye, MD, recommends cannabis-based vaginal suppositories that relax muscles and help relieve pain. As for lubes and serums meant to enhance sex, she says there isn't a whole lot of evidence yet, though some women, she says, "do report more sensation from a cannabinoid lubricant versus a conventional one."

Lubes and serums are meant to make things nice and slippery while absorbing into your genital skin and elevating the experience, or *getting your vagina high*. Lubes tend to be the more slippery of the two, while serums absorb a bit more efficiently. And, in case you were wondering, you don't get a head high or a body high from topicals alone. However, some women, like me, do experience a very localized and veeeerrry nice feeling on their genitals.

According to Manta, CBD lubes and serums tend to work best for easing inflammation and pain, and for promoting relaxation. THC lubes, on the other hand, are more pleasure-focused. The benefit to CBD products is that they're more widely legal and available, but Manta recommends a THC and CBD combo whenever possible. You can look for a combination product, or just DIY a 1:1 ratio with a few pumps from each bottle. As always, look for broad-spectrum or full-spectrum cannabis lubes and serums to make the most of the whole plant.

In case you were wondering, yes—your vulva and vagina (along with your uterus, fallopian tubes, and ovaries) have endocannabinoid receptors. And though a direct link between topicals and arousal has yet to be proven, anecdotal evidence from many happy women (including *moi*) points to the conclusion that your vagina can indeed get high.

So what does a vagina that's high on THC feel like? Increased blood flow (cannabis = vasodilator) is part of it, as is a tingly, fresh sensitivity to the clitoris, vulva, and vagina. (Hello, G-spot orgasms!) It's your vagina, 2.0—primed for pleasure, ready to be romanced. Weed moms, *it's good*.

My experience with CBD-only lubes hasn't been as pleasurable; to be honest, I feel somewhat numb after slathering on a CBD-only lube or serum. If I had pain with intercourse, I'd want to explore the CBD route more thoroughly. That's the cool thing about the legal cannabis marketplace: there's something for everyone. And if you're the quantitative type, I certainly recommend trying a few to compare and contrast, you know, for the sake of science. (Heads up: they can get pricey.) Just be aware, says Dr. Weiner, that it may take thirty to ninety minutes to feel the effects of topicals like these.

Even if your goal isn't to get your vagina high or to alter your sexual experience in any way, high-quality products are well worth it to improve the elasticity and health of your vaginal skin. Whatever product you choose, look for a simple and clean formulation with no impossible-to-pronounce chemicals; only the best for your vag, weed moms!

**Massage Oils:** In this category, you've got your CBD massage products, your THC ones, and your combos, which blend the two cannabinoids alongside other ingredients like essential oils. THC doesn't absorb into the bloodstream through the skin, so you won't get high. But massage in general is excellent foreplay, good for promoting pro-sex responses like circulation, pain relief, stress relief, pleasure, and trust. Giving or getting a CBD- or THC-enhanced massage may help reduce inflammation in your tissues and relieve achiness, too.

When it comes to sex, health, and wellness, I'm all about experimenting and combining—once you understand your limits and know how to calibrate your total intake, of course. You and your love can smoke a bowl (or just take a puff or two if you're new) and use a sexy serum, or try a low-dose edible and a massage. Or how about a bath à deux with a cannabis-infused bath bomb, followed by a 1:1 CBD to THC tincture to help you connect and get down? The possibilities are nearly endless! Still, it needn't feel like a multivariate equation; if you get a little high and have sex with someone you care about, that's plenty good enough.

**Q: Using cannabis gives me cotton mouth. Will it dry out my vagina, too?**

**A:** Dr. Tishler says that while cannabis doesn't dehydrate you overall, it does kind of slow down your salivary glands to produce that parched, cotton-mouth feeling. (FYI: sips of water remedy cotton mouth better than chugging.)

But cannabis causing a dry vagina? That's a myth, he says. The system involved in lubricating the vagina is unrelated to the salivary glands. Low estrogen, on the other hand, can definitely cause problems with lubrication and is often associated with menopause. Whether or not you think you need it, since becoming a mother I've found that *lube is always your friend*. Whether it's weed lube, a commercial brand, or plain old coconut oil— better to have too much than too little.

# CHAPTER 11

# PUFF, PUFF, PASS: CANNABIS AND YOUR SOCIAL LIFE

When I think back to the handful of times I smoked weed in college, it strikes me that the whole enterprise was skewed pretty heavily toward the male side of the spectrum. In my college town, at least, the guys in the Baja hoodies held the good stuff and all the paraphernalia; the young women who hung in the same circles were passed the joint or the pipe but weren't the ones packing bowls or acquiring buds.

In Northern California's Emerald Triangle, home to decades of outlaw weed culture, lots of women have grown, tended, harvested, and trimmed, but in so many cases, guys still run the show. Yep, in stoner culture, like in many other arenas, women have long done a lot of the work, but it's been a dude's game nonetheless.

Thankfully, all that is changing. From dispensary design to product offerings to the marketing campaigns you now see on social, there's a female side of the industry coming into focus. About one-third of cannabis companies are led by women, and, year over year, women's purchases take up more market share.

But we're not the only ones jumping on board. Older adults are a quickly growing demographic of cannabis enthusiasts, as are all kinds of new niche groups, like those in recovery from alcohol and an increasing number of athletes. It just makes sense that cannabis culture is growing to accommodate these other groups—and that's awesome because, while I can appreciate some classic stoner culture (*Half Baked*, anyone?), all in all it just doesn't feel like the perfect fit.

Today, you can find cannabis-centric events and gatherings for women (and, hopefully, for female-identifying and nonbinary folks, too!) in virtually every mid-to-large city with legal weed. You can find retreats, tours, and sumptuous vacations where you can meet and mingle with other women who toke. Check out #SisterSesh. You'll see.

But if socializing is usually squeezed into one- or two-hour increments max because *you're a mom*, you'll want to look a bit closer to home to find your weed-loving community (even if that community consists of you and a friend giggling over some OG Kush).

Early in my cannabis journey, I had the pleasure of attending High Court, a series of monthly events in San Diego hosted by MC Flow. She's an artist, a big-time weed enthusiast, *and* a mom who writes and raps with alternating hilarity and poignancy about all things cannabis. (On YouTube, check out "Welcome to the Dispensary" if you want to learn about cannabis while laughing your ass off, or "Oh, Charlotte," to understand the human-impact side of legalization while crying your eyes out.)

High Court was silly, with MC Flow crowned onstage as queen of the magical, weed-loving kingdom of Weestonia, and where Southern California musicians, storytellers, and comedians rubbed shoulders onstage with Jason Mraz, a surprise guest, one evening. A cannabis smoke and vape cloud emanated odorously from the venue, and looking around, I felt affirmed and honored to be among peaceful, cannabis-loving people—responsible adults with jobs, kids, and all the rest—who love to smoke a little herb, enjoy music together, and laugh. So·many of the participants were women out for a night of fun with female friends. My kind of scene.

## INROADS INTO OUR SOCIAL LIVES: WEED MOM SURVEY

Shannon Chiarenza, founder of WeedMama.ca, talks about how moms often lean on pharmaceuticals and alcohol to manage symptoms of anxiety, depression, low libido, or difficulty sleeping, while at the same time starting to awaken to the effects of those choices. "It's not like they're having a couple of drinks in a weekend—they're usually drinking a couple of drinks a night. That adds up—and it's just not good for you," she says, citing the bloating and stomach upset that often follow a night of drinking. Alcohol, as I've mentioned before, comes with a whole range of other side effects, such as a spike in cortisol and blood sugar instability as well as potential liver and cognitive problems with longtime overuse.

Comparing weed to alcohol, Shannon points out how easy it is with cannabis to enjoy yourself without getting wasted, and how, in the right dose, cannabis lacks side effects. "If used correctly—that is, not using too much—it makes you feel better. And then it wears off, and that's it," she says. That's why it's her go-to for relaxing and for socializing—though she prefers to use cannabis in smaller gatherings where others are also partaking. (More on that in a minute.)

In 2017, a Yahoo-Marist national poll titled "Weed and the American Family" found that 65 percent of Americans who had tried marijuana were parents, and 30 percent were parents with children under the age of eighteen.[128] I'd guess that, a few years and numerous legalization measures later, the numbers are probably quite a bit, ahem, *higher* than that.

In 2020, 47 percent of US cannabis consumers said they preferred the effects of cannabis to alcohol, and one in three survey respondents said they either drink less or have quit drinking entirely since cannabis became legal in their state.[129] Independent data backs that claim up, showing that per-person spending on alcohol declines an average of 12.4 percent in counties with legal access to cannabis.

I conducted my own informal survey while researching for *Weed Mom*. Forty-one moms who already use cannabis responded via an anonymous, online survey about their habits around weed, alcohol, and socializing. I offer their responses here with my publisher's permission and the caveat that I'm not a social scientist, nor are my respondents necessarily representative of all cannabis-loving moms.

In keeping with the abovementioned nonscientific survey methods, I'm gonna go ahead and break down the data into two categories: "Yeah, obviously" and "Wow, that's surprising."

### Yeah, obviously…

◊ Sixty percent of respondents have either quit drinking alcohol, or drink significantly less, since starting to use cannabis.

◊ Fifty-six percent frequently use cannabis when socializing, while an additional 40 percent use it socially at least sometimes.

◊ A full 92.68 percent of moms say they feel better the day after using cannabis than the day after using alcohol.

◊ Cannabis's legal status at the state and federal levels decreases moms' comfort around using it socially (33.33 percent each), as does the presence of their kids (51.28 percent).

◊ Social stigma around cannabis remains for 20.5 percent of these cannabis-loving moms.

### Wow, that's surprising…

◊ *None* of the respondents report drinking more alcohol since cannabis came into their lives (I anticipated the number would be low, but *zero?*).

◊ 36.6 percent say that cannabis is a better social drug than alcohol.

◊ 58.5 percent say that the question of whether they prefer alcohol or cannabis socially depends on what they're doing and whom they're with.

◊ Just 2.4 percent say that alcohol is a superior social drug to cannabis. Given how deeply entrenched social alcohol culture is in the US (from baseball games to Sunday barbecues to craft brewery tours to mommy's wine o'clock), this *is* surprising.

So, to summarize, it appears that alcohol isn't the only game in town for moms anymore. Plenty of weed moms consider cannabis and socializing a good match; many would enjoy cannabis socially more often if laws and social stigmas were to change in favor of cannabis (they are!). Alcohol generally makes people feel crappy the next day—weed doesn't.

# WEED MOM Q&A

### Q: What's the etiquette of social cannabis use?

**A:** Glad you asked! Cannabis culture has long been a sharing one, and COVID-19 has put a real harsh on that mellow. But assuming you're ever offered a joint or a pipe, feel free to partake or to politely decline. If you indulge, keep it to two puffs, then pass to the left. If you decline, you can still pass it on with a smile. No matter what's on the menu or who you're with, you're always welcome to join in the fun or sit out—cannabis folks are cool and respectful like that. And if you're the one holding, offering to share— and meaning it—is always the courteous thing to do.

Sharing your weed, not wasting others' weed, being a generally kind human, and knowing your limits are together the most important parts of socializing with cannabis. To explore this subject further, check out *Higher Etiquette* by Lizzie Post. (Yes, Emily Post's great-great-granddaughter wrote a book about pot. You're welcome.)

**Q: Is cannabis a good "social drug" (i.e., one that enhances the pleasure of talking and connecting)?**

**A:** My survey results indicate that—for the weed moms who responded, at least—yes, cannabis is a good social drug. But your enjoyment of socializing with cannabis will also depend on where you are, how you're consuming, and who you're with. What follows are my personal *yes, please* scenarios for social cannabis consumption:

◊ Walking and talking with a good friend who also consumes

◊ Attending a chill, canna-friendly event when I have a safe way home

◊ Having dinner or barbecuing at home with a group of people who know their limits

◊ Going to a party where some adults are drinking alcohol and others are consuming cannabis (as long as *all* adults are mindful not to become too impaired and to keep children safe)

And my *no thanks* scenarios:

◊ Going to a bar, a loud concert, a big festival, or any kind of crowded event

◊ Hanging out with a group in which everyone else is drinking

◊ Any time safety is a concern (e.g., I have to drive, or I'm unfamiliar with the people or the venue)

Shannon the "Weed Mama" tells me, "I prefer cannabis for smaller, more intimate conversations. It makes you a little more introspective, and you can have a different kind of conversation than with alcohol." She, like me, prefers not to use cannabis alone in a crowd because the vibe of the two substances is just different enough that it's uncomfortable to feel grooooovy while everyone else around you is straight-up buzzed.

Still, she says, "You can socialize with cannabis really well if you find the dose that's right for you." Remember, microdosing and moderate dosing are your friends. And while I'm the first to admit that it takes a wee bit of intrepidness to journey through the many realms of cannabis in search of all the right fits, I know that after a little time and self-experimentation, you'll find your sweet spot, and the right company, for those social seshes.

So what are the best social strains?

As always, the effects of the whole bouquet of cannabinoids, terpenes, and all the other good stuff in cannabis will be mitigated through your unique ECS, and so your personal faves will probably vary. That said, Super Lemon Haze and Strawberry Cough are both touted for their fun and chatty vibe. AC/DC is a CBD-dominant strain that may help ease social anxiety, if that gets you down. And many people find White Russian a delightful dinner party pairing that lends a healthy dose of openness and creativity to their verbal musings.

**Q: How can I meet other weed moms?**

**A:** If you don't have a lot of weed-lovin' friends, don't fret. In addition to #SisterSesh, follow hashtags with all kinds of iterations of "women" and "cannabis." There are tons of online groups and organizations, some of them for moms specifically—try a quick search with any variation of "cannabis and moms" on your favorite platform and you're bound to find some of them.

Natasha Best, the "Stoned at Home Mom," tells me that while "some of the moms' groups out there are really catty and just like, ewww," she's found the cannabis moms communities online to be supportive and nonjudgmental places to hang out. "I've never met a rude person in a cannabis moms group," she tells me.

Tokeativity is a women and women-identified community that hosts both online and in-person events with an empowered, accepting, badass kind of vibe. Duby and Weedable are two more social sites (not specific to women), and you can also check Meetup and Eventbrite for IRL opportunities to meet canna-folks. If your dispensary hosts classes or info sessions, that could be another place to seek out the like-minded; or you could always just do it the old-fashioned way and strike up a conversation with a potential new bud while waiting to pay for your bud.

If you happen to be in San Diego, check out Pink Sesh Society. Glowing Goddess Getaways are weekend retreats with the five "high" standards of self-love, inclusivity, empathy, good fun, and mindfulness. And if you're looking to dive headfirst into a heady mix of community, horticultural prowess, and cannabis commodification, head to the Seattle Hempfest, the Mile High 420 Festival in Denver, the Emerald Cup in Northern California, or the *High Times*–sponsored Cannabis Cup in Amsterdam; none of these are exclusively for women, though these days you can often find mixers and other events for women and women-identified folks.

**Q: How should I handle the cannabis conversation with the parents of my kids' friends?**

**A:** This depends, of course, on where you live, your co-parenting relationship, and your level of comfort with uncomfortable conversations. It's not particularly important to tell everyone in your life about your (responsible) love of cannabis. As long as you keep all in your house and your care safe, lock your stash, refrain from use when other kids are in your home, and never drive under the influence, it's really up to you if you want to spill these particular beans.

I tend to get out ahead of the conversation because what I do for a living means that, for anyone with an internet connection, there are only .36 seconds between my name and cannabis. Talking about a federally illegal drug with a near-stranger who may (or may not) soon be entrusting me with their child isn't *easy* exactly, but somehow it usually goes better than anticipated.

In the fall of my son's fourth-grade year, he made fast friends with a kid in his class who's smart and funny, like him. By the time they started asking to hang out on the weekends and after school, the kid's mom had friended me on Facebook. (Mind you, this was *after* we'd moved to a prohibition state.)

My son's new friend came from a church-going, military family from whom I'd sensed a pretty straightedge vibe, but, nonetheless, I told the mom my reasons for enjoying cannabis as medicine and pleasure, my commitment to being safe and responsible with kids, and the fact that I believe it will be federally legal before too long—all in a rather lengthy series of Facebook messages. But you know what? This straightedge, church-going, military mom living in a prohibition state seemed astoundingly unperturbed by the whole thing and allowed her kid to come hang out at our house regularly. Just a few years ago, this scenario probably would have gone down differently.

Amber Morelli, a divorced mom of a 16-year-old son and a sales manager in the Sacramento area, has had some experience coming out of the cannabis closet with the parents of her kids' friends, too. Amber enjoyed cannabis back in college, then quit for a long while after becoming a professional and a mom. Then, at a particularly stressful moment in her life, she discovered that low-dose edibles and vaping could profoundly improve her anxiety without side effects. Cannabis, she says, enabled her to let go of a stressful day at work and be present with her son in a way that alcohol didn't.

But even after starting to work a corporate job at cannabis company Pure Vape, she was reluctant to talk openly about it. "In the mother group I was surrounded by, I was highly uncomfortable sharing that. I was working in the industry for over two years before I said anything," she tells me. "It was my own fear that held me back," she goes on, "because I was afraid that kids wouldn't be able to come to my house, or that other parents wouldn't want me to drive because they'd think I'm high all the time."

It's difficult to think that our choices could affect our kids' friendships—but it's also real. Stigma against cannabis is definitely still a thing. So what did Amber do? She waited until her son was in high school and then went for it. Now, she says, "I don't whisper it. I say it out loud."

The moms in her group were actually more curious than judgmental, she says. She'd start by telling them she works for a cannabis company, and they'd often respond, "Wow, that's cool," and in the next breath, "But do you use it yourself?"

"Yes," she'd tell them, "I use it every day."

Their next question, inevitably, was, "Have I ever seen you high?" Because Amber is experienced enough to microdose edibles and to vape in quantities that don't interfere with her ability to function optimally, she'd admit to them that she often uses cannabis when watching her son's activities or while chaperoning him and his friends at Dave and Buster's.

That probably wasn't what the moms in her circle expected to hear. "The stigma around it," she says, "is that if you use cannabis, the only way to do it is to look like Cheech and Chong." So she took it upon herself to start having these conversations with other moms and to provide information about healthy ways to microdose for anyone interested. To her surprise, a lot of moms were.

They'd ask about remedies for anxiety and sleep—two of the most common wellness-oriented uses for women. Amber was, and still is, happy to share what she knows. But she's also quick to point out that the way she broaches the conversation, and her own behavior, has a lot to do with how people perceive and respond to the subject. She's not showing up to events stoned or waving a green flag around shouting, "Hey, I smoke weed!" Instead, she's informing people while reassuring them—moves that, honestly, feel very familiar to me as a public weed mom.

Amber's quite aware of the double standard between alcohol and weed within parenting circles. A few weeks after she told her son—but not her parent community—that she uses cannabis, they attended a pool party. Her son asked whether she was planning to take her vape pen to the pool. "I told him, 'I'm not going to do that—it's inappropriate,'" she recalls. But about halfway through the party, her son noticed that other moms had wine in their water bottles. He wondered why *that* was acceptable while stepping away to microdose wasn't.

Even though that was a few years ago, Amber says, "I'm definitely well aware that the stigma is still there." That's why she's a big proponent of #EndtheStigma—an internet campaign to do just that.

A couple years out, Amber's happy to report that she's not a pariah in her parent circles and kids still hang out at her house. But she's quick to point out that, even in the privacy of their own home, it's important to model moderate and responsible use. "If my son sees me take a low-dose edible or a Kin slip [a sublingual product]—or if he sees me hit my vape on Sunday morning with my cup of coffee when I'm off work—that is different to me as a parent than him seeing me hit a dab rig [a device for consuming highly concentrated cannabis] or take a bong rip."

# FOUR CATEGORIES OF FRIENDS

## FRIENDS WHO ARE DOWN

This one's easy peasy. You can enjoy cannabis freely, as a responsible weed mom, with friends who are down with Mary Jane. Just a couple of tips: 1) Be mindful of your state's laws around consuming in public spaces—it's usually *not* allowed in public unless you're at a festival or cannabis event that's been permitted that way, and using cannabis in state and federal parks is a big no-no; 2) If you're bringing your kids along to socialize, I recommend discussing the kind of usage you and your friends will choose to engage in and model. For instance, will anyone be consuming in front of children, and are you comfortable with that?

Like Amber, I believe that discreetly microdosing or moderate dosing is appropriate in a social situation with kids as long as you're still able to respond to emergencies and supervise in the capacity that's necessary given the age group and activities involved. See Chapter 6 for a list of low-risk situations where consciously enhancing can up your parenting game.

## FRIENDS WHO MAY BE DOWN

How you bring it up depends, of course, on your personality and your relationship with the friend or friends in question. At the right moment, you could try busting out your flower vaporizer or your favorite low-dose edible, which could spark a host of curious questions and some intriguing conversation, or even a spontaneous #SisterSesh.

## Weed Moms Speak on Alcohol, Cannabis, and Socializing

"In my opinion, alcohol numbs people, makes them tune out or say and do hurtful things they wouldn't ordinarily do. Cannabis can open you up to a greater depth of feeling and connection, and helps you tune in and appreciate the magic in the mundane." —*Sierra, mom of 2, Massachusetts*

"I am super-comfortable with socializing with cannabis and am very open about my uses and dedication to this plant medicine! And yes, I do use it with my child around. Now, my reservations are these: I will never compromise my safety by exposing myself to someone who chooses to condemn me based on something they simply do not understand or agree with. So for me it just comes down to discernment and being mindful of safety. I don't really drink alcohol, and cannabis has always been my go-to for letting go and enhancing experiences, especially social ones!" —*Stephany, mom of 1, Florida*

"I use cannabis both medically and recreationally because I choose not to drink alcohol or use drugs—or any substance for that matter that does not support my endocannabinoid system.... My method of administration is generally a combined water-soluble THC/CBD-infused beverage. I also enjoy tea with infused honey and an edible for a controlled, safe, fun recreational experience. Inhalation is something that I partake in; however, it is audience-dependent because some children associate smoking *anything* as the same as smoking cigarettes. I do not want children who do not have the cognition to witness me smoking, because, after all, smoking is smoking regardless of *what* you are smoking. I don't flaunt it, and I also don't hide it. Cannabis is a part of my life." —*Sherri Tutkus, RN, cannabis nurse and CEO of GreenNurse Group, mom of 3, Massachusetts*

"I have gotten into trouble with overconsumption of alcohol. Some terrible things have happened, including being raped while drinking, and I woke up hating myself. I love that I don't lose inhibitions with cannabis. In fact, I gain some, in a good way. There are never any regrets. I remember everything. I feel great the next day. It's just the better choice, as far as regular use, for me. I wish I could use cannabis publicly with my friends like I can with alcohol. I think that would make me consume even less alcohol." —*Erica, mom of 1, Massachusetts*

"I used to have a lot of shame around my usage of cannabis, and I think it had everything to do with the fact that it was socially *not* acceptable and was illegal—and if you talked about it, it had to be something kind of sneaky. But we're drinking martinis no problem in front of our kids, and that's completely normal! I always knew on a rational level that that was messed up, but I still had that feeling like, if I was using cannabis, I was doing something wrong. It's changing now, and I hope attitudes and norms do continue to evolve." —*Reya, mom of 1, Idaho*

"I hate pills and would much rather smoke some herb. I am not a drinker as I come from a family of alcoholics and don't wanna be like them." —*Anonymous mom*

"I 100 percent prefer to smoke over drink any day. I will definitely have a drink or two socially with friends, but I smoke daily." —*Jenn, mom of 2, Massachusetts*

Many of us weed moms work in the comparison to alcohol at some point in the conversation. It's not a perfect analogy, but a framework that most people can wrap their heads around. You can point out that with cannabis, like with alcohol, there's responsible use and irresponsible use, right and wrong moments to consume. You can talk about how cannabis can be both therapeutic or all about fun, and the ways it contributes to your social life a bit like alcohol, minus the hangover.

Think of yourself as a kindly ambassador from the land of responsible cannabis enthusiasts by answering questions, being open and honest, and refraining from pressuring anyone. We all have a role to play in the green revolution. #EndtheStigma.

## FRIENDS WHO AREN'T DOWN BUT DON'T JUDGE YOU

Sometimes you just know that a friend isn't going to be down with trying cannabis; maybe it's because of her faith, her job, or something she's said in the past. And once in a while, you might find that a friend who you thought would be interested just isn't into it. That's cool. We all know that friendships across differences like skin color, sexual orientation, gender identity, religion, personal history, and beliefs are a good thing. Since moving to a red state, I've even become friendly with a few Republican voters! As long as everyone's respectful, it needn't be an issue.

## FRIENDS WHO AREN'T DOWN, AND JUDGE YOU FOR BEING DOWN

Well, it all comes down to a choice: yours. Is the person a good friend? Does this person routinely judge you? And do you choose to accept shade for using a plant that, overwhelmingly, does more help than harm? Personally, I'm all done with taking on other people's emotional burdens. But the decision and the power, weed moms, is entirely yours.

# CHAPTER 12
# CANNABIS AND YO MAMA

"My mom was on fentanyl patches, Percocet, and Xanax for years," says cannabis nurse Jessilyn Dolan. Dolan's two kids always knew their grandma to shake and sweat, and to have a gray pallor to her skin. Of course, she couldn't drive on all those meds, and her quality of life suffered.

Utilizing her clinical and horticultural skills, Dolan was able to help her mother transition away from pharmaceuticals. "After almost a year of experimentation with three different kinds of cannabis oils," she says, "now my mom's driving—and she's not sweating and shaking like she used to."

Dolan's kids can clearly see the differences in their grandma's health after starting to use cannabis, and, importantly, they're old enough to know that she's actually much safer now. Dolan says those heavy-duty meds could have killed her—and now, she's managing her health with a plant.

Cannabis is, in fact, extremely helpful for many of the symptoms associated with aging, and older adults are the fastest growing cohort of cannabis users in the US today. A study spanning from 2006 to 2013 found a 57.8 percent increase in usage among people aged 50 to 65, and a whopping 250 percent increase for those over 65.[130] To clarify, that doesn't mean older adults are the *largest* category of users, just a quickly growing one. But this older contingent of cannabis enthusiasts aren't quite as visible or as vocal yet, perhaps owing to the years of stigma and anti-drug messaging they've lived with. "I can assure you that *lots* of older people are consumers," says Patricia Patton, aka "the Cannaboomer," who's the mother of an adult son, a grandmother of two, and the former director of finance and administration for the Belgian Tourist Office in North America. "But I can also assure you that we're not going to be smoking a joint and taking a picture of ourselves."

Even so, Amy Froebel-Fisher, VP of finance and accounting with a chain of New England dispensaries called Temescal Wellness, tells me, "Stigma is lessening." Firsthand, she's witnessed the profound shifts in attitude that accompany legal cannabis. "You can see that change toward acceptance within a five-minute window," she tells me. "People who have lived a lifetime with the stereotypes and the stigmas evolve so quickly....It's amazing to see someone my mom's age come in and be afraid to ask questions and talk to somebody...but once they talk and learn, they open up about what cannabis means in their life. They've been living under this stereotype for so long.... To see it break down in front of your face is amazing. When I leave," she tells me, "I'm in tears."

# HOW CANNABIS HELPS OLDER ADULTS

Research shows that about 39 percent of older adults take five or more prescription pharmaceuticals,[131] a phenomenon known as "polypharmacy," and those looking to taper or eliminate some of those meds may turn to cannabis, particularly in place of painkillers and sleep aids. A 2020 survey of 568 older adults at a geriatrics clinic in southern California found that 10 percent used cannabis in the last month, a majority considered themselves new users, and their top reasons for trying cannabis include pain, sleep, and anxiety.[132] Enhancing sexuality and lifting mood are other popular reasons older adults turn to cannabis.

# WHO ARE "OLDER ADULTS"?

"Older adults" as a category generally includes those over 65, though I want to be careful not to paint any generation or group of people with too broad a brush; differences in gender, race, sexual orientation, upbringing, and belief exist in every age grouping—and there are even generational differences between older adults. "We span a large number of years, but we're not all the same," says Patton. Many Baby Boomers—those born between 1944 and 1964—came of age during the Vietnam War and the countercultural ethos of the time; today, in their mid-fifties to mid-seventies, they may be more comfortable with cannabis use than those born before 1944; a number of Boomers have had experience with the plant already.

On the other hand, most members of the Silent Generation, born from 1925 to the early 1940s, lack previous experience with cannabis. Eloise Theisen, a California board-certified nurse practitioner specializing in cannabis and geriatrics, tells me that her average patient, at 76, is "right at the age where they missed the fun exploration of the sixties." As such, they're more likely to have misconceptions and fear surrounding its use.

# WHAT KINDS OF CANNABIS PRODUCTS ARE OLDER ADULTS USING?

Salves, creams, ointments, and all kinds of topicals are popular with older adults who are new to cannabis because "those products are familiar and feel a lot like what we're already using," says Patton. She also finds that her peers gravitate toward tinctures and gummies with higher CBD concentrations because many people find they lessen the psychoactive effects of THC while providing their own kind of relief. Vape is another option. "I need my lungs," says Patton, who prefers to avoid smoking cannabis.

Theisen mostly consults with older adults for symptom relief related to chronic illness or age, and usually starts the "how to consume cannabis" conversation with inhalation because it's a fairly simple and controllable way to medicate. If her patients are averse to inhaling, she'll suggest tinctures, though she tends to steer clear of edibles with older adults because the tasty factor make these "treats" a bit too easy to overdo. If a patient strongly prefers edibles, Theisen suggests they keep unmedicated treats on hand to satisfy the sweet tooth once they've consumed their dose.

# WHAT'S GETTING IN THE WAY OF OLDER ADULTS USING CANNABIS MORE?

According to a recent survey in Colorado, lack of access to quality information or direct guidance from a healthcare provider, combined with a reluctance to discuss cannabis (due to the stigma associated with it), were among the top barriers for older adults who may otherwise be interested in therapeutic cannabis use.[133]

Along those lines, Theisen tells me that, for older adults, "the challenge is that they don't really know where to start." The dispensary experience, whether medical or recreational, can be overwhelming for someone unfamiliar with the cannabis landscape. If an older person has taken consumption advice off the internet, or from friends or family, their first experience with cannabis may not have been a good one. Because older adults' needs and response times vary from those of younger folks, Theisen, who's treated over 6,000 patients with cannabis, tells me she often hears stories like, "My grandson brought me this brownie that helps him with sleep, but I tried it and it was *way* too strong!"

In her practice, Theisen provides a comprehensive treatment plan that includes information about risks and benefits, side effects, and possible prescription drug interactions as well as the logistics of where to go, what to buy, and how much to take. She checks in with patients after a few weeks to see how things are going and helps them adjust or recalibrate their plan when needed. "I really think," she tells me, "that that kind of comprehensive care is the key to success and longevity with using cannabis."

Another obstacle for older adults, Theisen tells me, is cost. If they're using cannabis as medicine—say, in place of a sleep aid—then the $85 cannabis tincture may feel unaffordable when compared to the $5 monthly cost of an Ambien prescription with Medicare. Patton agrees that there's a certain elitism and inaccessibility to the legal cannabis industry—at least in some parts of the country—and that those on a fixed income struggle with wanting to reduce their pharmaceutical intake while perhaps not being able to afford to do so.

# POSSIBLE DOWNSIDES FOR OLDER ADULTS

The good news is that recent research hasn't found cannabis use in older adults to be associated with cognitive deficits. By studying MRIs of users and nonusers over the age of sixty and administering computerized cognitive tasks, researchers at the University of Colorado Boulder found that both groups have similar amounts of gray and white matter in the brain and perform equally well, thereby concluding that cannabis use does not have a long-term effect on cognition.[134]

But cannabis use for seniors does come with other special considerations and potential downsides. Metabolism tends to slow with age, so older adults may experience stronger effects that last longer—but come on more slowly. That's particularly true with edibles, Theisen tells me, but can also apply to other ways of consuming; that's why older adults may benefit from smaller therapeutic or recreational doses of THC than younger people.

Dizziness and sleepiness are two common side effects experienced by older adults. While relaxation is certainly welcome at bedtime, daytime fatigue and dizziness can up the risk of falling. In addition, older adults taking multiple pharmaceuticals may experience more drug interactions or side effects with cannabis.

Because the number of variables that determine how cannabis will affect a person tend to increase with age, Theisen prefers to see older adults who are new to cannabis work with a qualified cannabis nurse or doctor before jumping in. To help, you can check out the Cannabis Nurses Network, American Cannabis Nurses Association, or search "find a marijuana doctor" to identify a practitioner.

# WEED MOM Q&A

**Q: I think cannabis can help my mom/dad/aunt/uncle/other older person in my life. How can I start the conversation?**

**A:** According to Patton, there are real generational differences when it comes to weed. For instance, she points out how—for those in mainstream careers from the 1970s onward—drug testing was prevalent, and there was a sense that you could get into big trouble if you enjoyed cannabis. Speaking on the EstroHaze podcast, Patton, who is Black, says, "The War on Drugs had *everything* to do with it, because, essentially, it tied drugs to bad behaviors, to illegality, to the idea that everything can be used against you." While that statement applies to all older adults, it's particularly true for people of color in her generation—and it certainly adds to their hesitancy in talking about cannabis and cannabis culture. "You millennials and Gen-Xers feel much freer about cannabis than we do," she tells me on the phone, "but still—it's important to have these intergenerational conversations!"

# CBD

"Because we can now see CBD in CVS and Rite Aid, that's one way to get into the conversation," Patton says. Indeed, the last few years have seen CBD's popularity spike so quickly and thoroughly that the nonpsychoactive cannabinoid has infiltrated products all across the health and wellness spectrum—and even introduced some folks to plant medicine for the first time. "I sometimes joke that CBD is a gateway to chamomile," says Dolan of CBD's popularity. Dolan has long worked with herbs and other plant medicines.

Popularity, of course, is a double-edged sword. Increasing visibility is a good thing because more people, including seniors, are trying and loving the cannabinoid; on the other hand, the proliferation of products in the absence of quality control means that it's pretty easy for consumers to find junk CBD.

Still, because CBD is having a moment, it's a great conversation-starter with the older adults in your life. You know, because—at its best—CBD has the potential to help with the kinds of things older people want, like sleep, pain, and anxiety *without getting anyone high*.

## TOPICALS

Topicals are another easy entry point because, with the exception of transdermal patches, they're also nonpsychoactive. Even THC-infused salves, creams, lotions, and rubs won't cause anyone to feel funny—but they may provide relief for those run-of-the mill muscle and joint aches, as well as for the chronic pain of arthritis.

## REFERENCE THEIR HISTORY OR THE SOCIAL HISTORY OF CANNABIS

You might also start a conversation about cannabis with the older adults in your life by asking questions about their experiences in the sixties and seventies. For instance, I was surprised to find out that my German grandmother, who passed last year at the age of ninety-one, once smoked "the Elephaaant"—as she referred, in her strong German accent, to the strain of large buds known as Hawaiian Elephant. According to a relative, my grandma laughed at everything for a few hours and then fell asleep; though her lifelong preference was for schnapps, not weed, she harbored no bad feelings about the plant. My point here is that, if you ask questions and show curiosity, your elders—from parents, to aunts and uncles, to grandparents (if you're lucky enough to still have them)—may have a story or two up their own sleeves.

## ANSWER QUESTIONS, DON'T LECTURE

If you decide to tell an older loved one (or anyone, for that matter) about your own cannabis journey, my recommendations are to keep the conversation simple and informative; you're an adult, so there's really no need to convince anyone to support your decisions as long as you're partaking responsibly, but it helps to open up about *why* you consume and the benefits you've enjoyed.

Or, if you've already shared about your own relationship with the plant and you think cannabis could help the other person as well, then you might offer some basic info (remember, help with pain, sleep, anxiety, and mood elevation are common needs for older adults) without telling anyone what *they* should do. In other words, be humble. Even though you love the person, and even though cannabis could maybe even help them—a lot!—respecting boundaries is definitely the way to weed mom.

Patton, who frequently fields questions from other Boomers, gets questions like, "How will I feel if I try cannabis?," "How do I get it?," "What kinds of questions should I ask?," and "Will I become addicted?" If you do have answers to these questions, you can kindly provide them; otherwise, try pointing the person toward solid reference books like *The Medical Marijuana*

Guide (2018) by Patricia Frye, MD, or *Cannabis Pharmacy* (2017) by Michael Backes, or even some of the (less profane) parts of this guide.

## INTRODUCE THEM TO PRO-CANNABIS MAINSTREAM MEDIA

If you're diving into the fun, weird world of online cannabis media, yay for you! But, unless your parent or aunt or granny is an unreformed hippie, I suggest leading the older people in your life to more mainstream sources of information and community.

When Dr. Sanjay Gupta flipped a one-eighty on cannabis back in 2013, millions of CNN viewers became aware of cannabis's potential for health and healing almost overnight. And though mainstream media attention has since shifted away to other pressing topics, you can still find numerous articles on the subject by Dr. Gupta. His multipart documentary, *Weed* is an inside look at how a skeptic with a conventional medical background became a believer, and as such, it's a great primer to watch together or recommend.

## SIMPLE SUBSTITUTIONS

The kind of cannabis use that enhances wellness without officially crossing the line into medical territory includes simple substitutions for OTC meds like ibuprofen, aspirin,[135] and salves. Easy-entry products, including topicals and CBD tinctures or gummies, are a solid means for an older person—or anyone for that matter—to feel out the legal cannabis marketplace without getting overwhelmed. "Ease them into it," suggests Patton, "and help them *not* to feel like they're doing something wrong."

Patton also suggests comparing the origins of the different kinds of substances we're comfortable putting into our bodies. We know very little, she points out, about the overseas labs manufacturing generic meds, but in many cases, we can learn firsthand (and even tour!) the farms and facilities in our own states that grow and produce cannabis products. Pointing out these kinds of inconsistencies may help people reexamine their beliefs and assumptions, she says.

# GET SOMEONE ELSE TO DO IT!

Theisen often gets new patients as referrals from other older adults who've had success with cannabis. Unfortunately, she tells me, "when we get advice or feedback from family members, we don't tend to take it as seriously as we do with a friend, or coworker, or healthcare professional."

No offense, but anyone else who's had a similar condition and treated successfully with cannabis may actually turn out to be a more credible source to your loved one than you are—especially if the person you're trying to convince is one of the humans who raised you. Theisen suggests bringing up the conversation casually, like, "My friend's mom is using cannabis and having a lot of success—would you like to talk to her about it?" Sometimes, weed moms, whispered suggestions are heard louder than shouted ones.

**Q: Do older adults want to get high? Or are they only interested in medicinal uses?**

**A:** It depends very much on the individual. You'll certainly find older people who enjoy a good toke and welcome the euphoria of being stoned, but you'll also find plenty of older folks interested in getting pain relief or better sleep while skipping the high. Still others have misconceptions about what moderate elevation with cannabis *actually* feels like, and they fear losing control or hallucinating.

Theisen tells me that, though many of her patients start by saying they have *absolutely no intention* of getting high, she responds by asking, "Okay, but do you want to feel more relaxed, more patient, more communicative with your spouse, and maybe laugh a little?" "Yes, of course," they tell her. Thus begins her patient education around how to consume cannabis in the right quantities to suit individual needs. "Your experience is related to your dose," Theisen teaches, but because that fact isn't well known yet, many people are overconsuming and coming to faulty conclusions about the way cannabis makes them feel.

In Patton's experience, too, the answer to the question of whether or not older adults want the elevated experience of cannabis often comes down to the way the question's framed. "I think that many older people are afraid of 'getting high,'" she tells me, "but at the same time, we want to live a richly textured, resilient life—and we're definitely open to feeling better." With the appropriate dose, cannabis can indeed help people feel more at ease in their bodies and minds. So whether you call that getting high or simply self-care, the fact is that while few older adults would choose to get stoned out of their gourds, a good many of them enjoy the subtle enhancement that goes along with feeling better. I mean, don't we all?

**Q: Should I take my mom/dad/grandma/favorite aunt to the dispensary?**

**A:** That depends.

Is the older person in good health? Is she or he taking pharmaceuticals? And what kind of experience or relief are they seeking?

"Cannabis is both an art and a science," Theisen tells me, and—because of the special needs of this group—she prefers that older adults work with a qualified cannabis nurse or doctor instead of wandering into a dispensary without a clear sense of the territory. "That's not to say that a properly trained professional couldn't guide an older adult," she tells me, but the lack of statewide standards when it comes to retail cannabis jobs means that your local dispensary may or may not provide budtenders with sufficient training to recommend the right products and consumption methods for older people.

But there are exceptions. If your loved one is in search of a pain-relieving topical or a quality CBD product, there's little harm in showing that person the lay of the dispensary landscape and chatting up the budtenders for intel on the best products. (Just be aware that it's possible for large doses of CBD, taken internally, to affect the absorption of certain medications, so have the person consult a practitioner if they're wanting to use CBD regularly).

Or, if your loved one remembers the sixties fondly and would like to take a trip down memory lane with the help of some "grass," you can offer to share your stash—following the *start low and go slow* motto. Remember, flower potency is off the charts these days, so start with one puff of the low to moderately concentrated stuff (15 percent THC and under) for inhalation, or a 1 to 2.5 mg THC edible to gradually reacquaint your loved one with weed.

**Q: What if my mom/dad/favorite aunt isn't cool with me weed momming?**

**A:** Citing the relative safety (especially compared to alcohol and other drugs) and the beneficial properties of cannabis, Patton believes that whatever stigmas remain in the older generation are completely wrapped up in prohibitionist attitudes and the War on Drugs. There's a glaring inconsistency in the fact, she says, that "so many of us are fine with ordering a beer at a restaurant or cracking a bottle of wine at dinner, but not with consuming a plant."

If you're using cannabis responsibly (see Chapter 6 for recs on when and where it's appropriate for parents to consume) and taking care of your own business (i.e., tending to yourself, your family, and your work in the world), and your loved one *still* disapproves, I see three possibilities:

Possibility #1: The person may come around if you give them time. As I've said over and over, attitudes are shifting—sometimes rapidly—as the legal cannabis regime rolls out. Quality information is increasingly available, which in itself helps dispel myths and change minds. Plus, last time I checked, the sky hasn't fallen on any of the adult-use states. So your loved one may just need a little time to catch up.

Possibility #2: The person may not come around on cannabis, but the two of you can kindly agree to disagree on the subject and love one another anyway. If weed is simply a nonstarter, I recommend letting it go. With mutual respect in the relationship, cannabis needn't become a wedge.

Possibility #3: "We all want our parents' love and approval," Patton tells me. "You want them to be cool with you being who you are." But sometimes, unfortunately, that just isn't possible (though I suspect that in this case, as with an intimate partner, the issues in the relationship probably go deeper than your use of the plant).

Ultimately, you don't need permission from a parent or older loved one as long as you practice consideration for others and ensure that cannabis doesn't infringe on your life roles.

## Weed Moms Speak on Talking about Cannabis with the Older Adults in Their Lives

"I am always able to test my audience by talking about my uncle, who had medical cannabis in San Fran in the nineties for AIDS. I talk about the medicinal aspects and eventually say I use it for my mental health and chronic pain....Most people who know me know I've used cannabis for decades so they sort of expect it. I talk about the fact that cannabis isn't physically addictive, and I talk about the benefits it has and some we think it *might* have....I talk about cancer patients. I talk about how I probably couldn't eat without it because I have constant stomach issues....I think I just try to make it human and connected to me." —*Erica, mom of 1, Massachusetts*

"I have had the conversation with family, friends, elderly people, mothers, ex coworkers, or anyone who is either curious or in pain. I decided long ago that in order to stop the stigma, I needed to shamelessly educate the benefits by sharing my story. The people who really seem to listen with an open mind and want to learn more are those in chronic pain—they are past the point of stigma if it means relief." —*Kristin, mom of 1, stepmom of 1, Connecticut*

"My father was raised in Naples, Italy, in a very poor and somewhat violent environment. His experience and knowledge of marijuana is directly tied to the mafia and drug rings. In understanding this, I am able to find points of conversation that may resonate with his view of and understanding of the topic and hope to offer seeds of thought to spark critical thinking and possibly see another side of the story....He has had a few years of terrible health due to excess over-the-counter and prescription medication taken throughout his life. I have really used this to help educate him on the benefits of a more natural approach to health and wellness, which includes the use of marijuana regularly....This leads me to think of my grandparents, very old-school Italian with little to no education. That is a population that I have realized I will never be able to get through to. So the way I approach that specific scenario is by respecting their personal limitations (conscious and unconscious) and choosing to leave the topic out of our conversations in a respectful manner." —*Stephany, mom of 1, Florida*

"You wanna hear their opinions, what they've experienced around it. You don't want to make them feel stupid for thinking the way they do, but you don't want them to judge you, either. I have a friend whose mom was completely against cannabis, didn't want *anything* to do with it...but she was experiencing some pain, and we talked to her about it. After a while, she was willing to try a THC elixir—and it helped! She became a firm believer." —*Megan, mom of 2, Montana*

# CHAPTER 13

# CANNABIS AND SELF-CARE: YOGA, MEDITATION, AND BEYOND

Self-care can take many, many forms but, in short, it's what you do that supports your health and well-being in body, mind, heart, and spirit. Sophie Saint Thomas, author of *Finding Your Higher Self: Your Guide to Cannabis for Self-Care* (2019), tells me, "I imagine us kind of like a plant. If we're not taken care of—if we're not nourished—we start to dry up." It doesn't really matter, she says, whether you're drawn to meditation, yoga, or long baths, or if you just need to binge watch Shonda Rhimes for three hours. Anything, she says, that helps "heal up those cracks and renourish you" is self-care.

Self-care helps shift you from the stressed-out-mom-on-the-go cortisol response of fight or flight (your sympathetic nervous system) to the mama's-chilling place of rest and digest (your parasympathetic nervous system). If you enjoy exercise, that's self-care. If spending a few minutes in prayer at the start of your day sets the tone for what's ahead, that's also self-care. If going on a hike or walking barefoot through the grass feeds your heart and soul, that's definitely the kind of thing I'm talking about. Nourishing your body with good food, hydrating well, and letting go of negative self-talk are also pieces of self-care. Hell, if you're a mom of littles, even closing the bathroom door counts!

Point is, there are many ways to care for the amazing, gorgeous, worthy, and unique being that is *you*; self-care needn't cost a lot of money or take much time, but it's vital nonetheless. "With all that we're responsible for," says Chrissy Hadar, cofounder and chief branding officer for the cannabis company Oregrown, "it's so important that mothers take care of ourselves."

Hadar, who's also the mother of a toddler, says, "Last Mother's Day, I was looking at cards for my nanny and my mother. And so many of them were surrounded by—I mean, really, the *whole premise* of them—was alcohol." At the company's three dispensaries (Portland, Bend, and Cannon Beach), Hadar sees moms looking to dip a toe in the waters of cannabis for self-care because—despite the persistent "mommy juice" and "wine o'clock" memes—they're waking up to the fact that cannabis promotes well-being and alcohol *doesn't*.

But even though cannabis is inarguably healthier, I'd never propose it as a simple one-to-one substitute for alcohol; there's just so much more to the self-care equation than consuming a substance—wonderful though it is. Still, conscious cannabis use can easily become part of a self-care repertoire because at its best, it helps grow our sense of physiological well-being as well as our empathy, patience, creativity, and presence, thereby contributing to the pursuit of that elusive thing called balance.

Sophie Saint Thomas tells me that using cannabis *in itself* doesn't necessarily constitute self-care; it's more about the plant's ability to help remove a layer of the judging, task-oriented mind so you can be present enough in your body to figure out what you actually need. "The euphoria cannabis provides," she tells me, "really allows you to drop into yourself so you can *actually do* your self-care and become re-nourished and glowing." Saint Thomas also points out the varied experiences—ranging from deep sedation to that blissed-out feeling to pain relief—by which cannabis may facilitate different kinds of self-care activities.

Jenn Lauder, who I interviewed in Chapter 6, shares that she's always been the kind of person who moves quickly and intensely through life. "Slowing down has been hard for me," she says. And at the same time, it's apparent to her that establishing certain limits around busyness and the always-on-the-move mentality is key to her happiness and productivity. Over time, she's developed what she calls "the self-awareness to know that I have to counter some of these tendencies of mine if I want to be my best self."

As such, cannabis is a natural fit for Jenn's self-care. "It lends itself so naturally to those rituals that are just about slowing down," she says, citing practices like deep breathing, meditation, yoga, or even enjoying a cup of tea. And since Jenn's been a longtime conscious user, she's learned that cannabis works a bit like meditation in that "it's not just benefiting you in the time that you're doing it." Instead, she finds there's a carryover that she's bringing into other parts of life, a "touchstone for the hard moments." For instance, if she's stressed at work, she's not going to duck out of the office to hit her vape; instead, cannabis and other self-care practices have taught her about peaceful presence in order to channel that feeling she *already* knows is in her capacity.

Another reason that self-care and cannabis may go so well together has to do with your endocannabinoid system. Movements that get your heart pumping—like running, hiking, and energetic styles of yoga—boost anandamide, the "bliss molecule," which, as you might recall, helps you feel amazing. All the while, your ECS is engaging to bring balance to areas as diverse as mood, appetite, digestion, sleep rhythms, and reproductive health. And since cannabis *also* helps regulate your ECS while relieving stress and boosting mood, many people find that combining it with activities like yoga, meditation, workouts, or other mind-body practices increases their sense of well-being.

# BEYOND RESPONSIBLE USE

By now, you've surely gathered that the most important piece of using cannabis as a mom is doing so responsibly—in a way that enriches your ability to live life well and care for yourself and your family. That means finding your *minimum* effective dose for relief or mood enhancement, and knowing when, where, and how frequently using cannabis will support your physical and mental well-being.

"I love, love, love being in nature with cannabis—like going on a nice, stony hike. That's a joy," says Reya, mom of a teen in Idaho. "But I'm not doing it every day because that would take away from the enjoyment." In other words, cultivating your long-term relationship to cannabis is all about finding your way to a place of moderation and mindfulness. This truly can benefit us moms in all things.

Sara Ouimette, LMFT, tells me how she came to her practice as a therapist who helps people renegotiate their relationships to cannabis by going through her own journey from unmindful to mindful use. There were times in her past, she says, when she used cannabis to escape her feelings. And while that may have helped her in the moment, eventually, it stopped working in her favor. So Ouimette chose to pivot to a different way of working with the plant that she still considers a helping and healing tool. "I started using it intentionally, more ceremonially," she relates, "and that changed everything." Microdosing is part of that shift for her because she gets more juice from cannabis in small enough quantities not to feel stoned.

Self-care with cannabis doesn't even have to include THC at all, says Hadar, who adds that nonpsychoactive stuff like bath bombs and skincare products can help you treat yourself. Particularly in stressful times—*like while sheltering-in-place with kids*—when avenues of self-care such as massage, in-person yoga, or hanging with a good friend aren't possible, moms can pivot toward at-home rituals that help us keep our sanity.

# WEED MOM Q&A

**Q: What are some self-care practices that pair well with cannabis?**

**A:** So many! Essentially, if you can do *whatever you already love* safely while incorporating cannabis, give it a whirl. You may find that you enjoy some enhanced activities, and not others. That's, of course, just fine. There's no one-size-fits-all to the whole question of self-care and cannabis, but here are some suggestions and starting points, and even a few practices to get you started.

Before we get down to details, a quick note about setting and circumstance: I strongly recommend setting aside solo, phone-free time to explore self-care with cannabis. Depending on where you are in your parenting journey, I know that can be really difficult to pull off. Whether you stay home with littles full time, balance your days between working and momming, or are a single parent, getting alone time that's responsibility-free *and* unplugged can feel the mythical purple unicorn of modern mothering. I get it. Thing is, nothing pulls you out of contemplation and inward focus like a toddler needing help with the potty or a tween raging from the next room about the internet connection. And phones—sheesh, don't get me started.

Do yourself a gigantic favor and choose a moment for bringing self-care and cannabis together when you can truly and safely be alone *sans* the kids and devices hell-bent on pinging you out of you-time. Even if that means waiting until everyone is asleep or at grandma's. Even if it's only for ten minutes. Carving out the space and time for your well-being *is* part of the practice.

# YOGA

For many years, my job as a yoga teacher and trainer was to help people breathe better, lengthen muscles, shed stress, and calm the busy mind. I've long believed that practicing yoga asanas, or postures, is a fantastic avenue for health and fitness. But it's not primarily for the physical benefit that I practice or teach; it's for the whole suite of life improvements that come along with getting on the mat, breathing purposefully, and cultivating a peaceful and present state.

In my yoga tradition—as in so many others—combining weed with the practice felt like utter sacrilege. Yoga, I was taught, is meant to increase your sensitivity, clarity, and focus, while drugs and alcohol steal those qualities away. The deepest insights and best opportunities for growth, I learned, come from a clear and unintoxicated mind. A *real* yogi or yogini does not indulge.

And there's plenty of truth in this way. Intoxicating and mind-altering substances do change, and potentially distort, perceptions of reality; self-restraint and abstinence can indeed help us along our spiritual path. But what of consciously altering our perception for a specific purpose? What of the deep insights that can be had by perceiving anew?

What of the ecstatic whirling of the Sufi tradition? Or the shaman-led use of psychedelics like peyote or ayahuasca that can open the heart and spirit to other ways of knowing, or heal a person of grief or depression? What of Rastafarians' ceremonial use of cannabis to feel the presence of Jah, and what of the cannabis drinks and potions that appear over and over in various streams of Indian yoga?

*Precisely*, I found myself asking at a certain point, *what about them?* So, just as I had to come to my own understanding of the plant back at the beginning of my canna-journey, I also had to deepen my understanding of the ways that cannabis could add to, or detract from, my long-running love of yoga.

Having treasured what yoga affords since discovering it in college, I've come to appreciate that yoga is a constantly evolving and shape-shifting path that's beautifully alive and vibrant—if I let it be. And, as you might recall from the beginning of this guide, when I let go of my expectations and biases about bringing the two together, something magical happened.

I still adore an enhanced home yoga practice because cannabis helps me attune to the subtleties of sensation and get deep into my groove. I find that microdosing or moderate dosing before practice—whether that's on my yoga mat, outside in the grass on a cool June day, or while breathing in the ocean air—works, paradoxically, to both elevate *and* ground me. I love how it feels and what it yields; but, just as Reya doesn't enhance every time she hikes because routine and expectation diminish pleasure, I don't use cannabis every time I practice yoga, either.

I'm certainly not the only one who finds cannabis and yoga deeply simpatico. Dee Dussault, founder of Ganja Yoga and author of *Ganja Yoga: A Practical Guide to Conscious Relaxation, Soothing Pain Relief, and Enlightened Self-Discovery* (2017), tells me that, because yoga's been on the scene for several thousand years, there have been many streams and many iterations of the practice that are quite different from the yogas we know today. There's evidence that some past yogis, particularly tantra practitioners, used cannabis sacramentally to elevate consciousness. "Yoga is *always* changing," Dussault tells me, "depending on the culture, the place, the time." She adds that throughout its long history, things have gone out of favor in yoga and then come back in.

The biggest benefit to combining yoga and cannabis, says Dussault, is that it helps people relax both mind and body. Mental benefits, she tells me, include decreasing anxiety and growing one's awareness of the moment, aka mindfulness or presence. And because it helps soothe tension while easing pain and inflammation, cannabis makes it more possible for people to practice yoga when they might otherwise just skip it. "If you're tight, if you're in pain—it's hard to even think about getting down on the floor," says Dussault. But with a little bit of cannabis, the body can feel looser and a little more amenable to stretch, movement, and mindful breathing. Indeed, says Dussault, who's taught Ganja Yoga since 2009 and trained hundreds of other yoga teachers in the style, "cannabis can make people *want* to do yoga."

Using the 15-Minute Enhanced Yoga Practice below as a springboard, feel free to explore the ways *your* body—with its unique genetics and biography—wants to move and breathe itself into greater aliveness. It's deeply ingrained in many of us who were socialized female to look outside ourselves for validation that our efforts are worthwhile and that we're doing it right. But try, with gentleheartedness for that part of you that still wonders whether your yoga practice, career, parenting style, relationship, or entire life looks the way it's supposed to, and *just trust yourself*. Your body is the temple here, not an ashram in India or a mountaintop yoga retreat center. Your inner Knowing is the guide.

# 15-MINUTE ENHANCED YOGA PRACTICE
## Elevating and Centering

◊ Decide how you would like to consume cannabis for this elevated yoga experience. Aim for a microdose, or a moderate one, so you can stay fully present.

◊ Take a deep breath. Set a simple intention for this period of practice, like to *be fully present to my mind and body*, or to *be kind to myself.*

◊ When you're feeling the effects of the cannabis, take a tall, cross-legged seat on your yoga mat. Use a blanket or cushion under your sitting bones if it helps you hold the seated posture with more ease. Place your palms on your knees—facedown for grounding, faceup for drawing in energy and inspiration.

◊ Close your eyes. Relax whatever muscles you don't need for sitting tall, like your jaw, throat, belly, and the muscles deep in your pelvis.

◊ Remind yourself of your intention, then begin long, slow deep breaths that allow your belly to expand as you inhale and soften as you exhale.

◊ If you know an alternate nostril breathing technique (Anuloma Viloma or Nadhi Shodhana), practice it for three to five rounds; otherwise, continue several rounds of belly breathing.

## Seated Spinal Movements

### To release tension in your neck, chest, and shoulders:

◊ Warm-Ups: Gently draw your chin toward your chest, pause, then lift your chin and gaze upward toward the sky. Repeat three times.

◊ More Warm-Ups: Roll your head from your left shoulder, down to your chest, and over to your right shoulder, forming a half-circle movement. Notice any tension or other sensations in your neck and trapezius muscles (where your neck and shoulders meet). Repeat twice more.

◊ Shoulder Opener: Clasp your fingers behind your back (or use a strap), bend your elbows, broaden your chest and collarbones and lift your heart center. Keeping your hands clasped or holding the strap, straighten your arms behind you without tipping your upper body forward. Press down and away through your knuckles while simultaneously lifting and expanding across your chest. Take two full breaths.

◊ Change the cross of your legs so that the other leg is in front or on top.

### To lengthen your side body:

◊ Seated Side Bend: Place your right palm on the floor near your right hip and slide it 1 to 2 feet away from your body. Reach your left hand up toward the sky on an inhalation, then reach that same hand and arm over toward the right while arcing your torso into a right-side bend. Keep your sitting bones well-grounded. Take two full breaths and change sides.

### To awaken your lower body:

◊ Warm-Ups: Extend your legs on the floor in front of you. Place your hands on the floor behind you to help keep your posture tall and your spine long. Alternately point and flex your toes and feel the awakening in your ankles, toes, and feet. Next, slowly circle both ankles in both directions. Wiggle every toe and feel your feet awaken.

◊ Cross-Legs Forward Bend, or Sukhasana, variation: Recross your legs and place your hands on the floor in front of your shins. Take a deep breath in, and as you exhale, slide your hands further away from you, and move into a cross-legged seated forward bend. You should feel a stretch around your hip/buttock area. Stay for three full breaths, then switch the cross of your legs once more, and repeat.

### To awaken your spine:

◊ Seated Twist: From your cross-legged seat, inhale and reach both arms up alongside your ears. Exhale and place your left hand on your right knee and your right hand on the floor behind you. Your spine will already be in a gentle twist, but you can increase the twist by actively turning your navel toward the right while keeping your lower body stable. Look over your right shoulder. Lengthen your spine on your inhalation, deepen your twist as you exhale. Hold for two to four breaths, then switch sides.

◊ Cat and Cow: Come to all-fours, aka table pose. As you inhale, bring your spine into an arched position where your tailbone and chin lift toward the sky while your belly moves closer to the floor. As you exhale, draw your navel in toward your spine, round your entire back, and tuck your chin and tailbone. Repeat five to ten times.

### To stretch and strengthen your legs:

◊ Standing Forward Bend, or Uttanasana: Stand at the front of your mat. As you inhale, sweep your arms out to the sides and overhead. Exhale and fold your torso forward over your legs as your arms reach outward to the sides in a t-shape and then down toward the earth. Stay two to five breaths in the forward bend while touching your fingertips to the floor (bend your knees if needed) and relaxing your neck. As you hang here and breathe, visualize the back of your legs (hamstrings) lengthening and the blood flow to your brain increasing. When you're ready, bend your knees and slowly roll yourself back up to standing.

◊ Goddess Pose, or Deviasana: Stand in the middle of your mat, facing the long side. Step your feet wide apart with your toes facing the corners of your mat. Bend both your knees as deeply as you can while sustaining an upright posture with your torso. Make sure that your kneecaps are pointing the same direction as your toes. Sweep both arms straight out to each side, parallel with your shoulders, then bend both elbows and spread your fingers wide. Hold for three to five deep breaths. This goddess is powerful and fierce, and she'll raise your heart rate, too!

◊ Downward Dog, or Adho Mukha Svanasana: Come to plank pose with your wrists directly under the heads of your shoulders and your fingers spread wide. Take a deep breath in, and on an exhalation lift your hips and buttocks toward the ceiling and stretch your heels down toward the floor behind you. Your body should form an inverted v-shape. Relax your head and neck and press your belly toward your thighs while your thighs press back toward the wall behind you. Stay for three to five breaths, or less if you're light-headed.

◊ Child's Pose, or Garbhasana: From Downward Dog, bend your knees and bring them to the mat. Press your buttocks toward your heels and rest your forehead on the floor or on your hands. Stay for three long, slow breaths.

◊ Check in with your body to see if continuing to move and explore will support your well-being, and if your body says, "Yes, please!," just follow along. Big or small, wild or precise, energetic or deeply chill—don't get hung up needing to "look like yoga" or fit the mold in any way. Savor the freedom that comes without expectation. Where exploration and self-compassion meet, you'll find the nectar of this practice.

◊ When you feel complete or simply need to move on with your day, rest on your back in Savasana, or Corpse pose, for at least five minutes.

# MEDITATION AND MINDFULNESS

"If you sit down and try to meditate, at first you can be very scattered, and the mind is jumping here and there. We call that the 'monkey mind,' or sometimes the 'antelope mind,' that's always going from one topic to the next," Swami Chaitanya tells me. "But with cannabis, you get more focus."

Swami, who's been meditating and using cannabis since the sixties, is a believer in the spiritual qualities of the plant and its divine origin as the goddess, Ganja Ma. Swami and his partner Nikki Lastreto, who together grow Swami Select cannabis in California's Emerald Triangle, honor Ganja Ma in all phases of the planting, cultivating, and harvesting process.

Nikki tells me that cannabis can give you a taste of the fruits of meditation, and thereby helps you access them a little more easily. "Cannabis is a teacher," she says, "because it puts you into that state of mind of knowing where you're going—so you can say, 'I've been there before, I know what that feels like.'" Whether you partake in cannabis before meditation or not, you can draw on past experiences with the herb to provide clues and signposts along the way. "It's like opening that door so you can go there again—," says Nikki, "a gateway for higher consciousness."

Just as we talked about in Chapter 10, cannabis can help you transition from one "operating system" to another—like from "work brain" to "mom brain," or "mom brain" to "sexy brain." Turns out, Swami tells me, that cannabis is *also* a wonderful tool for spiritual transitions, helping us shift away from our habitual mental patterns into a more imaginative and inspirational realm. But here, as in many things, the way you do it matters. Choosing cannabis to aid in meditation is a sacred act, according to Swami, "if your mental state, and the state of your intention are aligned."

# ELEVATED TRATAK, OR OPEN-EYE MEDITATION PRACTICE

◊ Choose a moment when you'll have at least five minutes of quiet, kid-free time. If you can meditate longer, great—but even five minutes will give you benefits.

◊ Find an object of beauty or meaning to you, such as a fresh flower, a candle, an OM symbol, or iconography from your own spiritual tradition; keep it nearby.

◊ Consciously choose your dose and method, then consume your cannabis. For meditation and self-inquiry, less is more.

◊ Take a comfortable seat on the floor, on a meditation cushion, or in a chair.

◊ Set a timer and state an intention or a simple blessing, such as, "May I be awake in my mind and peaceful in my heart."

◊ Take three long, slow breaths, and scan your body for any sensations—including discomfort. Consciously relax what you're able to.

◊ Set your object (flower, lit candle, etc.) a few feet in front of you at eye level, and focus your attention there. You needn't fix the object with a laser-like stare. Instead, try to relax your eyes and keep a soft gaze.

◊ When the mind wanders, gently bring it back using your visual sense as a way to focus your attention. Use the relaxation and sense of well-being cannabis helps create to enhance your meditation.

◊ Keep breathing and gazing. After a few minutes, you might close your eyes and see if you can continue holding the image in your mind's eye.

◊ When your timer goes off, take a moment to consciously deepen your breathing again, acknowledge your own effort, and rise from your meditation seat.

Meditation is, in essence, a simple practice—but it's also far from easy. Remember that wandering, busy minds are human minds. The trick is to notice the wandering and compassionately, consistently, draw your attention back to your object of focus. Don't worry if you find yourself doing that *over and over and over* again. "The only bad meditation," says Swami, "is the one you don't do."

If it's possible to carve out the space, meditating every day—even if only for a few minutes—will yield the richest benefit; consistency is more important than duration. Over time, many meditators find that they're drawn to sitting in stillness a bit longer, say fifteen to thirty minutes, and that as a result their everyday mind feels calmer, clearer, and less reactive than before.

Following years of meditation and sacramental cannabis use, Swami describes his spiritual experience as a paradox of all *and* nothing, "an empty fullness." "That's the thing with meditation," he says. "You can only talk about it up to a certain level of intensity and then the words just don't really express it much anymore." In other words, you have to experience it for yourself.

# CONSCIOUS EATING

The pleasure of tasting and eating is one of the most intrinsic we have, yet we often neglect it in favor of what's quick, convenient, or on our lists of *shoulds* and *supposed tos*. Years ago, I led conscious eating exercises with the undergrads I taught at American University. Some of them later told me that it was the most memorable part of the course because it asked them to reexamine their habits of treating food as a means to an end; it let them slow down and notice the pleasure inherent in nourishment.

To start, make a list of the healthy finger foods you love. For me, that's apples, berries, bananas, nectarines, peaches, apricots, citrus, seeds, nut butters, celery, carrots, cucumbers, hummus, olives, honey, and dark chocolate. Then, make a list of unhealthy foods you love, such as cheesecake, fudge, French fries, French bread, French cheese, Häagen-Dazs, and Pirate's Booty.

Next, choose three items from the "healthy list" alongside one from the "unhealthy list," and make sure you pick them up the next time you hit the grocery store or press "submit" on Instacart. (Obvious, but worth saying because I know a lot of moms who only buy favorite snacks for children or husbands or wives or *anybody else in their life who isn't them*.)

When you're ready to give conscious eating a try, make yourself a snack plate that entices the senses—nothing fancy, just a thoughtful arrangement of colors and flavors. (If you've ever painstakingly arranged chicken nuggets on a toddler's plate in hopes that he or she will find it fun or delightful, you can think of this as extending the same kind of care—just to yourself this time.)

Choose your dose and intake method, then consume your cannabis.

Once you're feeling pleasantly elevated, sit down at a table with your snack plate and tune into your senses. What does the food look like? Notice its colors, shape, and texture. Next, attune to your sense of smell. Do you notice sweet or earthy smells? Fruity or astringent ones? Are the scents sharp or mellow? Notice what, if anything, happens in your mouth as you take in the visual and olfactory qualities of the food; if your mouth is watering, for instance, it shows that your body's gearing up to taste, swallow, and digest.

Pick up an item from your plate and tune in to your sense of touch. Notice how it feels between your fingers. Is it smooth or bumpy? Dry or moist? What else do you notice?

Repeat the process with each item, if possible, while staying present to the visceral experience of being in such close proximity to food while not (yet) eating it. Notice if you're feeling anxious, or hurried, or distracted, or even weirded out. Any and all of those reactions are completely normal, but know that if you let it, cannabis can help you put aside your hang-ups (no shame, we all have them!) and immerse in the experience. Time passes differently when you're high, and the smallest of details can become absorbing. Plus, your senses of smell, sight, touch, and taste are wonderfully amplified.

Express your thanks for the food in whatever way feels natural, and as you begin to taste what you've prepared, keep a sense of curiosity and moment-to-moment attentiveness. Even though you've eaten the same foods before—perhaps hundreds of times—you've never before tasted *this* apple, *this* roasted almond, *this* wedge of Brie. Take small bites, chew slowly, and frequently pause to notice the sensations in your mouth, throat, belly, and entire being. I don't want to exaggerate, friends, but for me, the pleasure of consciously eating good food while high is a bona fide spiritual experience. I wish that for you, too.

That's the practice. It doesn't matter whether you eat a few bites or everything on your plate and more. If you're taking your time, deeply engaging with your sense of taste, and tuning in to your body's signals of hunger and satiety, then conscious eating can be a joyous and sensual delight.

# ENHANCING CREATIVITY

If you've ever been so engrossed in work or play that time slips by unnoticed while you're completely grooving in your zone, that's a flow state. Coined by the positive psychologist Mihaly Csikszentmihalyi, "flow" refers to a suite of neurochemical changes and brain activity that helps creatives create and athletes perform at their peak; it's also something that can arise spontaneously or be deliberately cultivated. Flow is a spectrum encompassing those easier-to-access states of "microflow" and dramatic, potentially life-changing moments of "macroflow."

In flow, we learn faster and enjoy ourselves more. We're immersed in what's sometimes called the "deep now," a place where past and future are secondary to *being* and *creating*—without expectation or the need to force specific outcomes. People who experience regular flow report better satisfaction with their lives as a whole. Flow, like weed, is legit awesome.

Cannabis use, in some ways, mimics flow. In both the cannabis user and the person in flow, the prefrontal cortex (tasked with keeping track of time and exercising judgment) quiets down. Cannabis and flow states also have alpha brain waves (most associated with relaxation and creativity) in common, as well as the release of the feel-good neurotransmitter dopamine and an activation of part of the brain called the striatum (related to motivation and the perception of reward). Recognizing the way cannabis helps stoke the imagination, creatives the world over—from musicians, visual artists, and comedians to actors, poets, and writers—have long used cannabis in their art.

Want to play around with accessing flow for creativity? First, make sure you've got some kid-and-responsibility-free time on your hands, choose your medium, then set up your paints, calligraphy pens, drum set, or what have you. Next, get your heart rate up for about twenty-five minutes, follow that with a cup (or two) of tea or coffee, and top it off with a low-to-medium inhaled dose of a strain of cannabis that has uplifting effects for you. The combination of aerobic exercise, caffeine, and THC—according to author and flow researcher Steven Kotler—is the quickest way to mimic the suite of neurochemical changes and brain activity that constitute flow. Fwiw, this combo is also called the "hippie speedball"; the name is *meh*, but the actual practice of it is nothing short of transporting. I highly (pun!) recommend.

# ENHANCING FITNESS

I'd like to start by acknowledging the tyrannies of "skinny" and "sculpted," and to emphatically state for the record that I choose not to contribute to them. It's my belief that moms—well, people, actually—of *all* sizes shouldn't be pressured to fit a culturally constructed mold or to be anything other than themselves in order to feel okay in their skin and be accepted out in the world. It's none of my business, or anyone else's, to pass judgment on your body, your fitness, or your goals.

And yet, I also happen to believe that fitness is an important piece of self-care—just maybe not in the ways we've been trained to think. "Right now, in our culture, there's a lot of attention to things like Cross-Fit or workouts done by celebrities playing superheroes," says personal trainer, yoga teacher, and parent, Karen O'Lone. But in her work with clients and students, O'Lone prefers the notion that fitness isn't about what it looks like on the outside—it's actually about longevity.

So, she tells me, the impressiveness of your workouts or your visible "results" pale in comparison to the real goals: being comfortable in your body throughout your life and being able to do the things you *want* to do as well as the things you *need* to do. Naturally, what we want and need to do with our bodies varies at different moments in life. For instance, says O'Lone, when you're a kid you probably want to run around; when you're an adult you want to keep up with your kids and have the energy for work and play; and when you're a grandparent, your needs may center on enjoying life without too many aches and pains. And so, because we all have unique genetics and biographies, exercise will look very different from person to person. "Sometimes the idea of fitness can get weighed down," O'Lone shares, "when really it's very simple: if you have a body, then you can have fitness."

Similarly, Sophie Saint Thomas emphasizes that self-care is something you do for yourself alone. "If you're working out," she says, "it's not because you're trying to look hot for someone else—you're doing it because it *feels* good."

Approaching fitness from that perspective, I believe that conscientious, low-dose cannabis use can lend a helping hand. Contrary to the lazy stoner stereotype, research shows that cannabis users exercise more often, which is a good thing for so many moms whose jobs and carpool schedules have us sitting the majority of our waking lives. Researchers at the University of Colorado Boulder found that four out of five survey respondents who use cannabis report doing so right before they exercise, and 70 percent of them said that cannabis makes exercise more enjoyable.[136] And that, the authors write, might have something to do with our old friend, the ECS. Anandamide circulates in the body with exercise,[137] and THC adds *more* feel-good chemicals to the mix; quite simply, it *feels great* to elevate a bit and move your body.

Other research shows that cannabis users have a lower BMI,[138] less insulin resistance, and more stable blood sugar than nonusers.[139] Again, I present this information not to advocate for low BMIs or any particular outward markers of fitness, but to add to the conversation. Other research, as previously mentioned, indicates that CBD has anti-inflammatory properties.[140] As such, it may also help your muscles recover better from exercise—like ibuprofen, but healthier.

So what kinds of fitness activities pair well with cannabis? Like I said at the beginning of the chapter, *anything* that you enjoy and can safely do while microdosing cannabis is a winner. That includes walking, easy hiking, dancing around your living room, light weight training, and of course, home yoga. Depending on a bunch of factors, it *could possibly* also include running or following along with a (low-risk) fitness class.

A good many surfers, skiers, snowboarders, rock climbers, mountain bikers, and other outdoor enthusiasts love weed—and cannabis culture thrives among them. But, in the interest of safety, I caution that Mother Nature is a beautiful, powerful force, and I'd recommend *against* combining cannabis with technical sports or activities that rely on quick instincts. Same goes for intense workouts like Cross-Fit, HIIT, or anything involving heavy weights.

What about after the workout? That's another story. Whatever activities you choose—and whether or not you incorporate cannabis—I encourage you to consider O'Lone's suggestion to "make fitness something that helps you live better, move better, and give better." Focusing on your well-being—not the outward pieces of it—*is* fitness for self-care.

# FOR SELF-AWARENESS AND INSIGHTS

Within the psychedelics community, "inner journeying" involves intentionally using psilocybin (magic mushrooms), LSD, or other substances for personal and spiritual growth. Because psychedelics can profoundly alter the ordinary mind state and shift perspective, some people find them extremely helpful for gaining new awareness and—ultimately—freedom. "Psychedelics aren't just about crazy colors," Michelle Janikian, author of *Your Psilocybin Mushroom Companion*, tells me. "They're about taking a closer look at your own mind—examining yourself, your behaviors, your reactions."

As I've mentioned before, in higher doses, cannabis can also be considered a kind of psychedelic in that it shifts the way we see the world and ourselves and facilitates the kind of introspection that real personal growth is based on; some cannabis journeyers find that the plant contributes to their process of healing from trauma or resolving unhealthy mental patterns.

Sara Ouimette, LMFT, who works with psychedelics integration, cautions that, while some people choose a higher-than-usual THC dose for journeying, it's important to understand your body's response to cannabis first; in other words, find the dose that facilitates the inner journey but doesn't overwhelm it.

And, of course, set and setting are important factors. Janikian describes the ideal set and setting as "being in a calm, chill, peaceful, supportive environment, and also having an open frame of mind" for exploring your inner landscape. A curated playlist—like soothing tunes or shamanic drumming—may also help facilitate the process.

Ouimette adds that thinking about your intentions for the journey can help you clarify the work to be done. She suggests contemplating questions like, "What are you hoping you might have some insight about? What are you wanting to cultivate in your life? And, do you have a particular question you're looking to answer in this journey?"

For everyday insights or help with decision-making, you may choose to take the cannabis-assisted journey alone, or with a safe friend. But for a deep dive—especially the kind that may lay bare unresolved trauma—Ouimette recommends finding a trusted guide or therapist to facilitate the process.

## Weed Moms Speak on Cannabis and Self-Care

"When using cannabis, I love to go on long walks with loved ones. I feel as though I can sink into the moment and really enjoy the fresh air, conversation, and laughter about anything and everything."
—*Nicole, mom of 2, California*

"Since becoming a mother, my ALL-time favorite leisure and "me" activity is sitting on my balcony alone and enjoying a joint. Then I draw a super-hot bath and choose an essential oil to add. I light a few candles and submerge myself totally under water, with only my nose out." —*Stephany, mom of 1, Florida*

"I've heard it spoken like this—that cannabis floods the time part of your brain, and you get this deep feeling of being in the now. It really does that for you. It slaps you right into the now. You have no interest in the past, no interest in the future. You're just kind of here. It allows you to focus. So it's really great for journaling, or drawing, or listening to music. It allows you to absorb yourself into what you're doing." —*Shannon Chiarenza, the "Weed Mama"*

"I've used cannabis recreationally since I was a teenager. But as more education surrounding the benefits of cannabis has surfaced, I've realized that being high isn't the greatest benefit. It's about being calmer and more relaxed, with heightened focus. Now that I'm older, I prefer cannabis in the morning before a hike or outdoor activity." —*Anonymous mom*

If you're working solo, the process is simple. Ensure that your set and setting will support you looking safely inward, set an intention, and consciously consume your cannabis. You may want to incorporate incense, candles, uplifting music, prayer, or anything else that helps you establish your space as a safe and nurturing one in which to look inward.

Then, keeping your intention or question as a touchstone, you can sit outside in an inspiring spot, spend time in nature, do yoga or conscious breathing, dance, or do whatever supportive practice calls to you at the moment. Let your mind free-float for a bit; there's nothing here to force or make happen. Periodically, check in with your body and breath to help anchor you in the present moment, and see what comes. As thoughts, feelings, or realizations about your intention or question arise, jot them down with pen and paper. Sometimes, it's *more* questions instead of answers that come—and that's okay, too. Try to let go of the need for a specific outcome, or a concrete answer, and trust the process instead.

"We are so accustomed to *not* feeling our feelings," Ouimette tells me, that they may bubble up when the space is opened for them. Even—okay, *especially*—those so-called negative feelings can be teachers; we needn't see uncomfortable emotions as bad necessarily, or something to avoid at all costs. "If anxiety or other unpleasant feelings come up," she tells me, "it can be a good time to contemplate the role of that emotion in your life—or whether there may be something you're not dealing with."

In Jungian psychology, the "shadow" is an aspect of the self that holds all our rejected and hidden-away parts, the pieces of our personality that shame us or scare us and that we therefore (consciously or unconsciously) disown. Cannabis, when used to journey inward, can also bring up shadow material, Janikian tells me. And when it does, we may choose—under the right circumstances—to stay with the feelings instead of running away from them, and to take note that there may be work to continue with a therapist or on our own after the journey.

Cannabis and Self-Care: Yoga, Meditation, and Beyond

*** 

I'll close this chapter with a long, not exhaustive, list of other self-care activities you may find wonderfully enhanced with moderate *and* mindful cannabis use: taking a bath, getting a massage, giving yourself a massage, dancing in your living room, walking and talking with a close friend, running, hiking, sketching, painting, creative writing, working with clay, making a collage, taking nature photos, practicing an instrument, listening to music, writing letters to friends and loved ones, snuggling with a pet, watching the sunrise or sunset, acknowledging difficult feelings, making a gratitude journal, consulting the Tarot, watching funny videos, making and enjoying DIY skincare, enjoying a cup of tea, standing in the rain, mirror-gazing, masturbating, creating a vision board, taking a nap, walking on the beach, finding shapes in the clouds, howling at the moon, gardening, and stargazing.

In short, self-care encompasses whatever you can think of that gives you joy, helps you make meaning, or simply provides a break from your routine and responsibilities. If you can do it safely, mindfully, and with self-compassion while incorporating cannabis, that's what I'm talking about.

So whether your self-care looks like a weekend retreat, an hour of yoga and meditation, or just a few minutes of alone time on your balcony, I encourage you to let cannabis show you the way to care for yourself in body, mind, heart, and spirit. And, on that note, I'll leave you with a thought from Michelle Obama, whom I admire greatly (and who has literally no clue that her words will appear in a book about weed): "To be a good parent, you need to take care of yourself so that you can have the physical and emotional energy to take care of your family."[141]

Yep. What she said.

# CHAPTER 14

# THE FUTURE OF CANNABIS

Public health researcher and cannabis expert Amanda Reiman, PhD, who lives and works in California, tells me that the three biggest positives of cannabis legalization concern criminal justice reform, normalization, and protections for people who work in cannabis.

Now that weed is legal in California, Reiman observes that the conversations around health, wellness, and the varied experiences this plant affords have become more nuanced, though she points out that normalization is a process, not an overnight accomplishment. Plus, industry jobs are now open to people—including moms—for whom illegality was too big a risk. The ability to have an aboveboard career in cannabis with regular pay and health insurance provides needed stability for workers and their families.

"We're not seeing the public safety indicators that cannabis legalization is having a negative impact on society," says Reiman. And the public seems to agree: polling data of over 32,000 respondents released by YouGov in May 2020 found that at least two-thirds of folks living in the adult-use states of California, Colorado, Illinois, Michigan, Nevada, and Washington say that the liberalization of cannabis policy has been successful.[142] In the spring of 2020, amidst nationwide retail shutdowns, cannabis businesses—even recreational ones—were considered "essential services" in a majority of states with established legal programs. And in numerous states that haven't yet fully jumped on the canna-bandwagon, some form of legalization—or decriminalization at the minimum—is on the table for voters or legislators.

Yep, there's no doubt about it: the tide of cannabis reform is moving steadily toward access and acceptance. But what, you may be wondering, will the future of cannabis look and feel like?

The immediate changes we're seeing in the cannabis space since COVID-19 came on the scene include:

◊ Increased popularity of edibles and tinctures

◊ Decreased flower and pre-roll sales

◊ Increased availability of delivery services and curbside pickup

◊ A pause on the practice of smelling and otherwise interacting with flower inside dispensaries

But well beyond pandemic-related changes to the industry, I'll pop on my fortune-telling hat here to submit my case about the future of cannabis in the US.

## Women in Weed Speak on the Future of Cannabis

"Pretty soon I think we're going to see cannabis playing a major role in treating cancer and cancer symptoms. I would love for providers to integrate cannabis into their healthcare plans, and to have the continuity of care around it. And, for parents, I'd like to see better legal protections, and, of course, federal legalization." —*Marissa Fratoni, RN, cannabis nurse and founder of* Holistic Nurse Mama, *mother of 2, Massachusetts*

"I think cannabis will become more and more mainstream and more and more a part of people's lives that doesn't need as much explanation. I'm hoping that it becomes a product that's embraced for its versatility and that people see it an option for recreation, or general wellness, or specific health issues." —*Jenn Lauder, founder of* Splimm, *mother of 1, Oregon*

"There are still people serving prison sentences for a plant that others are profiting off of, and that hypocrisy is *not* tolerable. I want to see equal representation and equal pay in a diverse industry that is led by people negatively impacted by the racist War on Drugs. So that people of color, minorities, LGBTQ leaders, and women have an equal say—if not more of a say—in the industry than Wall Street and the corporate cannabis hedge fund capitalists.

"Once it's really made safe, legal, and accessible to people— wherever they are—they'll understand that the drug war was truly propaganda invented by a government to control people....The stigma will so quickly fall away once they're able to interact with the plant." —*Mary Jane Gibson, former* High Times *culture editor, writer, actress, and host of* Weed + Grub *podcast*

# THE FUTURE OF CANNABIS IS...

## NORMALIZED

COVID-19–related quarantines radically shifted most Americans' working lives and family situations, at least for a time. Jenn Lauder shares how the realities of working from home, closely sharing space, dealing with new emotional and financial stressors, and the need to participate much more closely in educating children has all meant that increasing numbers of parents are leaning on cannabis for the purposes of health and self-care. "Its potential as a physical healer and something that can help us navigate a hard time is readily apparent right now," she shares. "Many of us are relying more on it now than in typical times as one way to make sure we're taking care of ourselves—and I'd be lying if I didn't say that cannabis is certainly something that's helping me stay sane in this time."

From a consumer perspective, Jenn acknowledges the deep irony in the fact that cannabis was very recently illegal everywhere in the US, and now, she says, "it's considered so essential that you can break quarantine to go to the dispensary." More than any other indicator, perhaps, this shows how deeply integrated cannabis is becoming in Americans' lives.

Amber Morelli of Pure Vape shares the industry perspective that the increasing availability of delivery, the cashless transactions potentially on the horizon, *and* the fact that many working Americans experienced a reprieve from the worry of workplace drug-testing meant that March through May of 2020 "have probably removed five or ten years of stigma."

We're at a moment, says Morelli, when people are reflecting on what is and isn't working in their lives and making healthier choices—like experimenting with the stress and anxiety-relieving benefits of cannabis—that perhaps they didn't have time or energy to investigate before. And those wellness-oriented shifts, she says, go hand in hand with cannabis for self-care. "I'm hearing from people now about their mental health, like 'oh, I'm doing yoga, I'm meditating, I'm journaling,'" she shares. "People are doing these things they *never* had time to do before, now that we've all been forced to slow down."

## GREENER

The DIY ethos is front and center these days. From backyard "victory gardens" to sourdough starters to the proliferation of at-home learning resources, the mediascape is newly rich with how to grow it, make it, and do it yourself. And, naturally, that extends to cannabis. Former *High Times* culture editor Mary Jane Gibson says many people are diving deeper into cultivation because being able to grow your own, to be self-reliant, and to take that step of interacting with the plant in the way of a gardener and a grower feels like an empowering aspect of the current zeitgeist.

And that's a beautiful thing because small-scale, local, and handmade stuff is intrinsically better for the health of the planet than highly packaged and manufactured products that come from far away. When choosing to DIY, or to buy and barter with our neighbors who DIY, we can step back from participation in industries that exploit people and the environment for economic gain. I'll add here that while it's true that cannabis is *already* more locally focused than most industries because of federal restrictions on interstate cannabis commerce, much of the packaging and hardware (like vape pens and cartridges) comes from overseas.

Hemp, too, is increasingly seen as part of the solution to the climate crisis. It grows well in many climates and—beyond its traditional uses for rope and textiles—can be manufactured into bio-plastics and bio-fuels. Indeed, according to hemp entrepreneur Morris Beegle, who's also the president of a hemp marketing firm called We Are for Better Alternatives, the nonpsychoactive variety of cannabis is "one of nature's best solutions for addressing climate change and making our world a cleaner and healthier place to live." Hemp is a regenerative crop that enriches soil while removing $CO_2$ from the atmosphere. As one of many solutions needed, Beegle says hemp addresses such problems as fossil fuel dependence, overuse of petroleum-based plastics, and deforestation.

## MORE JUST AND EQUITABLE

Many states with legal cannabis, including the large and populous state of California, wrote guidelines into the legal framework for expunging criminal records among those who'd previously been charged or imprisoned for cannabis offenses—people, who, as you can probably guess, are disproportionately Black and brown. The programs are slow and imperfect, but they're a start.

The conversation around equity is an incredibly important one in the cannabis space right now; we simply cannot allow the wealth-building opportunities of the industry to be monopolized by those with privilege and capital. Social equity programs reserve a certain percentage of retail and grow licenses for people from marginalized communities who've been—and still are—targeted in large numbers by the racist implementation of the War on Drugs. The city of Los Angeles, for instance, has one such equity program and a vibrant activist community working hard in the fight for fair implementation. Still, the program—along with similar ones in other cities and states—is flawed, and lots more needs to be done. In states that are just coming on board with legalization, or *will soon*, there's an opportunity to learn about what works and what doesn't in terms of social equity and racial justice in cannabis—and to do better.

## INCREASINGLY LEGAL

"I don't think we're going to see a 'one day all of a sudden cannabis is totally legal' kind of situation," Reiman, who's also been a policy manager at the Drug Policy Alliance, a lecturer at UC Berkeley, and a VP of community relations for cannabis brand Flow Kana, tells me. "I think we're going to see a slow acceptance by the federal government that states are making these decisions, and that the federal government should not get in the way." She predicts that bans on banking and interstate commerce will be gradually loosened, and that federal decriminalization, or a "hands-off" federal memo are all more realistic shorter-term possibilities.

"What helped end alcohol prohibition," says Reiman, "aside from the Great Depression, is the fact that so many states changed their laws around alcohol that it really wasn't tenable anymore for the federal government to maintain a prohibition position." And she thinks that we're approaching that territory on the medical side, if not yet on the recreational one. In the coming months and years, it's likely that an increasing number of states will look to cannabis legalization as a way to foster economic recovery from COVID, says Reiman. "So, if in a year we have twenty states with adult use, it's going to be harder and harder for the federal government not to make some kind of movement."

# CENTERED ON CONSCIOUS CONSUMERISM

When federal legalization—or significant movement toward it—*does* happen, the cannabis space will open up to multinational corporations with deep pockets. Believe me, even though mega-corps and hedge fund investors are *already* in the industry (particularly since Canada legalized at the end of 2018), federal prohibition has impeded their full-on involvement; many OG cannabis folks believe that's a good thing because small and mid-sized businesses have a chance to establish themselves without as much competition from mega-corps.

But even lacking federal legalization, norms that will affect the industry and its consumers for years to come are being shaped *at this very moment.* "We're in a marketplace giving us more choice than ever before," says Reiman, "and we need to do something positive with that." If you, like me, want to see sustainable, women-owned, and people-of-color-owned businesses do well in the cannabis space, now's the time to step up and support them. There are, in my view, few industries today where you can *be the change* as dramatically as you can in cannabis. Support craft cannabis grown on small farms by people who care about the Earth; support women-owned and people-of-color-owned retail ops and brands; and raise your voice for representation in cannabusiness as well as fair criminal justice reform. Again, five groups working on these issues are Equity First Alliance, Success Centers, Root and Rebound, the Last Prisoner Project, and National Bail Out. Remember that you, as a consumer and a person with a voice, can make a difference.

Mary Jane Gibson tells me minority-owned cannabusinesses have suffered disproportionately during the pandemic because many don't have the resources to weather the financial difficulty of the moment and—because of cannabis's federal status—aren't eligible for pandemic relief funds. "It's more important than ever," says Gibson, "to spend your dollars wisely—to seek out the minority-owned businesses, the women-led businesses, and to research the companies you're buying from."

## INCREASINGLY FEMALE

The opportunity for women to feel comfortable using cannabis openly "could really only come with legalization," Reiman tells me. "Legalization opened up this opportunity for women—and mothers especially—to look at cannabis as a viable alternative to sleep meds, anxiety meds, alcohol, and other substances that may *not* have been serving them but were available to them because they were legal."

According to Amy Froebel-Fisher, VP of finance and accounting at dispensary chain Temescal Wellness, market analyses show that female cannabis consumption is on the rise and female-focused products are quickly gaining market share. The proliferation of microdosing options and more discreet ways to consume means that, finally, larger numbers of women—including moms!—feel comfortable using the plant in ways that support their health and well-being.

# WHAT ISN'T CHANGING

By and large, weed people—and by that, I mean all who love and respect the plant—are good people, and the ethos of weed culture has long centered itself on sharing, compassion, community, self-reliance, and sustainability. Reya tells me that when she was undergoing chemotherapy for cancer, a grower friend would deliver huge mason jars stuffed with the most amazing bud on her doorstep, free of charge, to help her through that difficult moment. "He was like an angel," Reya tells me, and stories of this kind of generosity are as common in the weed world as blunts, joints, and bongs.

And though you needn't necessarily become a fan of weed culture to enjoy cannabis, its ideals, I believe, can help change the world for the better; in the words of Kathy Bates's character from the Netflix show, *Disjointed*, cannabis is "a miraculous plant that has the power to heal the sick, calm the afflicted, and usher in a golden age of people not being such dicks all the time." Right about now, that sounds pretty good.

✻ ✻ ✻

Over and over, as I interviewed doctors, scientists, policymakers, growers, retailers, and cannabis-loving moms, I heard the same thing: we've only just scratched the surface of what this plant can do. So here's my call to all the moms out there searching for avenues of healthier relaxation, happier parenting, and chilling TF out. You can—*we* can—use this plant responsibly to elevate and uplift ourselves along with our kids, families, and communities to push the culture toward a more humane place.

Because it's not just for our kids' *own* health and safety that we teach them about cannabis. When they learn the complex social and political history of the plant—when they gain the skills to think critically about policy, governance, and social justice—they'll become better citizens. Better policymakers. Better entrepreneurs. Better environmentalists. Better people. "This is what our world vitally needs more than anything," writes Jenn Lauder on *Splimm*, "—a generation of young people who can think for themselves and who have the intelligence, tools, and passion to make change."

As flawed as our world is, I believe in the resiliency of humans and in our ability, as Dr. Maya Angelou once urged, to do better as we know better. I believe in our kids and our future. And I believe in *you*, weed moms. You're my people. We got this.

# APPENDIX

## PRODUCT RECOMMENDATIONS

Note: I've personally tried, and liked, every brand or product listed here. I've bought some of them at a dispensary; others I've been sent as samples. I've received no money for endorsements of these products or brands, and, whenever possible, have prioritized women-owned and people-of-color-owned companies. While a few of these brands are multi-state operators, the majority of companies in the cannabis space today aren't—yet. I strongly encourage you to research the values and practices of any cannabis brands or retail operations you choose to support.

**Flower:** Flow Kana, Viola Brands, Bloom Farms, Cannabiotics, Karma, Lowell Farms

**Flower Vaporizers:** Firefly, Magic Flight, PAX

**All-in-One Vape Pens:** Dosist, Bloom Farms

**Edibles:** Satori, Wyld, Kikoko, Kin, Periodic Edibles

**Full-Spectrum CBD and/or CBD + THC Combos:** Bloom Farms, Make & Mary, Charlotte's Web, Care by Design, Papa and Barkley, Barlean's, White Fox

**CBD Isolate:** Nature's Elixir, Azuca (sugar base for cooking)

**Topicals:** Peak Extracts, Mary's Medicinals, Apothecanna, Make & Mary, White Fox, Brown Girl Jane

**Bath Products:** Canna Bath Co.

**Lubes and Intimate Serums:** Quim, Kiskanu, Foria

**Safe Storage:** Apothecarry

# NOTES

1  Rachael E. Thayer, Sophie York Williams, Hollis C. Karoly, et al., "Structural Neuroimaging Correlates of Alcohol and Cannabis Use in Adolescents and Adults," *Addiction* 112, no. 12 (2017): 2144–2154. doi:10.1111/add.13923.

2  However, it *is* possible to develop dependence to cannabis. For a thorough treatment of this subject, see Chapter 9.

3  A one-hitter is a teeny, tiny pipe used to smoke a small amount of ground cannabis flower.

4  J. C. Callaway, "Hempseed as A Nutritional Resource: An Overview," *Euphytica* 140, no. 1-2 (2004): 65–72, doi:10.1007/s10681-004-4811-6.

5  Marcela Mihoc, Georgeta Pop, Alexa Ersilia, Isidora Radulov, "Nutritive Quality of Romanian Hemp Varieties (*Cannabis Sativa* L.) with Special Focus on Oil and Metal Contents of Seeds," *Chemistry Central Journal* 6, no. 1, (2012), doi:10.1186/1752-153X-6-122.

6  It should be noted, however, that humans did in fact discover the medicinal and the mind-altering possibilities in the cannabis plant early in the relationship. See Chapter 3 for more information.

7  "2020 Cannabis Consumer Report," ICR & Spectacle Strategy, https://info.spectaclestrategy.com/cannabis2020.

8  Technically, the plants contain THCA and CBDA, the precursors to THC and CBD that must be heated before they can be utilized by the body.

9  McPartland, John M. 2018. "Cannabis Systematics at the Levels of Family, Genus, and Species," *Cannabis and Cannabinoid Research* 3, no. 1 (2018): 203–212. doi:10.1089/can.2018.0039.

10  I say this with respect for the many decent folks in law enforcement. Though there have indeed been many abuses of cannabis growers, users, and activists by cops and DEA agents over the years, the War on Drugs is a policy failure—not the fault of individuals.

11  Aakanksha Pant, et al., "Beta-caryophyllene Modulates Expression of Stress Response Genes and Mediates Longevity in Caenorhabditis Elegans," *Experimental Gerontology* 57, (2014):81–95, doi: 10.1016/j.exger.2014.05.007.

12  Shenlong Zou and Ujendra Kumar, "Cannabinoid Receptors and the Endocannabinoid System: Signaling and Function in the Central Nervous System," *International Journal of Molecular Sciences* 19, no. 3 (2018): 833, doi:10.3390/ijms19030833.

13  Ethan B. Russo, "The Case for the Entourage Effect and Conventional Breeding of Clinical Cannabis: No 'Strain,' No Gain," *Frontiers in Plant Science* 9 (2019), doi:10.3389/fpls.2018.01969.

14  Thaddeus E. Weckowicz, et al., "Effect of Marijuana on Divergent and Convergent Production Cognitive Tests," *Journal of Abnormal Psychology* 84, no.4 (1975): 386–398, doi:10.1037/0021-843x.84.4.386.

15  Li Liu, et al., "Fermented Beverage and Food Storage in 13,000 Y-Old Stone Mortars at Raqefet Cave, Israel: Investigating Natufian Ritual Feasting," *Journal of Archaeological Science: Reports* 21 (2018): 783–793, doi:10.1016/j.jasrep.2018.08.008.

16  Jan M. Keppel Hesselink, "Kambô: A Shamanic Medicine - Personal Testimonies," *Juniper Online Journal of Case Studies* 8, no. 3, (2018): doi:10.19080/jojcs.2018.08.555739.

17  Steven Kotler and Jamie Wheal, *Stealing Fire, How Silicon Valley, the Navy SEALs, and Maverick Scientists Are Revolutionizing the Way We Live and Work* (New York: Dey Street Books, 2017).

18  Meng Ren, et al., "The Origins of Cannabis Smoking: Chemical Residue Evidence from the First Millennium BCE In the Pamirs," *Science Advances* 5, no. 6, (2019): doi:10.1126/sciadv.aaw1391.

19  Ethan B. Russo, et al., "Phytochemical and Genetic Analyses of Ancient Cannabis from Central Asia," *Journal of Experimental Botany* 59, no. 15, (2008): 4171–4182, doi:10.1093/jxb/ern260.

20  Martin A. Lee, *Smoke Signals: A Social History of Marijuana—Medical, Recreational, and Scientific,* (New York: Scribner, 2012).

21  Frank Luther Mott, *American Journalism: A History 1690-1960,* (New York: McMillan, 1962).

22  "The Early Years," The Drug Enforcement Administration, https://www.dea.gov/sites/default/files/2018-05/Early%20Years%20p%2012-29.pdf.

23  Lee, *Smoke Signals.*

24  Lloyd D. Johnston, et al., "Monitoring the Future: National Results on Adolescent Drug Use: Overview of Key Findings," *FOCUS* 1, no. 2 (2003): 213–234, doi:10.1176/foc.1.2.213.

25  Michael Gabay, "The Federal Controlled Substances Act: Schedules and Pharmacy Registration," *Hospital Pharmacy* 48, no. 6 (2013): 473–474, doi:10.1310/hpj4806-473.

26  Raymond P. Shafer, *Marihuana: A Signal of Misunderstanding,* (New York: New American Library, 1972).

27  "Drug Overdose Deaths," Centers for Disease Control and Prevention, https://www.cdc.gov/drugoverdose/data/statedeaths.html.

28  Dan Baum, "Legalize It All," *Harper's Magazine,* last modified April 2016, https://harpers.org/archive/2016/04/legalize-it-all.

29  Michelle Alexander, *New Jim Crow,* (New York: New Press, 2020).

30  "Making Economic Sense," Drug Policy Alliance, https://www.drugpolicy.org/issues/making-economic-sense.

31 "Highest to Lowest - Prison Population Rate," World Prison Brief, https://www.prisonstudies.org/highest-to-lowest/prison_population_rate?field_region_taxonomy_tid=All.

32 "Marijuana Arrests by the Numbers," American Civil Liberties Union, https://www.aclu.org/gallery/marijuana-arrests-numbers.

33 Justin McCarthy, "Two in Three Americans Now Support Legalizing Marijuana," Gallup, last modified October 22, 2018, https://news.gallup.com/poll/243908/two-three-americans-support-legalizing-marijuana.aspx

34 Andrew Daniller, "Two-Thirds of Americans Support Marijuana Legalization," PewResearchCenter, last modified November 14, 2019, https://www.pewresearch.org/fact-tank/2019/11/14/americans-support-marijuana-legalization.

35 Referring to cannabis as "420" is based on a story of five northern California high school dudes in 1971 who met at 4:20 p.m. to scour the Marin County coastal lands for a fabled weed patch.

36 Michelle Sexton, et al., "A Cross-Sectional Survey of Medical Cannabis Users: Patterns of Use and Perceived Efficacy," *Cannabis and Cannabinoid Research* 1, no. 1 (2016): 131–138, doi:10.1089/can.2016.0007.

37 Philippe Lucas, "Medical Cannabis Patterns of Use and Substitution for Opioids & Other Pharmaceutical Drugs, Alcohol, Tobacco, and Illicit Substances; Results from a Cross-Sectional Survey of Authorized Patients," *Harm Reduction Journal* 16, no. 1 (2019): doi:10.1186/s12954-019-0278-6.

38 National Academies of Sciences, Engineering, and Medicine, "The Health Effects of Cannabis and Cannabinoids: Current State of Evidence and Recommendations for Research," Washington, DC: The National Academies Press.

39 Emanuela Mazzon and Sabrina Giacoppo, "Can Cannabinoids Be a Potential Therapeutic Tool in Amyotrophic Lateral Sclerosis?," *Neural Regeneration Research* 11, no.12 (2016): 1896–1899, doi:10.4103/1673-5374.197125.

40 Martin R. Tramer, et al., "Cannabinoids for Control of Chemotherapy Induced Nausea and Vomiting: Quantitative Systematic". *BMJ* 323, no. 16, (2001), doi:10.1136/bmj.323.7303.16.

41 "Any Anxiety Disorder," National Institute of Mental Health, https://www.nimh.nih.gov/health/statistics/any-anxiety-disorder.shtml.

42 "Major Depression," National Institute of Mental Health, https://www.nimh.nih.gov/health/statistics/major-depression.shtml.

43 T. Rubino, et al., "CB1 Receptor Stimulation in Specific Brain Areas Differently Modulate Anxiety-Related Behaviour," *Neuropharmacology* 54, no. 1 (2008): 151–160, doi:10.1016/j.neuropharm.2007.06.024.

44 Prakash Nagarkatti, et al., "Cannabinoids as Novel Anti-Inflammatory Drugs," *Future Medicinal Chemistry* 1 no. 7 (2009): 1333–1349, doi:10.4155/fmc.09.93.

45 Sexton, et al., "A Cross-Sectional Survey of Medical Cannabis Users," 131–138.

46 Esther M Blessing, "Cannabidiol as a Potential Treatment for Anxiety Disorders," *Neurotherapeutics* 12, no. 4 (2015): 825–836, doi:10.1007/s13311-015-0387-1.

47  Scott Shannon, "Cannabidiol in Anxiety and Sleep: A Large Case Series, "*The Permanente Journal* 23 (2019): doi:10.7812/tpp/18-041.

48  Kimberly A. Babson, et al., "Cannabis, Cannabinoids, and Sleep: A Review of the Literature," *Current Psychiatry Reports* 19, no. 4 (2017): doi:10.1007/s11920-017-0775-9.

49  T.V. Zanelati, et al., "Antidepressant-Like Effects of Cannabidiol in Mice: Possible Involvement of 5-HT1A Receptors," *British Journal Of Pharmacology* 159, no. 1 (2009): 122–128, doi:10.1111/j.1476-5381.2009.00521.x.

50  Karina Genaro, et al., "Cannabidiol Is a Potential Therapeutic for the Affective-Motivational Dimension of Incision Pain in Rats," *Frontiers In Pharmacology* 8 (2017): doi:10.3389/fphar.2017.00391.

51  D.C. Hammell, et al., "Transdermal Cannabidiol Reduces Inflammation and Pain-Related Behaviours in a Rat Model of Arthritis," *European Journal of Pain* 20, no. 6 (2015): doi:10.1002/ejp.818

52  Wei Xiong, et al., "Cannabinoids Suppress Inflammatory and Neuropathic Pain by Targeting A3 Glycine Receptors," *The Journal of Experimental Medicine* 209, no. 6 (2012): 1121–1134, doi:10.1084/jem.20120242.

53  Lucas Elms, et al., "Cannabidiol in the Treatment of Post-Traumatic Stress Disorder: A Case Series," *The Journal of Alternative and Complementary Medicine* 25 no. 4 (2019): 392–397: doi:10.1089/acm.2018.0437.

54  Aisling O'Neill, et al., "Normalization of Mediotemporal and Prefrontal Activity, and Mediotemporal-Striatal Connectivity, May Underlie Antipsychotic Effects of Cannabidiol in Psychosis," *Psychological Medicine*, (2020): 1–11, doi:10.1017/s0033291719003519.

55  Linda A. Parker, et al., "Regulation of Nausea and Vomiting by Cannabinoids," *British Journal of Pharmacology* 163, no. 7 (2010): 1411–1422, doi:10.1111/j.1476-5381.2010.01176.x.

56  Jeff Jones and Lydia Saad, "Gallup" (Gallup Poll Social Series: Consumption Habits, July 12, 2019), https://news.gallup.com/poll/263147/americans-say-cbd-products.aspx.

57  Marcel O. Bonn-Miller, "Labeling Accuracy of Cannabidiol Extracts Sold Online," *The Journal of the American Medical Association* 318, no. 17 (2017): 1708, doi:10.1001/jama.2017.11909.

58  Maya A. Farha, "Uncovering the Hidden Antibiotic Potential of Cannabis," *ACS Infectious Diseases* 6, no. 3 (2020): 338–346, doi:10.1021/acsinfecdis.9b00419.

59  Mahmoud A. ElSohly, "Changes in Cannabis Potency Over the Last 2 Decades (1995–2014): Analysis of Current Data in the United States," *Biological Psychiatry* 79, no. 7 (2016): 613–619, doi:10.1016/j.biopsych.2016.01.004.

60  "Top 10 Ways People Are Consuming Cannabis in 2019" BDSA, last modified July 26, 2019, https://bdsanalytics.com/top-10-ways-people-are-consuming-cannabis-in-2019.

61  Sarah S. Stith, et al., "The Association Between Cannabis Product Characteristics and Symptom Relief," *Scientific Reports* 9 no. 1 (2019): doi:10.1038/s41598-019-39462-1.

62  Not all cannabis is "craft," or grown with care by small farmers. But that's the kind of weed I choose to support.

63  "The Health Effects of Cannabis and Cannabinoids: The Current State of Evidence and Recommendations for Research," The National Academy of Sciences, Engineering, and Medicine.

64  "Outbreak of Lung Injury Associated with E-Cigarette Use or Vaping," Centers for Disease Control and Prevention, https://www.cdc.gov/tobacco/basic_information/e-cigarettes/severe-lung-disease.html.

65  Ellena Badrick, "The Relationship Between Alcohol Consumption and Cortisol Secretion in an Aging Cohort," The Journal of Clinical Endocrinology & Metabolism 93, no. 3 (2008): 750–757, doi:10.1210/jc.2007-0737.

66  Melanie C. Dreher, et al., "Prenatal Marijuana Exposure and Neonatal Outcomes in Jamaica: An Ethnographic Study," Pediatrics 93, no. 2 (1994): 254–60.

67  Emily Lee, et al., "The Impact of State Legalization on Rates of Marijuana Use in Pregnancy in a Universal Drug Screening Population," The Journal of Maternal-Fetal & Neonatal Medicine, (2020): 1–8, doi:10.1080/14767058.2020.1765157.

68  Lihi Bar-Lev Schleider, et al., "Real Life Experience of Medical Cannabis Treatment in Autism: Analysis of Safety and Efficacy," Scientific Reports 9, no. 1 (2019): doi:10.1038/s41598-018-37570-y.

69  "Monitoring the Future Study: Trends in Prevalence of Various Drugs," National Institute on Drug Abuse.

70  Drug Enforcement Administration, "Drugs of Abuse: A DEA Resource Guide," 2017.

71  Benjamin Chadwick, et al., "Cannabis Use During Adolescent Development: Susceptibility to Psychiatric Illness," Frontiers in Psychiatry 4 (2013): doi:10.3389/fpsyt.2013.00129.

72  Gabriella Gobbi, et al., "Association of Cannabis Use in Adolescence and Risk of Depression, Anxiety, and Suicidality in Young Adulthood," The Journal of the American Medical Association Psychiatry 76, no. 4 (2019): 426, doi:10.1001/jamapsychiatry.2018.4500.

73  Nicholas J. Jackson, et al., "Impact of Adolescent Marijuana Use on Intelligence: Results from Two Longitudinal Twin Studies," Proceedings of The National Academy of Sciences 113, no. 5 (2016): E500–E508, doi:10.1073/pnas.1516648113.

74  Jean-François G. Morin, et al., "A Population-Based Analysis of the Relationship Between Substance Use and Adolescent Cognitive Development," American Journal of Psychiatry 176, no. 2 (2018): 98–106, doi:10.1176/appi.ajp.2018.18020202.

75  Randi Melissa Schuster, et al., "One Month of Cannabis Abstinence in Adolescents and Young Adults Is Associated with Improved Memory," The Journal of Clinical Psychiatry 79, no. 6 (2018), doi:10.4088/jcp.17m11977.

76  Ken C. Winters and Chih-Yuan S. Lee, "Likelihood of Developing an Alcohol and Cannabis Use Disorder During Youth: Association with Recent Use and Age," Drug and Alcohol Dependence 92, no. 1 (2008): 239–247, doi:10.1016/j.drugalcdep.2007.08.005.

77  "Underage Drinking," Centers for Disease Control and Prevention, https://www.cdc.gov/alcohol/fact-sheets/underage-drinking.htm.

78  Claire Gorey, et al., "Age-Related Differences in the Impact of Cannabis Use on the Brain and Cognition: A Systematic Review," European Archives of Psychiatry and Clinical Neuroscience 269, no. 1 (2019): 37–58., doi:10.1007/s00406-019-00981-7.

79  "Healthy Kids Colorado Survey and Smart Source Information," Department of Public Health and Environment, https://www.colorado.gov/pacific/cdphe/hkcs.

80  "Youth Marijuana Use, Attitudes and Related Behaviors in Oregon," Oregon Health Authority, https://www.oregon.gov/oha/PH/PREVENTIONWELLNESS/MARIJUANA/Documents/fact-sheet-marijuana-youth.pdf.

81  "Monitoring the Future Study: Trends in Prevalence of Various Drugs," National Institute on Drug Abuse, 2019.

82  Sasha Simon, "What Is Harm Reduction?" last modified March 30, 2020.

83  "Monitoring the Future Study: Trends in Prevalence of Various Drugs," National Institute on Drug Abuse, 2019.

84  E. L. Engelsman, "Dutch Policy on the Management of Drug-Related Problems," *Addiction* 84, no. 2 (1989): 211–218. doi:10.1111/j.1360-0443.1989.tb00571.x.

85  Kathrin F. Stanger-Hall and David W. Hall, "Abstinence-Only Education and Teen Pregnancy Rates: Why We Need Comprehensive Sex Education in the U.S.," *Public Library of Science O* (2011): doi:10.1371/journal.pone.0024658.

86  Sasha Simon, "What Is Harm Reduction?" last modified March 30, 2020.

87  "Debunking The 'Gateway' Myth," Drug Policy Alliance, https://www.drugpolicy.org/sites/default/files/DebunkingGatewayMyth_NY_0.pdf.

88  Ralph E. Tarter, et al., "Predictors of Marijuana Use in Adolescents Before and After Licit Drug Use: Examination of the Gateway Hypothesis," *American Journal of Psychiatry* 163, no. 12 (2006): 2134–2140, doi:10.1176/ajp.2006.163.12.2134.

89  Substance Abuse and Mental Health Services Administration, U.S. Department of Health and Human Services, "Reports and Detailed Tables from the 2017 National Survey on Drug Use and Health (NSDUH)," Tables 1.1A.

90  "Monitoring the Future Study: Trends in Prevalence of Various Drugs," National Institute on Drug Abuse, 2019.

91  Frank M. Tims , et al., "Characteristics and Problems Of 600 Adolescent Cannabis Abusers in Outpatient Treatment," *Addiction* 97, no. 1 (2002): 46–57, doi:10.1046/j.1360-0443.97.s01.7.x.

92  R.B. Laprairie, et al., "Cannabidiol Is A Negative Allosteric Modulator of the Cannabinoid CB1 Receptor," *British Journal Of Pharmacology* 172, no. 20 (2015): 4790–4805. doi:10.1111/bph.13250.

93  Ethan B. Russo, "Taming THC: Potential Cannabis Synergy and Phytocannabinoid-Terpenoid Entourage Effects," *British Journal of Pharmacology* 163, no. 7 (2011): 1344–1364. doi:10.1111/j.1476-5381.2011.01238.x.

94  Reto Auer, et al., "Association Between Lifetime Marijuana Use and Cognitive Function in Middle Age," *The Journal of the American Medical Association Internal Medicine* 176, no. 3 (2016): 352doi:10.1001/jamainternmed.2015.7841.

95  Celia J. A. Morgan, "Impact of Cannabidiol on the Acute Memory and Psychotomimetic Effects of Smoked Cannabis: Naturalistic Study," *British Journal of Psychiatry* 197, no. 4 (2010): 285–290, doi:10.1192/bjp.bp.110.077503.

96  Susan A. Stoner, "Effects of Marijuana on Mental Health," Alcohol and Drug Abuse Institute, 2017, https://adai.uw.edu/pubs/pdf/2017mjanxiety.pdf.

97  Carrie Cutler, et al., "A Naturalistic Examination of the Perceived Effects of Cannabis on Negative Affect," *Journal of Affective Disorders* 235 (2018): 198–205, doi:10.1016/j.jad.2018.04.054.

98  Kelly A. Sagar, et al., "Joint Effects: A Pilot Investigation of the Impact of Bipolar Disorder and Marijuana Use on Cognitive Function and Mood," *Public Library of Science ONE* 11, no. 6 (2016): e0157060, doi:10.1371/journal.pone.0157060.

99  Elizabeth Tyler, et al., "The Relationship Between Bipolar Disorder and Cannabis Use in Daily Life: An Experience Sampling Study," *Public Library of Science ONE* 10, no. 3 (2015): e0118916, doi:10.1371/journal.pone.0118916.

100  Melanie Gibbs, et al., "Cannabis Use and Mania Symptoms: A Systematic Review and Meta-Analysis," *Journal of Affective Disorders* 171 (2015): 39–47, doi:10.1016/j.jad.2014.09.016.

101  Shaul Lev-Ran, et al., "Bipolar Disorder and Co-Occurring Cannabis Use Disorders: Characteristics, Co-Morbidities and Clinical Correlates," *Psychiatry Research* 209, no. 3 (2013): 459–465, doi:10.1016/j.psychres.2012.12.014.

102  Sven Andréasson, et al., "Cannabis and Schizophrenia: A Longitudinal Study of Swedish Conscripts," *The Lancet* 330, no. 8574 (1987): 1483–1486, doi:10.1016/s0140-6736(87)92620-1.

103  Wayne Hall and Louisa Degenhardt, "Cannabis Use and the Risk of Developing a Psychotic Disorder," *World Psychiatry* 7, no. 2 (2008): 68–71, doi:10.1002/j.2051-5545.2008.tb00158.x.

104  F.M. Leweke, et al., "Cannabidiol Enhances Anandamide Signaling and Alleviates Psychotic Symptoms of Schizophrenia," *Translational Psychiatry* 2, no. 3 (2012): e94–e94, doi:10.1038/tp.2012.15.

105  Marta Di Forti, et al., "The Contribution of Cannabis Use to Variation in the Incidence of Psychotic Disorder Across Europe (EU-GEI): A Multicentre Case-Control Study," *The Lancet Psychiatry* 6, no. 5 (2019): 427–436, doi:10.1016/s2215-0366(19)30048-3.

106  Samy I. McFarlane, "Cannabis and Myocardial Infarction: Risk Factors and Pathogenetic Insights," *Sci-Fed Journal of Cardiology* 1, no. 1 (2017): doi:10.23959/sfjc-1000004.

107  Elizabeth A. Penner, et al., "The Impact of Marijuana Use on Glucose, Insulin, and Insulin Resistance Among US Adults," *The American Journal of Medicine* 126, no. 7 (2013): 583–589, doi:10.1016/j.amjmed.2013.03.002.

108  Divya Ravi, "Associations Between Marijuana Use and Cardiovascular Risk Factors and Outcomes," *Annals of Internal Medicine* 168, no. 3 (2018): 187–194, doi:10.7326/m17-1548.

109  Donald P. Tashkin, "Effects of Marijuana Smoking on the Lung," *Annals of The American Thoracic Society* 10, no. 3 (2013): 239–247, doi:10.1513/annalsats.201212-127fr.

110  Mark J. Pletcher, et al., "Association Between Marijuana Exposure and Pulmonary Function Over 20 Years," *The Journal of American Medical Association* 307, no. 2 (2012): 173, doi:10.1001/jama.2011.1961.

111  "2020 Cannabis Consumer Report," ICR & Spectacle Strategy https://info.spectaclestrategy.com/cannabis2020.

112  Michele Baggio, et al., "Helping Settle the Marijuana and Alcohol Debate: Evidence from Scanner Data," *SSRN Electronic Journal* (2017) doi:10.2139/ssrn.3063288.

113  Tod H. Mikuriya, "Cannabis as a Substitute for Alcohol: A Harm-Reduction Approach," *Journal of Cannabis Therapeutics* 4, no.1 (2004): 79-93, doi:10.1300/j175v04n01_04.

114  Celia J.A.Morgan, et al., "Cannabidiol Reduces Cigarette Consumption in Tobacco Smokers: Preliminary Findings," *Addictive Behaviors* 38, no.9 (2013): 2433–2436, doi:10.1016/j.addbeh.2013.03.011.

115  Vicky Katsidoni, et al., "Cannabidiol Inhibits the Reward-Facilitating Effect of Morphine: Involvement of 5-Ht1areceptors in the Dorsal Raphe Nucleus," *Addiction Biology* 18, no. 2 (2012): 286–296, doi:10.1111/j.1369-1600.2012.00483.x.

116  Jillian L. Scavone, et al., "Impact of Cannabis Use During Stabilization on Methadone Maintenance Treatment," *The American Journal on Addictions* 22, no.4 (2013): 344–351, doi:10.1111/j.1521-0391.2013.12044.x.

117  Claudia Calpe-López, et al., "Cannabidiol Treatment Might Promote Resilience to Cocaine and Methamphetamine Use Disorders: A Review of Possible Mechanisms," *Molecules* 24, no. 14 (2019): 2583, doi:10.3390/molecules24142583.

118  Calpe-López, et al., "Cannabidiol Treatment Might Promote Resilience."

119  "Is Marijuana Addictive?" National Institute on Drug Abuse, last modified April 8, 2020, https://www.drugabuse.gov/publications/research-reports/marijuana/marijuana-addictive.

120  "Alcohol Facts and Statistics," National Institute on Alcohol Abuse and Alcoholism, https://www.niaaa.nih.gov/publications/brochures-and-fact-sheets/alcohol-facts-and-statistics.

121  "Overdose Death Rates," National Institute on Drug Abuse, https://www.drugabuse.gov/related-topics/trends-statistics/overdose-death-rates.

122  "Available Treatments for Marijuana Use Disorders," National Institute on Drug Abuse, https://www.drugabuse.gov/publications/research-reports/marijuana/available-treatments-marijuana-use-disorders.

123  Andrew J. Sun and Michael L. Eisenberg, "Association Between Marijuana Use and Sexual Frequency in The United States: A Population-Based Study," *The Journal of Sexual Medicine* 14, no. 11 (2017): 1342–1347, doi:10.1016/j.jsxm.2017.09.005.

124  Becky K. Lynn, et al., "The Relationship Between Marijuana Use Prior to Sex and Sexual Function in Women," *Sexual Medicine* 7 no. 2 (2019): 192–197, doi:10.1016/j.esxm.2019.01.003.

125  Carolin Klein, et al., "Circulating Endocannabinoid Concentrations and Sexual Arousal in Women," *The Journal of Sexual Medicine* 9, no. 6 (2012): 1588–1601, doi:10.1111/j.1743-6109.2012.02708.x.

126  Don Wei, et al., "Endocannabinoid Signaling Mediates Oxytocin-Driven Social Reward," *Proceedings of The National Academy of Sciences* 112, no. 45 (2015): 14084–14089, doi:10.1073/pnas.1509795112.

127  While it may seem like "hippie-dippie baloney" (to quote the LEGO movie) if the thought of looking at yourself in the mirror and saying *I love you* sounds hard, that might mean you need it.

128  Weed & the American Family," Marist Poll, http://maristpoll.marist.edu/yahoo-newsmarist-poll/#sthash.vqLr9jKU.dpbs.

129  "2020 Cannabis Consumer Report," ICR & Spectacle Strategy, https://info.spectaclestrategy.com/cannabis2020.

130  Benjamin H. Han, et al., "Demographic Trends Among Older Cannabis Users in the United States, 2006–13," *Addiction* 112, no. 3 (2016): 516–525, doi:10.1111/add.13670.

131  Christina J. Charlesworth, et al., "Polypharmacy Among Adults Aged 65 Years and Older in the United States: 1988–2010," *The Journals of Gerontology Series A: Biological Sciences and Medical Sciences* 70, no. 8 (2015): 989–995, doi:10.1093/gerona/glv013.

132  Kevin Yang, et al., "Cannabis Use for Anxiety Among Older Adults," *The American Journal of Geriatric Psychiatry* 28, no. 4 (2020): S81–S82, doi:10.1016/j.jagp.2020.01.108.

133  Julie Bobitt, et al., "Qualitative Analysis of Cannabis Use Among Older Adults in Colorado," *Drugs & Aging* 36, no. 7 (2019): 655–666, doi:10.1007/s40266-019-00665-w.

134  Rachel E. Thayer, et al., "Preliminary Results from a Pilot Study Examining Brain Structure in Older Adult Cannabis Users and Nonusers," *Psychiatry Research: Neuroimaging* 285 (2019): 58–63, doi:10.1016/j.pscychresns.2019.02.001.

135  Referring here to aspirin use for pain relief, not for blood-thinning properties.

136  Sophie L. York Williams, et al., "The New Runner's High? Examining Relationships Between Cannabis Use and Exercise Behavior in States with Legalized Cannabis," *Frontiers in Public Health* 7 (2019), doi:10.3389/fpubh.2019.00099.

137  P. B. Sparling, et al., "Exercise Activates the Endocannabinoid System," *Neuroreport* 14, no.17 (2003): 2209–2211, doi:10.1097/00001756-200312020-00015.

138  Yann Le Strat and Bernard Le Foll, "Obesity and Cannabis Use: Results from Two Representative National Surveys," *American Journal of Epidemiology* 174, no. 8 (2011): 929–933, doi:10.1093/aje/kwr200.

139  Elizabeth A. Penner, et al., "The Impact of Marijuana Use on Glucose, Insulin, and Insulin Resistance Among US Adults," *The American Journal of Medicine* 126, no. 7 (2013): 583–589, doi:10.1016/j.amjmed.2013.03.002.

140  Thorsten Rudroff and Jacob Sosnoff, "Cannabidiol to Improve Mobility in People with Multiple Sclerosis," *Frontiers in Neurology* 9 (2018): doi:10.3389/fneur.2018.00183.

141  Morgan Whitaker, "Michelle Obama Talks Nutrition and 'Wakeup Call' Moment in her Family's Past," September 10, 2015, https://www.aol.com/article/2015/09/10/michelle-obama-talks-nutrition-and-wakeup-call-moment-in-her-familys-past/21234056.

142  Linley Sanders, "States with Recreational Marijuana Laws View the Legislation as a Success," last modified May 13, 2020, https://today.yougov.com/topics/economy/articles-reports/2020/05/13/recreational-marijuana-poll?utm_source=twitter&utm_medium=website_article&utm_campaign=recreational_marijuana.

# ACKNOWLEDGMENTS

I extend my heartfelt thanks to the many women quoted in these pages. Your words help illuminate what it's like to be a conscious and uplifted weed mom.

I want to thank my husband for allowing me to share some of our personal and marital challenges in these pages and for holding down the fort while I locked myself in our bedroom to write this book during a freaking global pandemic. Baby, I definitely wouldn't have been able to get this project done without your support, and neither would I want to.

I also want to thank my mom for throwing her lot in with us during the lockdowns and for bringing good humor to our lives at a very difficult moment. Thanks, Mom, for taking over bedtime duties, watching funny animal videos with the kids, and for all the dishes.

The irony of writing a book about parenting and cannabis is that I had to take a few steps back from actual parenting to get this done. I want to thank my two incredible children for their patience with me while I skipped family movie nights and phoned it in on pandemic homeschooling. I wrote this book to help make a better world for you and all the kids of your generation.

A million thanks, Dad, for always being in my corner, even when what I do worries the heck out of you.

Thanks to my talented writing group, Genevieve, (the other) Danielle, Corinne, and Jessica. You championed this project from the very beginning. And Riki, a big hug for reading and astutely commenting on many chapters. There are so many more friends, healers, and allies I wish I could name here.

Many, many thanks to my agent, Jessica Faust of BookEnds Literary, for believing in this project and for taking on a new author. Thank you to my editor at Ulysses, Ashten Evans, for helping this book take shape and for your grace and professionalism. Last, I bow deeply to the entire team of editors, artists, and other book geniuses at Ulysses who helped bring this work into the world, including, but not limited to, Claire Chun, Renee Rutledge, Kate St.Clair, Tyanni Niles, Jake Flaherty, and Lilith Stepanyan.

# ABOUT THE AUTHOR

**Danielle Simone Brand** is a journalist covering the cannabis and parenting spaces—and their many overlaps. A few years ago, she wouldn't have self-described as a "weed mom," but she's found her sparkle in writing about cannabis to inform, uplift, and occasionally challenge her readers while helping push the conversation toward a more progressive place. She holds a BA from Dartmouth College and an MA from American University, and has worked as a yoga teacher and trainer, a staff writer, and a researcher on issues of international conflict resolution. She lives with her husband, two kids, and a barky terrier in the Pacific Northwest.

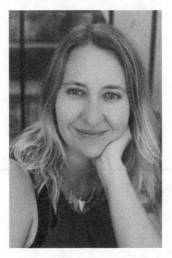

# 100 MARATHONS

# 100 Marathons

## Memories and Lessons from Races Run around the World

Jeffrey Horowitz

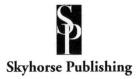

Skyhorse Publishing

Skyhorse Publishing books may be purchased in bulk at special discounts for sales promotion, corporate gifts, fund-raising, or educational purposes. Special editions can also be created to specifications. For details, contact the Special Sales Department, Skyhorse Publishing, 307 West 36th Street, 11th Floor, New York, NY 10018 or info@skyhorsepublishing.com.

Skyhorse® and Skyhorse Publishing® are registered trademarks of Skyhorse Publishing, Inc.®, a Delaware corporation.

Visit our website at www.skyhorsepublishing.com.

10 9 8 7 6 5 4 3 2 1

Paperback ISBN: 978-1-62636-045-7

Library of Congress Cataloging-in-Publication Data
Horowitz, Jeffrey.
My first 100 marathons : 2,620 miles with an obsessive runner / Jeffrey Horowitz. p. cm.
ISBN 978-1-60239-318-9 (hardcover : alk. paper)
1. Marathon running—United States. 2. Marathon running—Training—United States. 3. Long-distance runners—United States—Anecdotes.
4. Horowitz, Jeffrey. I. Title. II. Title: My first hundred marathons.
III. Title: My first one hundred marathons.
GV1065.2.H67 2008
796.42'520973—dc22
2008028945

Printed in the United States of America

To all those who have inspired, challenged, prodded, and pushed me over the years, but most of all to my wonderful wife, Stephanie, for her encouragement and patience, and for bringing Alex Michael into the world.

# CONTENTS

# Foreword

I sat down to write a book about running, but ended up writing something else.

After running marathons for nearly 20 years, from the Atlantic to the Pacific and across the world from Antarctica to Africa and Asia, there were plenty of good stories to pick from. But as I began to write them down, I discovered that running isn't something that we do; running explains who we are. It shapes the way we view the world and our place in it, and reflects our values, our dreams, and our work ethic.

As the stories unspooled, I found, too, that some of them weren't about running and racing at all, at least not directly. They were about life. There were moments of joy, but also moments of sadness and loss. One reader emailed me saying that the book surprised him because, as he put it, "running books aren't supposed to make you cry." But that's life, isn't it? Running is life is laughter is sorrow is joy is loss. It all becomes one seamless whole.

It would be easy to say that this book is just about my life. That's certainly true, in a way. But I aimed for it to be more than that. It's an invitation. Every runner has a story to tell, and I hoped that my book would resonate with other people, reminding them of their own experiences that were waiting to be shared. I wanted to start a conversation. I wanted people to write me messages saying, "Hey, I loved your book, but let me tell you my story."

I got my wish. I never expected that my book would be popular enough to lead to action figure spin-offs and themed Happy Meals, but I was thrilled to receive a steady stream of emails from people who found my book interesting, entertaining, and thoughtful, and who then had something they wanted to share with me in return. I'm grateful to all of them.

I also found that my editor was right: readers really would be interested in having training and racing advice mixed in along with the stories. Many of the emails I received thanked me for those tips, and asked for follow-up advice. I'm grateful, too, for the chance to help other runners, just as I had been helped so many times with sound advice from my own friends and mentors.

One unexpected question that came from a number of readers, though, was what would I do now that I had reached my goal of running 100 marathons?

I found that perplexing. I would keep running, of course! What else would I do?

Since completing my 100-marathon quest, I've returned to many of my favorite races, but I've also traveled far and wide, running marathons in Florence, Milan, Sydney, and Madrid. I've run a marathon on an indoor 200-meter track in Virginia, and a marathon starting at midnight in the Nevada desert. I've run in a 5-day stage race in the Himalayas in the shadow of Mt. Everest, and in the 3-day TransRockies Run. I also ran in a 100k Ultramarathon in Cairo, Egypt, where I was chased by a pack of wild dogs, had rocks thrown at me by unimpressed teenagers, and was either guarded or threatened by armed villagers, depending on who I asked.

I still seek out these racing adventures, but as my life moved more from Me to We, as my wife and I raise our son, I've slowed down the pace a bit. I still scan the web for interesting new races, and I still haunt those familiar running trails and paths as before, but I find more and more frequently now that I'd rather stay at home with my wife and help our son grow into a young boy than dash off to add another marathon to my list. But still, the marathon continues to have meaning for me. I'm now more than halfway towards my next centennial milestone, and with any luck, I'll be able to continue past that, collecting marathons and adventures for years to come.

More marathons, more stories, more life.

Jeff Horowitz, 2013

# Out the Door and Around the Block

There is an old proverb that says a journey of a thousand miles begins with a single step. Sometimes, though, a quick trip to the emergency room begins that way, too.

That was my story. It was 1985. Ronald Reagan was president, New Wave was on the radio, and I had just moved away from home for the first time. I had come down to Washington, D.C., from New York City, for law school. After a rocky start, I found a good roommate, settled in, and acquired a love for my new hometown. I had always been overweight—"husky" was the euphemism the clothing stores seemed to like—but now I had added some new padding around my middle, and I was determined to do something about it. A new body for my new life. Except that as a grad student, I was barely getting by on my meager savings and student loans, living on spaghetti and tuna fish, and using furniture I'd built from of cinder blocks and boards. There wasn't much spare cash for a health club, personal trainer, chef, or a masseuse. But running fit the bill. I already had sneakers and shorts, so all I needed to do was head out the door and begin. Simplicity itself.

I started off with a few slow laps around the block where I lived in Arlington, Virginia. As out of shape as I was, I still immediately recognized how right it felt. I'd played sports as a kid growing up in Queens, New York, but I never excelled; I wasn't what anyone would call a naturally gifted athlete. But I was persistent, which was a trait that cut me out to be a good distance runner. Soon, my runs lengthened into laps around a small park, and then out-and-back runs down the street toward the Potomac River. Reaching my turnaround point, I gazed across the water at the spires of Georgetown University.

In those moments, I was filled with a sense of possibility. Running cleared the day's cobwebs from my mind and focused my thinking, and gave me time and space to sort out anything that was bothering me, or to detach and think of nothing at all. It had also started to reshape my body. Those new extra pounds fell away, taking some of the older, more stubborn fat along with them. Running also made me more aware of my body's needs; I quickly realized that I could only be as good as the fuel I took in, so I started to avoid all of the greasy and sugary foods that had found their way into my diet.

As the months passed, I realized that, little by little, I was actually turning into a real runner. I had never run any races, and I hadn't been on any track teams, but now I felt that I was not just some guy trying to stay in shape. I was an athlete.

If I was going to do this, then, I had to do it right. It was time for me to shelve those ratty old Pro-Keds I'd been running in and upgrade to some real running gear, which is what led me one day to a local sporting-goods store, where I eyed the shoes displayed on the back wall and tried to make sense out of the little information cards that fell out of them. Judging the technology diagrammed on those cards, you would have thought that the shoes had been to the moon and back.

I ended up taking home a pair of gray hi-tech marvels, my first true running shoes. They set me back $69, which seemed wildly extravagant.

As soon as I got home, I laced them up and went out for a run, hoping that I hadn't foolishly wasted my month's eating budget. I didn't expect miracles; all I wanted was that they at least would feel, well, *different*. And they did. Oh, how they did! Suddenly I had spring in my step, and I felt like I could run forever.

Armed with my fancy new shoes, I ran down the street toward the river, but this time I didn't stop. I crossed Key Bridge into D.C., and then followed the river south. I passed the Watergate Hotel and the Kennedy Center for the Performing Arts—a fancy building on the site of an old brewery—and crossed back into Virginia at the next bridge, completing a five-mile loop.

I was hooked. As my runs took me farther, I started wondering what I could do with my newfound love of running. I'd always been the kind of person who hated half steps; once I found a passion for something, I wanted to dive into the deep end of it. It wasn't that I ever needed to prove anything; I just wanted to fully and completely experience whatever it was that intrigued me. And now, that thing was running. I'd have to pursue that passion wherever it led me.

In hindsight, it's also obvious to me now that running provided the perfect counterpoint to sitting at a desk studying law. The mind-numbing tedium of studying left my body aching for some outlet. I didn't understand it at the time, but our bodies need attention and encouragement as much as our minds. They are not meant to be kept quiet, preserved like a specimen in a jar. We are meant to *move*. When we forget that we are not just intellectual, emotional, and spiritual beings, but also animals, we do so at our peril.

As a dedicated runner, then, the obvious next step would be to enter a road race. The idea of having a number pinned to my shirt—a very public declaration that I was a runner, an athlete—was thrilling. But which race? Most new runners start out with a 5K or 10K, but those races were shorter than my training runs. They just couldn't capture my imagination, couldn't give me that intoxicating mix of fear and excitement that I craved. I needed something big.

I knew the answer, of course: the marathon. Growing up, I lived in the shadow of the New York City Marathon. Even though I had never run more than a few miles at a time back then—and even then just barely—I felt that someday I would run that distance. Now, all these years later, the time had come to run a marathon. I would be David, throwing myself against the Goliath of running. If I came out victorious, I would truly understand what it meant to be a runner.

Luckily, one of the best marathons in the country was in my backyard—the Marine Corps Marathon, held the last weekend of every October. It starts at the Iwo Jima Memorial in Arlington, taking runners on a grand tour of D.C. and northern Virginia, circling the Pentagon, the Capitol, the Smithsonian, and the Jefferson and Lincoln Memorials before returning to the Iwo Jima Memorial for the finish. Since its course included some of my new training routes, it was easy for me to imagine running the race. I was nervous, but the more I thought about it, the more reasonable this crazy idea seemed to be.

The mailing of an application is itself a very symbolic and important act. As I wrote the check, sealed the envelope, and dropped it in the mailbox, I felt the solemnity of the moment, and a new seriousness of purpose. *I'm in for it now*, I thought. Even now, decades later, when online registration has mostly replaced the mailing of applications, I pause before clicking the final button that will commit me to a race. *Are you sure you want to do this?* But I knew then—have always known, in those kinds of situations—what I was getting myself into. I wasn't worried about it. It was simply time to get to work.

I began by increasing my weekly mileage, with the goal of building up to a 21-mile run three weeks before the race. In 1986, there wasn't the flood of training advice that runners today have to wade through; there was really very little good information available at all. There was

Jim Fixx's book on running, a few other training books, and a couple of running magazines. I read as much as I could, and more or less sorted my way through it by trial and error.

Sometimes this involved more error than I liked to admit. Once, after a good 15-mile run, I decided to run 15 miles every day, on the reasonable—though entirely wrong—assumption that if a little is good, more must be better. After a week of this, my muscles ached and I was tired to the bone. Obviously, my 15-mile-a-day plan wasn't a good idea.

Despite my blunders and setbacks, my training advanced, and finally I completed my last long run. I had met my training goal. I was ready for the marathon! Elated, I went on a short celebration run the next day with my roommate. We followed a horse trail into the woods—not my usual route—and early into the run I rolled my foot on a rock. I felt a sharp pain in my ankle, and I knew instantly that I had sprained it badly. I considered stopping, but I thought that managing pain was part of being a marathoner, so I decided to keep running.

Bad idea. There's often a very fine line between bravery and stupidity and on that Sunday morning in October 1986, I crossed it. After running 6 more miles, I made it back to my room, slumped in an easy chair, gently removed my running shoes, and inspected the damage. My ankle had turned as dark as thunderclouds, and was quickly swelling up to double its normal size. I phoned my girlfriend Kathleen and quietly, humbly, asked if she could drive me to the emergency room. Kathleen had no love of running, but she knew from the sound of my voice that this was serious. She came right over.

My short little celebration run had landed me on crutches. I was out of the marathon. I had thrown all my hard work out the window. I had blown my once-in-a-lifetime opportunity. I was devastated.

The death of a dream is a sad and painful thing. Eventually, I reconciled myself to my loss, and focused on just returning to a regular running routine. Once again, though, I demonstrated my capacity for stupidity by rushing my recovery and reinjuring my ankle. Once. Twice. Three times. Little by little, I managed to parlay a simple sprain into a six-month layoff.

Finally, showing a glimmer of wisdom, I left my ankle alone until it felt completely healed, and then left it alone some more. Eventually, I was able to return to a regular, pain-free, modest running routine.

As the weeks went by, though, I found myself thinking again about the marathon. It was like an old lover you swore you'd never call again, but whose number you kept. I began increasing my weekly mileage, waiting for the pain to come, but it never did. Finally, one day I wrote another check and sealed another envelope. I was going back to the Marine Corps Marathon.

In the final weeks before the race I was cautious to a fault, refusing to run off-road, step on cracks, or walk under ladders. I was rewarded by making it to the race day healthy and whole. Before the race even started, I had already accomplished my goal.

There were things that I still had left to learn, however. As I walked to the starting line near the Iwo Jima Memorial, I saw a woman standing just a few feet from the roadway, near a tree. She was carefully holding back her shorts to one side as she crouched slightly in the direction of the tree. It took me a moment to realize what she was doing. She was peeing. Right there, in front of 13,000 runners and their families and friends. Even more startling, though, was the fact that no one around her seemed the least bit surprised. She could have been blowing her nose for all they cared.

It was a revelation. I wasn't yet familiar with running culture, with the fact that runners are endlessly fascinated with their bodies—how they work, how they look, what goes into them, and most importantly, what comes out and when. And they were not the least bit shy about discussing all these issues with anyone at any time. Remember: I had done most of my training alone at that point, so I was like a feral child, a Tarzan among socialized runners.

Then the starting cannon roared—a Marine Corp Marathon tradition—and I had no more time to think about such things. The crowd surged forward. We began to run, and then suddenly, inexplicably, came to a full stop. Bodies crashed into one another. After a few moments of awkward shuffling, the crowd moved forward again, and we were able to settle into a regular running pace.

I was confused. What had just happened? There was open road in front of us. Why the sudden traffic jam? I didn't know it at the time, but that stop-and-go phenomenon happens in almost every big race. And I still don't know why. But I've learned not to let it bother me.

I ran cautiously, hoping to save enough energy to get me through the final few miles. We ran south to the Pentagon before returning north and crossing Key Bridge into D.C. We ran past the historic row houses and shops of Georgetown, and along the riverfront to the Lincoln Memorial, where we turned eastward toward the Smithsonian museums and the Capitol. I thought about how this route must seem for the out-of-town runners; even as a resident, I often have moments—as I did during the race—where I'm startled by how beautiful D.C. is.

I passed the halfway point at the U.S. Capitol feeling surprisingly strong. With 13 miles behind me, I decided to take a calculated risk—I picked up the pace. Streaking downhill past the Smithsonian museums, I passed the Jefferson Memorial and turned south toward lonely Hains Point, a pointy spit of land—landfill, actually—that juts out into the Potomac River.

This would be the make-or-break point for many runners. Hains Point brought with it miles 19 and 20 of the race, where the dreaded Wall lurked. If a runner had not properly prepared his or her body during training to burn fat, then it would be somewhere around this point where the supplies of blood sugar in the body—glycogen—would be used up. When that happens, a runner feels like someone just cut his or her power cord. Even well-trained runners who don't face this problem still find this stretch of road difficult because so many miles have been conquered, but there are still so many miles yet to come. This is the point where mental toughness weighs in. It's no wonder that veteran runners say the marathon is really two races: the first 20 miles, and the last 6.2.

I didn't know all of this at the time, which was probably a good thing, since I couldn't worry about something I wasn't expecting. But as I approached the turnaround at the tip of Hains Point, I felt my energy wane and my willpower slip. I was suddenly so tired of running.

Then I saw him. Or rather, heard him. A lone fan, standing beside his open car trunk at the tip of Hains Point, was blasting the theme from *Rocky* on his car stereo. Suddenly, adrenaline surged through my veins, and I felt new life in my tired legs as I followed the course back north for the final few miles to the finish line.

Before I could claim my finisher's medal, however, there was the 14th Street Bridge, a long, wide, rolling overpass that would take us from D.C. to Virginia. I later learned to call this stretch the Anvil of God, since, on a warm day, the sun can pour heat down on a runner along this stretch with unrivaled cruelty.

On this day, though, I had come too far to be denied, and I conquered that last obstacle and then raced the final few miles toward the finish line at the Iwo Jima Memorial. I passed the final mile marker—Mile 26!—and followed the course up a short, steep incline toward the memorial. Spectators massed along the retaining fence cheered as I followed the course as it circled the memorial, eager for a glimpse of that glorious finish line.

But where was it? Those final two-tenths of a mile seemed to stretch on forever. But finally, there it was: the finish line. I crossed it, and turned toward one of the marines to accept my finisher's medal. "Outstanding," he said. And I had to admit, it was.

I had run the second half 15 minutes faster than the first half, an impressive negative split, as I later learned to call it. I felt both brilliantly alive and bone tired, something I'd never before experienced, but that I completely enjoyed. I even liked the soreness that overtook my legs over the next few days. My friends were horrified watching me hobble downstairs backward, but I knew that every ache meant that I had faced my fear and doubt and won. I had run a marathon.

Having reached that milestone, I turned toward a few others that were on my calendar. In 1988, I graduated from law school, passed the bar exam, and began working as an attorney with the federal government. Instead of making D.C. a quick stopover, I was settling down as a permanent resident. And instead of being a distraction from my studies, running became my lifestyle. Perhaps if I spent less time in front of a computer, I wouldn't have become so devoted to it. Or maybe I was genetically predisposed to run. Either way, I found myself figuring out how to fit my running into my new work schedule. I woke up before dawn to run, brought my gear to the office for a quick lunchtime workout, and ran on weekends. Whatever it took, I made it work.

Three years later, I ran the Marine Corps Marathon again, no longer burdened with a fear of the unknown, but instead looking for another hit of that exhilarated/exhausted feeling. After another successful run, I turned homeward, toward New York City. I was finally ready to check off that boyhood goal.

On race morning, I stood shoulder to shoulder with 20,000 other runners in Staten Island, at the foot of the Verrazano Bridge. The gun went off, and we all surged up the mile-long climb to the apex of the bridge, jostling for a little elbow room along the way. After cresting, I found myself warmed up and energized for the mile-long descent. It was the fastest mile I'd ever run. And I still had 24 more miles to go. I quickly realized how monumentally stupid I'd just been, and how I'd pay dearly for it later in the race.

I settled down into a slower pace and made my way through Brooklyn and Queens, and then climbed the Queensboro Bridge to Manhattan. As I descended on the far side—at a comfortable pace, this time!—I began to hear a mysterious low roar. I was almost on the Manhattan side, but I still couldn't see where the noise was coming from. Then I saw it: a solid mass of people, five or six deep, straining the barricades, screaming like they had lost their minds. I was dumbstruck.

The party continued up First Avenue, as people lined the streets, hung out windows, crowded onto balconies, and stood on rooftops, all cheering like mad. I felt like an astronaut in a parade. It shot a bolt of lightning into me. I ran effortlessly up toward Harlem.

That's where my earlier foolishness hit me. This time I was the one who felt as though someone had cut my power cord. I was reduced to walking. Suddenly, a huge man jumped out of the crowd and rushed toward me. I braced myself, but he just yelled, "I didn't come out here to see you walk!" Believe me, I was back to running in no time flat!

From there, it was on to the Bronx, into neighborhoods that I had never seen in all my years living in New York. Then it was time for the homestretch down Fifth Avenue and into Central Park. My mother and younger sister were waiting for me near the finish line, and had talked other bystanders into cheering for me as I came into view, but I was so focused on the finish line that I never heard a thing. No matter. Just knowing they were there, watching for me and cheering me onward, gave me the extra strength I needed.

Finishing that race meant a lot to me. It taught me that I could overcome adversity during a race, and also that I had a lot yet to learn about running this thing.

In March of 1993, I ran my fourth marathon, in Virginia Beach. After the race, in the hotel corridor, I met an older runner who told me that he had just run his thirty-fifth marathon. I was astonished.

The number seemed impossible, like Joe DiMaggio's consecutive-game hitting streak. I was sure that this guy was a different breed of runner.

I expected to feel tired after the Virginia Beach marathon, but instead, I craved more. There was something about the marathon that called to me, that captured my imagination, that left me feeling a sense of accomplishment like I'd experienced nowhere else. I wasn't sure if it was a good idea to run another marathon so soon—I hadn't heard of anyone else doing something like that—but I felt fresh and strong, and was certainly motivated, so I ran the Pittsburgh Marathon two months later, where the scorching heat reduced me to walking most of the last few miles. My suffering there was alleviated by the sight of one late-night reveler in leather pants and boots, who, after stumbling out his door and squinting at the bright daylight, looked at all the runners streaming past and asked someone, "Where are they all going?"

I ran two more marathons that same year, still electrified by the experience. Like a child who's discovered how to walk, I was amazed at what my body could now do. It was as if I'd walked through a doorway into a brand-new, beautiful room that I hadn't known was there. I even began to earn a reputation at work as being an avid marathoner; I became known as *that running guy*.

The marathons then came in bunches, like a blizzard following a few errant snowflakes. I ran six in 1994, including one in Philadelphia, where I found myself desperate at one point to relieve myself, but without a Porta-Jon or bush in sight. Spectators lined the streets, but I had little choice but to use a light post as my bathroom stall. Looking over to my left, I saw a policeman. He just looked the other way. This road racing was a funny business.

By 1995 people had begun calling me "obsessed," but I thought of myself as just being enthusiastic, and I continued running and racing. I traveled back and forth across the continent, and overseas as well. In 1998, in Madison, Wisconsin, I reached marathon number 35, and I realized that I was now like the older runner I had met a few years earlier in Virginia Beach. Like him, I was now a different breed of runner.

But what kind of runner was I now? I had proven beyond any doubt that I could run a marathon, and yet the marathon distance still intrigued me. Rather than slaking my thirst for racing, each marathon left me wanting more. I knew that I could simply keep running and racing, but that alone wouldn't be enough. I had entered my first marathon because I needed a goal to focus my training. Now I needed a similar goal to focus my racing. I had proven to myself that although I might not be the fastest runner in the field, I was one of the most durable. So my challenge would be to find out exactly how durable I was. If thirty-five marathons once amazed me, what would be a suitable goal now?

*100 marathons*. As soon as I thought of it, I knew that I had the right answer. Even if it was an arbitrary number, it was beautiful. It seemed complete. Ninety-nine marathons cried out for one more; 101 marathons seemed a stop on the way toward another goal. But 100 was perfect. It was also a number that would, in its audacity, seem insane even to other athletes. Totaled up in miles, it described a course heading west from my home in Washington, D.C., all the way to Carson City, Nevada. It was a feat of running that most people couldn't imagine, but it was something that I really felt that I could do. The thought of it also scared and exhilarated me, which meant, of course, that it was just the kind of challenge I was looking for.

In fact, as I discovered, I wasn't the first person to take on and beat such a challenge. Still, the club of people who have run 100 marathons is a pretty select one, and even if that weren't true—even if hundreds of thousands of other runners across the globe had done it—it was not something *I* had done. And that was the point. Ultimately, it was going to be a challenge not of the human spirit and body, but of *my* spirit and body. And so I committed myself to it.

Then, seemingly way too soon, it happened. It actually took eighteen years, but it happened. One hundred marathons. 2,620 miles of racing. Finished.

Here are the memories and lessons of those eighteen years of marathon racing. My first 100 marathons. Compressed within these pages are the joys and agonies of all those long miles, and, I hope, some of the knowledge that came from making a habit of pushing myself beyond pain and fear and doubt.

When I talk about my marathons, I feel like a child who can't wait to show his birthday gift to his friends. "See this? Isn't it the coolest thing you've ever seen?" After almost two decades, I think it still is, and by the time you've reached the end of this journey, I hope you'll see why.

## Running Tip #1

### *Getting Started*

- *Get proper gear.* Buy shoes in a proper running store, where they can identify your particular needs. And avoid cotton clothing; cotton stays wet and makes you colder if you're cold and hotter if you're hot.
- *Warm up.* Start each run with a 5-minute walk or slow jog. Running too hard too soon will only make for a miserable run.
- *Breathe smoothly.* Find a pace that allows you to talk while running. Runners who run out of breath don't run very long.
- *Stay relaxed.* Keep your shoulders low, and swing your arms smoothly, with your hands near your upper hip.
- *Don't overstride.* Your foot should land directly under your body.
- *Don't be too ambitious!* Keep your mileage increases to no more than 10 percent from week to week.

# Why Run the Marathon? First Lap

Looking back, I could see that once I put on my first pair of running shoes and set out down the street, it was probably inevitable that I would want to run a marathon. Like a Little League baseball player dreaming of the major leagues, distance runners dream of the marathon.

It didn't necessarily have to be that way—I'm told that there are runners out there who are content to do their training and never pin on a race number. Regular training, as opposed to racing, brings all the proven benefits of weight control, cardiovascular health, and improved emotional outlook, and all with as little work as three sessions of 20–30 minutes a week. And many runners who choose to race are often content to just run 5Ks and 10Ks. But that wasn't good enough for me, or for almost a half-million other people in the United States every year who are drawn to the marathon. Why? At some level, it isn't good enough to just say that it seemed like a good challenge, that it felt right, that it was hard but fun.

It's a simple question, really, so there should be a simple answer: Why run the marathon?

Perhaps the answer is in our desire to be part of something bigger than ourselves, to connect with history and become a part of it. The marathon, after all, is the most famous and storied of all footraces. Here's the original story, in a thumbnail sketch, taken straight from Herodotus (more or less): Sometime around 490 BC, Darius the Great of Persia amassed a huge army and moved to conquer each of the Greek city-states, which had not yet united into a single power. The cities fell one by one, and soon only Athens and Sparta remained independent.

Darius landed some 30,000 soldiers at the plains of Marathon and prepared to attack Athens. Athens gathered a force of 10,000 soldiers to meet them under the leadership of Athenian general Miltiades, who immediately sent a runner named Phidippides to Sparta, some 150 miles distant, to ask for help. The Spartans were celebrating a religious holiday, and would only send warriors once the festival ended five days later. Phidippides raced back and relayed the news to Miltiades, who decided to strike alone before the Persians became fully prepared. The Athenians flanked the Persians and then encircled them, hacking their way through toward the Persian center. Once the carnage had ended, Darius's army had suffered some 6,400 casualties, while Miltiades had lost a scant 192 men. More or less.

News of the victory was delivered by a *hemerodromoi*— an "all-day runner." And that was the end of that. Except that centuries later, in the retelling, it was Phidippides who raced the 25 miles from the battlefield to Athens, shouted *"Nenikékamen!"*— we are victorious!"—and then dropped dead.

More or less.

Well, the battle certainly happened, as a large burial mound on the modern plains of Marathon silently confirms. And runners were certainly used as messengers. As for the rest, well, we'll never know for sure.

Now flash forward: the modern Olympic Games were being held in 1896 in Athens, and among the events planned was a 25-mile footrace called a marathon, held in commemoration of Phidippides's legendary run. The race ended with a dramatic and rousing victory for the Greek runner Spiridon Louis. Witnessing the first Olympic Games was a young Bostonian who was so enamored of the marathon that upon returning home, he convinced his athletic club to host a similar marathon race. Thus was born the Boston Marathon, the oldest annually held marathon in the world. But the marathon race wasn't yet a set distance; it wasn't yet the race we know today.

By 1908, the Olympic movement was firmly established, and the Games were being held in London. The royal family, apparently impressed by the fortitude of the distance runners, wanted to witness the race finish from the royal box. Accommodating their wishes added another mile and 385 yards to the 25-mile race distance. And that's how we ended up with the strange total of 26.2 miles for the marathon race.

The marathon, as an established race, is now over a century old. We have seen barefoot champions and computer chips in racers' shoes, and the erosion of racial and gender biases. We have also seen record times drop to seemingly inhuman levels, with the current world's best mark at 2 hours, 4 minutes, 26 seconds for men and 2 hours, 15 minutes, 25 seconds for women.[1]

---

1 These records were set by Haile Gebrsellasie of Ethiopia in the 2007 Berlin Marathon and Paula Radcliffe of Great Britain in the 2003 London Marathon.

Amazing stories. Captivating figures. Triumph, elation, tears, and disappointment. It's all there. Perhaps, then, we marathoners race to become part of this great tradition, to become part of an unbroken line of history stretching back to those brave Athenians, to share in the glory.

Perhaps, except that most modern marathoners probably don't know all of this history when they toe the line on race day, and in truth, it would have little impact on their choice to race a marathon even if they did. And glory? No. Except for the lucky few elite runners, modern marathoners do not race for fame or fortune. We toil in obscurity, part of the mass of bobbing heads that fill a city's streets on a Sunday morning once a year. Our friends and family will tire of congratulating us after several days have gone, and our names and finishing times will eventually be lost to history.

So, again, why run the marathon?

Maybe the answer is not in the history of the race, but in the moment, in the here and now of conquering the racecourse. Few of us ever find ourselves enjoying the adulation of the crowds, and having thousands of people screaming encouragement and calling your name is an adrenaline rush of the first magnitude. That would certainly get most people out of bed in the morning.

Some people misunderstand the attraction of cheering, though. An administrative assistant in my office once decided to write a short piece about my running for our newsletter. I started by explaining to him the thrill of Boston and New York. During everyday life, I told him, you rarely know exactly where you stand. You might be doing great at work and in your relationship, or you might be doing badly, but most often it's hard to tell. Life is filled with mixed signals, and anything can change in a second, often with little explanation, and no one cheers you on if you do the right thing. But when you run a marathon, life is wonderfully and beautifully simple. You run 26.2 miles as fast as you can, and you get a medal if you finish. Along the way you have hundreds or thousands of people telling you what a great job you're doing and how great you look. What's not to love about that?

My interviewer nodded appreciatively and diligently took notes. When he left my office, I felt like an evangelist who had just brought someone new into the flock. *He gets it,* I thought.

Then the newsletter came out, and I quickly turned to his article. "Jeff is going to run the Boston Marathon this month," it began. "He said he does it for the attention." Ugh.

But while the cheers of the crowd are a good motivation for a great many people, a few hours of cheering hardly seems a good return on the months of sacrifice and effort that preceded it. Cheers also cannot fully explain my own marathon odyssey, because few of my marathons attract runners by the tens of thousands. Some of them cannot attract even 100 racers. Instead of being cheered by hundreds of thousands of spectators and fans at these races, I'm often only quietly observed only by a few hardy volunteers shivering by their refreshment tables. On those days, far from the boisterous crowds, the question remains: Why the marathon?

The failure to be able to explain my running passion became a problem for me. The more I was asked the question, the more I realized that I needed an answer, if only for my own peace of mind. I came to fear that perhaps I wasn't running *toward* something, so much as I was running *away* from something. One day I watched a report on television about a man who overcame his addiction to drugs and alcohol by running a marathon every weekend. The interviewer marveled at the amazing transformation, but I wasn't so impressed. It sounded to me only that the man had traded one set of addictions for another. I had seen people like that, and the results were never good. Eventually, the wheels would come off, and some debilitating injury would end their marathon streak. Usually the person would then lurch off in another direction, and become addicted to something else. I felt that my own enthusiasm was much different, but how could I be sure?

What I needed were some tests, some indicators that I had not wandered off onto dangerous ground. I found one while racing in St. Louis in 1997. During the course of 26.2 miles, you tend to notice the other runners around you. It's not uncommon for strangers to congratulate one another at the finish line, or to strike up a conversation and offer encouragement during the race to pass the time. In St. Louis, I realized that the man next to me had matched me stride for stride over several miles.

"Nice pace," I told him. "You're looking strong."

"Thanks," he replied. "I need to be fast. I told my wife that I wouldn't do this anymore. She thinks I'm out getting the newspaper."

I'm no marriage counselor, but even I could see trouble there.

From that exchange, I spotted a potential test: I would simply ask whether I had ever tried to hide my running. Although the answer wouldn't say much about why I was running, it would, hopefully, prove that whatever the reason was, it wasn't a bad one.

I probed my memory, and found my answer: I hadn't lied about my racing.

I then asked myself a second question: had I ever forced myself to run? Sure, there were some days where it was a bit tough getting out the door, but I generally looked forward to my runs, and enjoyed them. There was a moment in just about every run where I felt strong and eternal; not exactly the mythical "runner's high," but a comforting sense of well-being that made all the difficult parts of the run worthwhile. Skeptics say it's simply the result of an endorphin and adrenaline cocktail that my body concocts for me, but that seemed such a spiteful way of describing it, like describing love as a product of certain glandular secretions. When I feel it, it feels great, and that's good enough for me. Of all of life's great pleasures—sex, a great meal, a glorious sunset— a good run has to be near the top.

Such pleasure hardly ever comes without a price, however. If the pleasure of running is truly chemical, it's possible to become addicted to those chemicals. Evidence of such addiction isn't hard to find; many runners insist on hitting the roads despite aching joints and strained muscles. It seems like they had somehow lost sight of the fact that running is supposed to make them feel better, not worse. It's important to be dedicated enough to train hard. However, as I learned—the hard way—it's even more important to be dedicated enough to know when to stop.

I discovered the next test in my third attempt at the Marine Corps Marathon. After finding success in 1987, I decided to try again the following year. I had a difficult training cycle, though, and had dramatically cut back on my running in order to relieve an ache in my knees. My injury disappeared, but as I stood at the starting line before the race, I was nervous that my sacrifice left me unprepared for the race.

I flew through the early miles in the race, and I began to think that I had worried needlessly. But the first lesson of the marathon is not to put too much stock in how you feel at any one moment, since there is plenty of time for things to change. Sure enough, an hour later I was struggling badly. Like a car that has run out of gas, but is still rolling, I shuffled onward toward the finish. Doubt crept into my thinking for the first time, and I began to realize that I would soon have to make a tough decision.

At mile 17 I looked down at my feet, and saw that they were hardly moving, with 9 miles still left to go. I was exhausted, and I suddenly knew that the time had come. I dropped out of the race. I stepped over to the curb and just stopped. It was an odd sensation. Just stepping off the course is a temptation that nips at the heels of every runner who finds himself or herself in distress, but the desire to stay on the course is so great that most of us would rather risk a complete breakdown and injury than take those few steps to the side. But when I did it, it felt as though I no longer even had a choice. I was through, and I knew it. To confirm that point, my muscles stiffened and cramped as soon as I hit the grass.

I should have been upset about my failure, but I wasn't. I knew I had fought as valiantly as I could, but that it was simply not my day. Elite runners drop out of races all the time to save their bodies from unnecessary punishment. But even as I was heading home, I began to analyze why it had happened. Being at peace with my decision to drop out didn't mean that I ever wanted to repeat that experience.

In the years since that day, I have looked back on that DNF (Did Not Finish) as a benchmark of sorts. It was proof that I knew when it was time to quit. Since then, every time I pass mile 17 in a race, I think of that failure, and remind myself that I would always struggle to run the best race that I could, but that in the end, I would not push myself into the danger zone out of sheer stubbornness. I knew that as much as I wanted to finish every race that I entered, I would never be unmindful of the cost. After overcoming injuries and setbacks, I would not sell my running future for a fleeting moment of personal glory on race day. I would not force myself to run.

Still, simply refraining from lying about my racing and avoiding injuries hardly sounds like a ringing endorsement for a lifestyle choice. I was hoping for something that would be a little more useful, that would get to the heart of my running. Ultimately, I found it, and it was a simple thing.

Crossing the finish line, as I had explained to countless people, was a wonderful, life-changing experience, and its glory is never diminished by the number of times I've done it. If anything, my earlier DNF only made each marathon finish that much more precious to me, since I had been forced to realize how much could go wrong in preparing for and racing a marathon. I came to realize that if ever I should cross a finish line and feel disappointed over my time and my performance, the marathon would no longer be a transcendent event for me. It would have lost its meaning, and devolved into drudgery and work. When that happened, I knew that it would be time for me to quit.

So far, though, that day had not yet come, and each marathon finish was a life-affirming event for me, whether I ran my best times or my worst, because in each marathon I did my best, and that was cause enough for celebration.

With those thoughts in mind, I gave myself a clean bill of mental health, reassured that I was not running for the wrong reasons. But still, I had not really answered the question why. But why does anyone do anything? Why do painters paint and singers sing? I realized that I would not be able to answer this question all at once, so I put it away to ponder another time, and went out for a run.

# A New Quest

$B$y the end of 1995, I had run eighteen marathons, but my life had changed quite a bit. As an attorney with the National Labor Relations Board, I protected employees' rights to act together to improve their working conditions. It was an interesting job, exposing me to stories from a great number of people from all walks of life, and giving me an opportunity to help people who had been treated unfairly. But as much satisfaction as I got from that job, I was still enthralled by my running. At work, it was frustrating to see how many people I couldn't help—or couldn't help enough—and there were days when I wondered how much I had really accomplished.

With running, however, my achievements were clear, and the joy I took in my running wasn't tempered by any misgivings or compromises. Little by little, running spilled over into all the corners of my life; even the drawers in my office were filled with energy bars and running clothes.

And I had still not yet become bored of the marathon. I had braved an arctic cold front in Delaware that brought windchill temperatures below zero and froze sweat into icicles hanging from runners' headbands and caps. I had completed marathons in eleven different states, from Virginia to Nevada, plus D.C. It occurred to me that with a little organization, I could run a marathon in every state. The thought quickly settled comfortably in my mind. It was an elegantly simple and daunting challenge. Fifty states, fifty marathons. An added bonus to my goal of running 100 marathons, there for the taking.

As it turned out, just as with my 100-marathon goal, I hadn't been the first person to imagine this quest, either. There was actually an informal club of runners who had set this goal for themselves, and some of them were even working on their second tally. Rather than feeling diminished by this fact, however, I felt comforted. Nothing confirms our sanity more than finding out that there are people out there crazier than ourselves. Membership in the club was open to runners who had completed marathons in ten different states. I was eligible, so I joined the club. I was now an official marathon lunatic.

During the six years that I'd been racing, I also had seen my best time, my Personal Record time, drop from 3 hours, 45 minutes in my first marathon, to 3 hours, 35 minutes. Ten minutes may not sound like much, but it felt like a monumental achievement to me.

My dream for the marathon, my fantasy goal, was to qualify for the Holy Grail of road racing, the Boston Marathon. Boston was special to me not only for its storied history, but also for its elitism; it was the only marathon in the country for which you had to prequalify. There are no slow, novice racers in Boston, at least not officially, because having a race number itself means that you have already finished a marathon in qualifying time. The required times vary according to age and gender, as explained on the race Web site. I was in the most challenging group: men under 35 years of age. To toe the line in Boston, I would have to run a marathon in 3 hours 10 minutes or less. That was 25 minutes faster than I had run a marathon in six years of racing. Impossible. Or so I thought.

Qualifying is not actually the only way to the start line for the Boston Marathon. The Boston Athletic Association donates a certain number of race numbers to designated charities, which give them to runners who have met a designated fundraising goal. I was so sure that I would never qualify for the race that I managed to get a number this way. So I ran Boston, but I did not have the "Boston Marathon experience." I hadn't qualified, and I didn't have the kind of speed or toughness to run Boston the way it deserved to be run. Rather than a race, my marathon there felt more like a long training run. It just didn't feel right. I swore to myself that if I ever lined up at the start of another Boston Marathon, it would be because I had earned it, and deserved to be there. Until that happened, in my mind, I had never really run the race.

I kept running, and my times did improve. I posted 3:21:28 in Chicago in October 1995, and then 3:19:41 in the Mayor's Midnight Marathon in Anchorage Alaska in June 1996. That race wasn't held at midnight, as its name promised, but it might as well have been. There really isn't any darkness in Alaska in June. There is daylight, twilight, then daylight again. It was a confusing place for someone from "the Lower 48." There were none of the telltale signs of gathering evening. At one point I realized that it was late evening only because all of the stores had closed. Apart from that, it looked like high noon.

I couldn't help having a bit of fun with this; I called my mother and told her that I was calling from a pay phone in a park in the dead of night. Being a native New Yorker, Mom feared the worst. "Get out of there!" she told me, her voice rising. "Don't worry, Mom. I'm just watching a softball game right now, under clear blue skies."

I returned from Alaska still nine minutes from qualifying for Boston. It might as well have been nine hours for all it mattered. I was sure that I had pushed my body to its limit; it had gone about as fast as it would ever go.

Then I discovered track workouts. I had always trained alone, but I knew that running didn't have to be that way. I found out about a running club in D.C. that held track workouts every Wednesday at Georgetown University, and one day after work I showed up at the track, curious and eager. By the time it was over, I felt like I had stepped from the black-and-white world of Kansas into the splendor of Oz. I had discovered speed work.

Speed work, also called interval training, conditions the body to run faster by alternating hard repeats of shorter distances with slower recovery laps. Done correctly, it avoids the injuries that come with added stress from hard running, while making the most of the beneficial adaptations caused by hard running. It was as different from running long miles as riding a supercharged motorcycle is from taking a leisurely drive in the country.

I loved it. On the first day I showed up for training, I was near the back of the pack during the workout, but in the following weeks I slowly moved up toward the front. We ran different workouts every week—quarter-mile intervals, half miles, miles. Each one was an adventure. Ironically, the trick was not running too hard, since sprinting improves short distance speed, but doesn't prepare the body to run faster for longer distances. It took wisdom and experience to know how fast to run, and little by little, I learned.

The coach who called out our weekly workouts assured us that speed work would not only improve our race times but also familiarize us with pacing, as we learned to associate given effort levels with particular clock times. If I had any doubts about this claim, they were dispelled when I ran with a woman who told me her exact goal for each repeat, and then proceeded to run each interval within a second or two of her goal, without ever looking at her watch. She did it by feel alone.

I was impressed. That was the kind of runner I wanted to be.

I met other runners as well at the track: men and women, old and young, fast and, well, less fast. I joined them for food and beer after the workouts, and met them for long Sunday morning runs. There was Camilla, Yvonne, Stewart, Darryl, and two Beths, both of whom were fast runners. I was discovering that running didn't have to be a solitary sport; there was a running *community*.

One day on the track, I tried to block out the discomfort of hard running by thinking about West Virginia. A marathon was being held there that coming Sunday, and I was debating whether I wanted to drive out there to run it. In addition to adding to my overall marathon total, racing in West Virginia would also add to my total of states, since I hadn't entered a marathon there yet. That was the positive side. I would have to drive out there alone to do it, though. That was the negative.

By the time the workout was over, I still hadn't decided what to do. As I stretched and gathered up my gear, another runner told me in passing that he was debating running a marathon that weekend himself. It was June, when few marathons are held because of the heat. Could he be thinking about West Virginia? He was. Would he be interested in going out there together and splitting the driving? He was. That's how I met Dave Harrell.

Dave was more than twenty years older than me. He had come to marathoning later in life, but like me, had taken to it with a passion. He had run a dozen or so marathons, all over the mid-Atlantic and North-east. He ran with an easy, gliding style, an economy of effort that enabled him to win or place in his age group in many of the races in which he competed.

Dave, however, differed from me in one important respect: his racing strategy. Not one for subtlety, Dave started each race with the intent to run as fast as he could for as long as he could. While most runners start off conservatively and then try to maintain or even increase their speed over the miles, Dave liked to jump out in front early, which he usually paid for with great suffering in the final few miles. It was an unorthodox style, strange to see and difficult to match, uncommon in a runner with Dave's experience. But that was how Dave liked to run, and he wasn't going to change.

The race in West Virginia was called the Ridge Runner, and true to its name, it started with two daunting climbs in the first mile up a ridge, with another long ascent late in the race, and a fast, painful descent at the end. At the crack of the starter's gun, I was surprised to see Dave take off like a bat out of hell. I had thought we might run together, at least for a while, but upon seeing the road rise up in front of me, I decided to let him go, and concentrated on hauling myself up to the top of the ridge. As the race wore on, I found myself feeling stronger, as I usually did at some point midway through my races, and I picked up my pace. It was a beautiful course, and I enjoyed the views all the way through to the end. I flew down the final descent and crossed the finish line, and finally found Dave, who had already crossed the line before me. As I soon learned, he had only crossed it some 41 seconds before I did.

Dave and I didn't know each other well at this point, but that didn't stop us from talking trash. I thought it was obvious that if I had known that he was less than a minute in front of me, I would have sped up and caught him. Unbelievably, Dave insisted that if he knew I was right behind him, he would have sped up and left me in the dust. By the time we made it back to our hotel, we had decided that there was only one way to resolve our dispute: a 40-yard dash. Never mind that we just ran a difficult marathon. Our competitive fires were lit, and there was no other way to douse them.

So, still wearing our race clothing, now whitened with a salt residue from our sweat, we marked out the course in front of the hotel: from here to that second streetlight. *Go!* I ran as fast as I could, but I was horrified to see Dave pull a step in front of me. Laughing and yelling, I lunged forward and grabbed at his singlet, but he evaded me and made it to the finish first. Again. Grrrrr! No hard feelings, though; it had all been in fun, and we went into our hotel to clean up and check out.

On the ride home, and later at the track, Dave and I talked about our race goals. I suggested to Dave that given his past marathoning experience, and his ambitious plans for the future, all it would take for him to also complete the fifty states would be a bit of organization and planning. With his volume of racing, if we timed it right, Dave and I might also reach 100 marathons together. Dave rolled it around in his mind for a moment, then grinned. I had found a racing partner.

I don't know what drove Dave to run with such dedication. It wasn't something we ever spoke about. Sometimes those kinds of questions are the hardest to answer; I still wasn't even exactly sure why I took to long-distance running like I had. At the least, it was a good balance to the hours I spent at a desk. I've heard it said that running is like meditation, since the rhythm of the legs and the breathing can lull one into a quiet, thought-free state. I've experienced that, but I've also experienced moments of deep, focused thought, where I worked through problems and issues that have arisen in my life. Perhaps my love of running came from one of these things, or perhaps it came from them all. Or, perhaps, it came from something else entirely. I couldn't exactly say.

I don't know if Dave wondered about these things. If he did, he never told me. We did most of our communication with our legs, over hundreds and hundreds of miles. We both knew, without ever saying it aloud, that each of us had recognized that there was something perfect about the marathon, something that made it one of the most important things in our lives. We understood this about each other. There was nothing more that needed to be said. Any other questions that I had, I would have to answer on my own.

## Running Tip #2

### Ten-Week Speed Program

It's been said that there are as many running programs as there are coaches. Here's mine. Give it a chance, and remember to do a 1-mile warm-up and cooldown.

- Week 1—4 X 880m (half-mile) @ 10K race pace/moderately hard (15–20 seconds faster than marathon race pace), with a 440m slow recovery between each repeat
- Week 2—6 X 880m @ 10K race pace/moderately hard, with a 440m recovery
- Week 3—440m (quarter mile), 880m, 1320m (3-quarter mile), 880m, 440m @ 10K race pace/moderately hard, with a 440m recovery
- Week 4—8 X 880m @10K race pace/moderately hard, with a 440m recovery
- Week 5—10 X 440m @ 5K race pace/hard, with a 220m recovery
- Week 6—3 X 1760m (1 mile) @ 10K race pace/moderately hard, with a 440m recovery
- Week 7—2 X 2 miles @ 10K race pace/moderately hard, with a 440m recovery
- Week 8—1 X 1760m, 1 X 2 mile, 1 X 1760m @ 10K pace/moderately hard, with a 440m recovery
- Week 9—10 X 880m (half mile) @ 10K pace/moderately hard, with a 440m recovery, 5 minute rest after repeat number 5
- Week 10—4 X 1760m @ 10K race pace/moderately hard, with a 440m recovery

# The Magical Year

By 1996, I had worked in the same office for eight years. I enjoyed working for the Labor Board and wanted to stay there, but I also wanted to do something different. So I became an appellate litigator for my agency, defending its decisions before the U.S. Courts of Appeal. The first time I stood up at the podium to argue a case was a nerve-racking moment. The courtroom seemed huge, and was subtly designed to impart an aura of importance to the proceedings, as well as intimidate all who entered. As I looked up at the three judges who would hear my case, my heart felt like it was about to rip through my body. And then I began to speak. "May it please the Court, my name is Jeff Horowitz, and I represent the National Labor Relations Board."

Suddenly, calmness came over me, and I felt completely at ease as I laid out the facts and the law for the judges, answering their questions and deflecting any criticism. It only lasted 10 minutes—average for an appellate argument—but when it was over, I felt an incredible sense of power and release. I loved it. Some attorneys in my office loved the grind of writing the briefs we had to submit, and dreaded oral argument, but I was the opposite. I liked the immediacy and danger of appearing in court.

It was almost as good as finishing a marathon. Almost. But compared to the adrenaline rush of the marathon finish line, it was no contest. Racing was my drug of choice.

Still, I had a lot to learn. In May, I flew to Cleveland for the old Revco Marathon. Having already run twenty-one marathons, I thought myself invincible, so I went out for Chinese food the night before the big race. Spicy eggplant. It turned on me at about mile 14 of the course the next day. Of course, there were no portable toilets anywhere in sight just then, and as I snuck down a dark alleyway, clutching the biggest leaves I could find, I swore that I would never take any chances again.

So, I was not invincible. Lesson learned.

Even with all my mistakes, I was still doing an awful lot right, and I had my breakthrough year in 1997. I had been doing speed work regularly, and was doing my long weekend runs with a fast bunch of guys. I felt quick and strong, and as the 1997 racing season, I felt an upsurge of confidence. I knew with great certainty that I would set a personal record every time I raced.

I was right. I ran a 5K in under 20 minutes, a 10-mile race in 62 minutes, and a half-marathon in 1:27. In late September, I ran marathon number 30 in East Lyme, Connecticut, in 3:12:57. Only 3 minutes separated me from the Boston Marathon. I began to believe it was possible.

I was scheduled to run my next marathon three weeks later in Detroit. It was a well-organized race with potential: a fast, flat course, not too big a field. I drove out there with my running buddies, who were also racing, and patiently waited for the race. We went to a University of Michigan football game, toured the city, ate, and rested. Finally, it was time to run.

The Detroit Marathon actually started in Canada, and boasted the only underground mile in marathoning, as runners were herded through a tunnel back to the United States. As with every marathon, the air seemed to crackle with energy as we waited for the race to start. My friends and I began as a pack, hoping to run together for as long as possible. As we ran, I happened to notice one woman in particular, running directly in front of me. My eyes traced down her long blond hair to her blue running tights, stretched taut over her lean body. Her stride was beautiful, and utterly mesmerizing. After a few seconds that seemed like an eternity, I sheepishly looked away. Glancing left and right, I saw that a row of five or six guys, including my friends, all had their eyes glued to the same spot. As if on cue, we all looked up, noticed each other, and broke into embarrassed laughter.

The early miles flew by. I separated from my friends and surged forward, settling into my target pace. As I moved into the second half of the race, I felt strong and was running well. I suddenly understood the pressure of having an ambitious time goal; every mile marker brought a quick recalculation of pace and split times. I counted down miles and counted seconds, and I knew that I had none to spare. In my previous thirty marathons, I was able to run relaxed, losing myself in the joy of the moment and in my thoughts, but not in Detroit. I spent precious energy trying to concentrate on the task at hand, to keep focused for mile after mile, hour after hour. It was excruciating. I used to daydream about being an elite runner, trading my desk for a schedule of full-time training and racing. It used to sound like heaven, but not any more; I realized that being a professional runner must be hard work.

With a mile to go, I was still on pace to qualify for Boston. I was tired and my muscles ached, but I knew that I only had minutes of pain left, and a lifetime to recover. *I could do this*, I thought. Being a marathoner meant that you were the kind of person who kept running when other people would quit. I was a marathoner. I would not quit. I pushed as hard as I could, my mind focused only on the rhythm of my running. Finally the finish line was in view. Flying across, I checked my time. 3:08:59. I had done it! A new personal best, and a qualifying time. I was going to return to Boston, and no one could say that I didn't deserve to be there.

But my big year wasn't over yet. I decided to risk mailing in an application for a race I wasn't sure I could even finish: the JFK 50 Mile. The name alone scared me. I had never before run an ultramarathon, and the thought of nearly doubling my longest race distance seemed insane. That, of course, is exactly what drew me to it. As intoxicating as it is to finish a marathon, something irretrievable is lost when that goal is first achieved: the fear that you cannot do it. The excitement that goes with that uncertainty is gone forever. After the finish line is crossed, the only question that remains for the future is whether you can do it again, or do it faster. Usually that's a good thing, but I found myself missing the unknown, missing the fear. When I mailed in my 50-miler race application, I felt a deep nervousness that I hadn't felt in years. After returning from Detroit, I gave myself a little recovery time, and then committed to myself to training with a fresh sense of urgency.

I did have several factors in my favor. First, I was already an accomplished marathoner, which meant that my body had become adept at relying on fat to fuel my running, instead of just glycogen. I had covered enough miles to make this adaptation, so I was confident that I would have an easier time transitioning to an ultramarathon than a beginning recreational runner would have transitioning to a regular marathon.

The second factor that calmed me was my realization that the longer the race distance, the less important it was to cover the target distance in training. This was reassuring; I wouldn't have to do a 50-mile training run in order to prepare for a 50-mile race. From everything I had read, the consensus seemed to be that a 35-mile run would give me a sufficient endurance base to conquer the JFK. Running 35 miles sounded much easier than running 50, which made this whole enterprise seem much more possible.

Still, 35 miles is still a long way to run by yourself. I would have to plan a way to get access to the supplies I would need. One option would be to just carry the food and drink I'd require, but that didn't sound too appealing, since I was looking at a 5-hour session. Another option would be to map out a route and stash food and drink on the course, but that didn't seem like a great idea either, since I couldn't be sure that the stuff I'd left out in plain view hours earlier would still be there when I really needed it. What I really needed, I thought, was to have refreshment stops, manned by volunteers, just like they have in the marathon. That's when the obvious solution hit me: I would use a full marathon as a training run, making full use of the course support throughout, and simply add another 9 miles of running at the end. Brilliant.

The race I chose was the Vulcan Marathon in Birmingham, Alabama, which was scheduled just three weeks after the Detroit Marathon, and just three weeks before the JFK. In addition to the perfect symmetry of this timetable, racing in Birmingham would add Alabama to the list of states I had run. I talked Dave into joining me—getting him to agree to run a marathon was like talking a kid into eating candy—and we flew down to Birmingham together.

Being from the Northeast, I thought sophistication ended at the Mason-Dixon line, but I discovered that Birmingham had beautiful neighborhoods, golf courses, and thriving shopping districts nestled within the city's boundaries. It was a good lesson to learn: there was a lot about this country that I knew nothing about.

On race day, Dave and I decided to abandon our all-out approach to marathoning, and instead committed ourselves to finishing the race together—no small accomplishment with pedal-to-the-metal Dave!—with a goal finish time of 3:30. I knew this meant that we'd both have to show restraint at different times, but as the race unfolded, I knew that we were doing the right thing. Not only was I reserving enough energy to continue running after I crossed the finish line, I was also enjoying having Dave as my companion throughout the race. Our shared racing goals had created a special bond, and the Vulcan Marathon seemed a fitting celebration of our brotherhood.

When the finish line came within view, we tried our best to cross the line at exactly the same time—3:31, within one minute of our goal. The official race Web site ended up awarding Dave the win by a few seconds, which led to endless ribbing. But that was later. After crossing the finish line, I still had work to do. I collected my medal and set out back on a street parallel to the course.

I was feeling surprisingly spry, and after running about 4.5 miles, I reversed course and dove back into the crowd of marathoners heading toward the finish line. It was a strange experience for me, since I was surrounded by runners who I never really got to see before: the back-of-the-pack runners who usually finished in 5 or 6 hours. As I weaved though them, I got more than one confused look from people who must have been wondering how I could be running so hard and still be so far back. I got more puzzled looks and comments from the aid station volunteers who recognized me from my first pass. I just shrugged and smiled and raced onward. When I got to the finish line, I veered off the course, and fought off the well-meaning and urgent directions of volunteers who tried to guide me into the finisher's chutes. I pulled out my medal and smiled. I had finished another marathon, but more importantly, I believed that I was ready for the JFK.

The JFK 50 Miler is legendary among ultramarathoners. It was inaugurated in 1963, after President Kennedy challenged his military staffers to complete a 50-mile hike in a single day. The race quickly grew into one of the largest ultramarathons in the country, with a starting field of 700–1,000 runners. That's a lot of crazy people in one place.

They would have to be fast, too; the JFK has a finishing cutoff time of 14 hours, with several checkpoints. Runners who failed to reach the checkpoints within the cutoff times would be removed from the course.

But for those who completed the race, there would be glory and bragging rights: according to the race Web site, less than one-tenth of 1 percent of Americans have completed a 50-mile race. Elite company indeed.

I thought about this as I lay down the night before the race. I kept thinking about the number 50. Suddenly, I just couldn't see any way that I could possibly finish the race. It was just too long. I'd been fooling myself; I'd never make it. Then I thought of something my mother had once told me: gambling is wrong, she said, but if I wanted to bet on something, I should bet on myself. Something clicked for me when I thought of that. I would take a chance on me. With that, I drifted off to sleep.

The JFK 50 Miler is held in Hagerstown, Maryland, conveniently located just a few hours from where I lived. On race day I woke up well before dawn and drove to the start, where I found a large group of mostly older, often heavier runners milling about at the local school, which served as the race day headquarters. It was a different sort of racing crowd than I expected. I thought everyone would look lean and sinewy, their bodies worn down to just the essentials. Instead, I saw some a lot of portly runners who looked to me like they might not even be able to make it around the block. We filed over to the race start in the darkness, and at the blast of the starter's gun we began our journey.

The race began on city streets, and as we ran, I eavesdropped on the conversations around me. These runners, even the heavier ones, talked about having run the JFK numerous times, and other ultras as well. These were experienced guys. At that moment I decided to stop judging them by their shape, and instead credit their accomplishments and try to follow their lead. When they began to walk on the upgrades, I followed suit, and when they paused at aid stations and ate the sandwiches and soup that were offered, I did that, too. This wouldn't guarantee me success, but it would put the odds in my favor.

The race soon led us onto the Appalachian Trail. I wasn't an experienced trail runner, but I thought that the trail portions chosen for the race would surely be the easiest available. Oh, was I wrong. The trail meandered up and down on rough, uneven paths, over rocks, boulders and exposed branches. I was soon acquainted with the agony of stubbed toes and sore ankles. I became so focused on my foot placement that I failed to see a thick, low-lying branch in my path. I ran smack into it headfirst. Everything flashed bright white, and I could hear a distant voice asking if I was okay. I mumbled "yes," and hoped it was true.

Eventually, we left the trail, and ran onto the C&O canal towpath. I was familiar with the canal from the portion of it that ends in D.C. While I had never been this far out on it, I knew that it would be a flat, hard-pack dirt path. We were to run 26 miles on it, almost a full marathon. I was already sore and tired, and doubted if I would be able to finish the race, but I was determined not to drop out unless things got much worse. They would have to pull me off the course for failing to hit the cutoff times. Otherwise, I'd keep moving forward.

The race became an exercise in myopia; I tried to forget how much road lay before me, and concentrated only on getting to the next mile marker, and the next aid station. At each station I swallowed down as much food as I could handle, and then shuffled forward. My pace dropped to little more than a fast walk, but I was not alone. Others around me were in the same condition, or worse. One runner was so disoriented that he failed to notice a hip-level barrier that we had to circle. He hit it full-stride and flipped over onto his back. Undeterred and uncomplaining, he slowly arose and resumed running, mechanically but relentlessly.

The mile markers came and went, conveying impossible-sounding information. Mile 30, mile 31, mile 32. At mile 35, a strange thing happened; I began to feel better. I stopped taking walk breaks, and picked up the pace. By the time I exited the canal for a final 8 miles on the roads, I had sped up to a respectable 8:30-per-mile pace. Darkness descended as I raced those final miles, and when the finish line loomed before me, in front of a local high school, I looked up at the clock and smiled in disbelief. Nine hours 24 minutes. I had run all day, from predawn to nightfall. Even as I collected my medal, I couldn't believe I had done it. There was still the long drive home, though, and the fact of my race set in firmly as my legs ached and my muscles sagged. I had never felt so tired and sore, not even after my very first marathon. I would need weeks to fully recover physically, and almost as long to recover my desire to race.

So what to make of this? What was I to do with an ultramarathon finish? Could I add it to my list of marathons? After all, it was *at least* a marathon. That seemed fair enough. But even as I wrote it down, I knew it couldn't stay on the list. I was committed to running marathons, and that's a precise distance. I was free to run any other distance also, but they could not be included on the list. I could not add four 10Ks together and call them a marathon, and neither could I divide my marathons into eight separate 5K-plus finishes. My totals would be precise and beyond question; I had officially run thirty-two marathons and one *ultra*marathon.

The JFK 50 brought an end to my 1997 racing campaign. There were still adventures to be had in my future, exotic journeys and great races, but there would never again be a year for me quite like 1997.

## Running Tip #3

### *Form Drills*

Drills break down the running motion into distinct movements and improve running efficiency, form, and speed. Once a week, find a 50-meter stretch of road or track. Warm up and do each of these drills 2–4 times, taking a 30-second recovery between each repeat.

- *Butt kicks.* Take short steps while kicking your heels up as high as you can. This drill strengthens the hamstrings, a primary muscle group used in running.
- *High steps.* Take short steps as you pick your knees up as high as they can go. This drill strengthens the calves and hip flexors, which is the area where the bottom of your abdomen meets your leg—a muscle group that's crucial to the running motion, and emphasizes proper running posture and the lift-off phase of running.
- *High Skips.* Swing your arms strongly and skip as high as you can. This drill helps build explosive power in your running stride to improve hill-running and a strong finishing kick in your racing.
- *Stiff-legged Running.* Also called "soccer kicks." Run on your toes, keeping your legs locked out as straight as possible the entire time. This drill will also strengthen the hip flexors.
- *Strides.* Don't sprint; run hard but in control, with an emphasis on monitoring your form. This drill gives you a chance to work on any inefficiency in your form, and prepares your body for the next phase of your workout—your actual distance run—by lengthening your stride.

# Pain, Fear, and Faith

As my marathon total climbed, I found that people weren't asking me why I ran out of admiration now so much as with concern. Many of them had seemed to become suspicious about my running. They began calling me obsessed, in that "I'm joking but you should really think about this" kind of way, and seemed to assume that my running enabled me to avoid dealing with some deeper, darker issues. They said that I must be running away from something.

I didn't think that was true. Running wasn't an escape; if anything, it was a lantern in the dark, a mirror showing me things about myself that I had to face. I could no sooner run away from my problems than I could run away from my own body; when I ran, there was only the road, my thoughts, and time. Eventually, inevitably, I would have to think about anything troubling me. Perhaps it was the rhythm of my footsteps that calmed me down and sharpened my thinking, or perhaps I just reacted well to the rush of endorphins, but whatever the reason, when I ran I saw things more clearly, and could see answers to questions that seemed insolvable only hours before.

Do you remember that poem, "Footprints in the Sand"? Sure you do. You've seen it on automobile air fresheners and on cheesy plaques at every truck stop you've ever wandered into. It goes like this: A man looked back on the path he'd traveled all his life and saw that although the Lord often walked by his side, during the most difficult times, there was only one set of footprints in the sand. The man turned to the Lord and asked, "Why did you abandon me when I needed you the most?" The Lord answered, "Oh, my son, it was then that I carried you."

I hate that story. Not just because it's the worst kind of corny, dime-store religious palaver, although that's exactly what it is; I hate it because it turns me to mush. Every time I read it, my heart rises into my throat and my eyes begin to moisten. Good god, that's actually happening to me right now. I just can't help it, and it's infuriating.

My running reminds me of that story. During the hardest times of my life—when I lost loved ones, when my heart was broken, when I was studying for the bar exam, and whenever I felt alone in the world—running was there for me, providing some relief from my troubles, putting things in perspective and letting me see that the road always continued onward. My running carried me and sustained me.

I've always thought that everyone should have some activity in their lives in which they can become so immersed that they lose track of time. When that happens, when there is no past or future, but only the present, you can find a little bit of that most rare commodity: a little peace of mind. When I relax on a long run, I can get to that place, and in that relaxed state, I can see answers to the problems in my life, and put things in perspective.

This is especially true on my longest runs. During a shorter run of six to eight miles, I know that I'll be finished within an hour, give or take a few minutes. That run becomes a small part of the day's plan, and during the run, I find myself looking ahead to what I need to take care of next when the workout is over, and sometimes I get impatient to be finished so I can get on with the day's chores. But on an 18- to 20-mile run, I know that I'll be on the road for hours, and when I'm finished, I'll be in no mood to rush off to tackle other projects and run errands. The long run becomes the 500-pound gorilla sitting in the middle of a room, completely impossible to ignore. On those days, I give in to the gorilla, and settle into a comfortable pace, knowing that there is nothing else that I need to concern myself with other than putting one foot in front of the other. Any impatience that I might have had during shorter runs disappears. On the long days, there's just me, the road, and endless time.

Not that running is always a pleasure. Running, especially marathon racing, also brings pain. During the last miles of a marathon, my quadriceps muscles are often aching, my hamstrings might be complaining, my calves are possibly cramping, and even my shoulders are fatigued. None of this surprises me; in fact, all of it is entirely expected. I think of these aches and pains as old friends come to visit. I even welcome them, since they signal to me that I'm back in familiar territory, and that the end of the race must be near.

I don't usually talk about these aches and pains with nonrunners, though, because I don't think they'll understand. It's not that marathon runners are masochists—at least not in the traditional sense, and certainly not most of them. It's just that pain means something else to us than it means to most other people. To a runner, pain is a sign of achievement; it's proof that we've expended the maximum effort. When our sides ache from oxygen debt and our legs burn with lactic acid build-up, or when we spend the days after a hard race hobbling pitifully up and down stairs, we know that we had run as hard as we possibly could. The pain, then, is not a cause for concern; it's a cause for celebration. And when we feel perfectly fine after finishing a race, we hear a little voice inside asking us whether it might be true that we could have run faster than we did. In fact, one of my running fantasies is to collapse immediately after finishing a marathon, having used my very last measure of energy to throw myself across the finish line for a new personal best. That would be a perfect race.

But I don't actually enjoy the pain. It's not fun to cool down after a race and discover that your body has stiffened up so much that you could no longer easily or painlessly step down from the curb to the street. Nor is there easy rest for a weary body when every toss and turn in the middle of the night brings complaints from sore muscles, and every attempt to stand up from a chair takes minutes rather than seconds. This kind of pain is humbling; it's disruptive not only to a regular workout routine, but to any kind of normal life. It's a deep-to-the-bone kind of soreness that I would never have known if I had never run a marathon.

The memory of these aches leads me to look down at my legs with pity at every starting line, since they don't know yet what hell I'm about to put them through. But after an hour or two of running, they'll figure it out, and brace themselves for the familiar challenge. If they could speak, perhaps they would tell me not to worry. They understand that this pain is fleeting; we have weathered it before, and we can weather it again. Just get on with it, they would say.

Actual injuries are an entirely different story. There is no long-time runner who hasn't experienced their share of sprains, strains, fractures, and tears. Get a group of runners together, and before long they'll start talking about their injury histories, like war veterans comparing battle scars. During those moments, it might be easy to believe that runners don't mind being injured, but that's dead wrong. If the storytellers are smiling, it's only because the injuries are healed, or because they're trying not to let their frustration show. Dealing with an injury is often a greater test of a runner's resolve than any grueling workout or race.

Once I began to run marathons on a regular basis, many of my friends predicted that my bones would turn to dust, and I'd be crippled within just a few years. Some doctors said much the same thing.

The injuries that I sometimes struggled with only seemed to confirm their predictions. After overcoming that bad ankle sprain in 1986, I suffered a sequence of regular setbacks over the next few years. At one point I had terrible back spasms and had to undergo physical therapy, and another time I developed pain in my knees due to tightness in the muscle and connective tissue that runs along the outside of our legs, called the ilio-tibial band. On a less serious but no less painful side, I also developed awful-looking blisters during my early races. I tried to prevent them by slathering my feet with petroleum jelly, or wrapping each toe with medical tape. In desperation, I once both wrapped and jellied my feet. Not a good idea. By race's end, I was left with a slippery mass of balled up tape jammed in the front of my shoes.

Another time, I felt a blister developing on my right pinky toe early in a race. Being an old pro by this point, I pulled over to an aid station and wrapped tape around the toe. Problem solved. I jumped back in the race and ran smoothly for the next 19 miles, but after crossing the 26 mile marker, with the finish line within sight just up ahead, I suddenly felt a very painful pop in my right foot. I was quickly reduced to a hobble, and I was sure that I had torn a ligament in that pinky toe. After pulling myself across the finish line, I staggered straight to the medical tent, where I sat down and pulled of my right shoe. The end of my sock was covered in blood. I pulled off the sock, and then had a medical technician carefully cut the tape along the length of my toe. I slowly pulled the tape back, and gazed at what I saw underneath. The toe was a raw stick of meat. Stuck on the tape was my skin and toenail. Slowly, it dawned on me what had happened. I had developed a blister underneath the toenail, and finally, at mile 26, it popped violently, unhinging both the nail and the surrounding skin. Luckily, it didn't feel as bad as it looked, but whenever I want to make someone cringe, I pull that story out from my bag of tales.

Eventually, I found the right combination of treatments to get my feet safely through my races, and eventually they seemed to just toughen up and blister less frequently. My other injuries also healed and disappeared, leaving me wiser. I began to see my body as a kind of minefield which I could traverse only by stepping carefully around the spots where I knew explosives lay. *Not there! You'll get a sore knee if you do that. And that will hurt your back!*

Despite all of those training and racing woes, however, I came to realize over the years that I was actually a very durable runner. I had a stable stride an unusually large vastus medialis—the muscle above the kneecap that helps hold the kneecap in place. Like most other runners, I still had to work on my flexibility and strengthen the muscles in my back and abdominal areas, but I had come to realize that while I might not be the fastest runner in the field, I was built to keep running.

Still, if I have a different relationship to pain than most nonrunners, I also have a different collection of fears. Preparing for and running the JFK 50 Mile led me to consider again the role of fear in running, since, for the first time in a very long while, I had ventured outside of my comfort zone into unknown territory. By that time I was very confident that I could run a marathon. After all, I had already run thirty-two of them. But I was very worried about the JFK 50. I felt a fear of failure that I had not felt in years. It was a feeling that was unsettling and disturbing, though not entirely unpleasant.

Fear, like any stress, is a double-edged sword. Unhealthy and paralyzing in large doses, it's also essential for achievement, and leads to the cathartic hormonal release that we all find so pleasurable. This is the fear that we seek out and pay for with every horror movie and roller-coaster ride we experience. But runners live with a more common brand of fear, cousin more to insecurity than to terror. This is the fear that whispers in our ear that past achievement matters little because our bodies are no longer in the condition they were in a few months or even weeks ago. This is the fear that gains traction with every disappointing workout and slow training run we endure. It is the fear that undermines our confidence day by day, replacing it with gnawing doubt.

Runners, like many other people, seek to conquer our fears by clinging to ritual. We have our lucky socks and hats, our favorite old shirts and shoes. We swear by our food choices, our race-morning routines, and our prerace warm-up. Some of these rituals are rooted in experimentation that would make a scientist proud, while others are shrouded in superstition and faith. For example, I personally would never wear a race's shirt before finishing that race. It's a *finisher's* shirt, after all, and wearing it before you cross the finish line could result in a powerful jinx. It just makes sense. Or, at least, it does to me. But however established, these rituals and superstitions hang on with the tenacity of a pit bull, because to a runner, preparation is everything, and if we repeat the exact details that led to past success, then that success can be replicated. We convince ourselves that there will be no failure, no shame, no heartbreak on this day, because we have done everything right. With all the necessaries attended to, success should follow, as surely as night follows day. Fear is conquered.

In a larger sense, though, our fear is not about a single training session, or a particular race. It is about our mortality; it is about our knowledge that there is a limit to our improvement. We know that eventually, inevitably, age, the swiftest runner, will catch us and hang on our backs. Our legs will slow, our finishing times will climb like the temperature on a sweltering day, and we'll realize that we're one mile closer to the end of our life's race. We run every workout and race under this cloud. Just as running fulfills the promise of life, it contains within it the seeds of decline.

But we need not give into this fear. With every strong workout, every fast lap, every personal best, we push the darkness back. To do so requires determination, and yes, pain. Speed workouts hurt, racing hard hurts, but we do it. We do it to push away the fear, to hold onto the illusion of immortality one more moment. To live fully, completely.

With experience, we can learn not to despair with every slow run, secure in the knowledge that a great workout will likely soon follow. Even an occasional bad race won't be the harbinger of doom. Eventually, we know, decline will set in. But not today, not here, not now. I will muzzle this fear, and cover the Earth in great hungry strides, cheating time and decay with every step for as long as I can.

As I pondered these thoughts, I began to see the human body as something of a divine instrument, and running itself as an expression of faith and an affirmation of the wonder of life. This was my private belief, though, and I wasn't eager to make a public declaration of it. Religion was, I felt, a private matter, and I wasn't interested in expressing my views to anyone who might not be interested in hearing about them.

Not everyone else agreed. I once heard about Catherine Ndereba, the great four-time Boston Marathon champion and 2004 Olympic silver medalist, when she graciously spoke to a small crowd of runners before the Barbados Marathon in 2003. She was open and warm, and everything you could hope for in a celebrity.

But Catherine began her talk by thanking God for her accomplishments, and referred again and again to her faith as the source of her power. I shifted uneasily, and I thought I saw others do the same. We weren't interested in talking about religion; we wanted to talk about running, and questions from the crowd steered her away from religion by asking her instead about her training schedule and her views on her competitors. I respect Catherine's beliefs, and admire her great ability, determination, and courage, but I didn't much like being preached to.

I came to feel uncomfortable with another expression of faith in the running community as well: those runners who literally wear their beliefs of their sleeves. I began seeing slogans like "With God All Things Are Possible" splashed across their shirts, followed in short order by others bearing biblical quotes and psalms. Not what I would do, but it really wasn't any of my business. But then one day I passed a runner with a shirt declaring "Jesus is my coach." Really? What speed work does Jesus recommend for marathoners? Does Jesus believe in effort-based training, or does He use a stopwatch? Does Jesus recommend supplements? Of course, I said none of those things to him; I didn't want be rude or offensive. But flip declarations of faith are, in my view, little more than advertising slogans, and I don't like them.

There is a role for faith in running, as in all of life. All runners have faith, of one kind or another; it's what enables us to try going beyond the limits that we once thought would stop us. But all runners know, too, that faith is only the safety net; real achievement comes from our own sweat, from our conscious choice to sacrifice and work hard. Making choices is the foundation for all morality, and rather than relying on faith to guide us in our actions, we should fashion our actions to reflect our faith. Running, to me, is what the cathedral was to the masses in the Middle Ages: a visible declaration of the wonder of creation. For me, running is the best expression of a runner's faith. Through pain and injury, and success, we are who we are, and become who we want to be.

My quest continued.

## Running Tip #4

### *Dealing with Injuries*

Injuries happen. The trick is not just to avoid injury, but to respond intelligently when you feel one coming on. If you respond quickly and correctly when you develop a problem, you'll be back running at 100 percent in almost no time at all. Generally, cutting back on training, and stretching, strengthening, and icing the area will help. Thinking that you could just bully your body into submission, however, will *not* work. Trust me, I know.

Here's a short list of the most common training ailments, with suggested treatments. As with any injury, if symptoms persist for more than a week or two, worsen, or if the pain feels sharp rather than dull, you should see a doctor.

- *Black toe.* The toenail turns black, and sometimes falls off. This is a sign that your shoes are too small, and the toe is jamming against the front of the shoe, resulting in bruising of the nail bed. The fix? Buy shoes that are at least a half size or more larger than your dress shoes.
- *Knee pain—on the front.* This is probably patella tendonitis, and is caused by excessive movement of the knee cap over the knee joint. Insufficient muscle strength in the front of the upper leg—the quadriceps muscles, particularly on the inner side—is usually to blame. Do leg strengthening exercises such as squats, leg presses, or lunges.

→

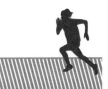

- *Knee pain—on the outside.* Called iliotibial band syndrome, this is an inflammation of the muscle and connective tissue running from the upper front hip bone (ilium) down along the outside of the leg, over the outside of the knee, down to the kneecap and calf (tibia bone). Tightness causes the IT band to rub against the outside of the knee, causing pain. Treat with ice and self-massage, and stretch until you feel tightness in your hip and backside.
- *Knee pain—on the back of the knee.* This is often caused by tightness in the hamstrings. Stretch your hamstrings and do self-massage.
- *Pain on the heel or arch.* This is likely plantar fasciitis, an inflammation of the connective tissue in that area. A common indicator of plantar fasciitis is pain in the arch first thing in the morning. Treat with gentle stretching and icing.
- *Pain on the front of the lower leg/shin.* Likely shin splints, a result of training too intensely too soon, especially on hard surfaces. Ice by massaging the area with a frozen cup of water, holding the open end on the affected area. Strengthen the area by doing "duckwalks"—walking once a day back and forth across a room on your heels with your toes up in the air for 5–10 minutes.

# Mountain Madness

In the summer of 1998, I was just over a third of the way to my 100-marathon goal—close enough to claim to know what I was doing, but far enough to still not be able to imagine actually achieving it. When I sat down and thought about all the miles and races before me, I felt farther away from my goal than ever. I realized that the only way to keep on my path was to ignore that I was on it; by refusing to acknowledge how far I had to go, I would be able to keep putting one foot in front of the other. It was the same strategy that I used in each race I ran. As I told people, I never imagined running 26.2 miles at a time—I saw myself as running a single mile twenty-six times in a row. Somehow, it that made all the difference. But now, to reach the ultimate finish line, I would have to extend this trick to years, not just hours.

Some runners seem to maintain their motivation through familiarity, returning to the same races year after year, like salmon returning to their spawning grounds. They find comfort in running familiar ground, and take pride in not missing a single edition of their favorite races. Or perhaps they discover new, subtle things about the course every time they run them, like a Shakespearean scholar who finds new meaning and artistry with every reading of *Macbeth*.

That's not me. I have run certain marathons multiple times—Boston, New York, and the Marine Corps Marathon—but by and large I want to see something new and different every time I race. For me, there's no greater way to experience a new place than on the run, and there's no better way to distract myself from pain and fatigue than by running down unfamiliar roads. That's really why I began to travel to run in the first place.

Of course, not all races are created equal; some are more exotic and challenging than others. And then there are some that some races that are so far off the beaten path that it seems misleading to simply call them marathons. The Pikes Peak Marathon is one such race.

Pikes Peak is a 14,110-foot-high granite mountain in central Colorado, thrusting skyward from the city of Colorado Springs, with the smaller town of Manitou Springs hugging its eastern flank. The fledgling United States gained title over the mountain in the Louisiana Purchase, and it was named for Zebulon Pike, the man President Jefferson sent to survey the southwestern border of the new territory in 1806. Pike tried to scale the mountain, but was turned back by a blizzard. The summit was finally conquered in 1820, but the surrounding area wasn't settled for another fifty years. In 1873, the U.S. Army built a weather station on the summit, and by 1888 a toll road had been built to the top. A cog railroad was soon added, and by 1901 the first automobile climbed the peak. In 1918, a hiking trail to the top was completed, named the Barr Trail, for the father and son team who constructed it.

Once it became possible to reach the top, human nature being what it is, people began to challenge each other to race to the summit. An auto race was held in 1916, and then, on Sunday, June 28, 1936, twenty-five men and two women lined up for the first Pikes Peak footrace. Nineteen made it to the top. Twenty years would pass before another such race was attempted.

On Friday, August 10, 1956, fourteen runners lined up to race once more to the top, this time in honor of the 150th anniversary of Zebulon Pike's mission. According to legend, the race was the result of a bet between smokers and nonsmokers. As it turned out, no one fared especially well, as only four people made it to the summit. But the race had touched something in people's imagination, and this time it would not die. It was held again the following year, and then again, until it became an established event. Slowly the field of participants grew from a handful of lunatics the first several years, to several hundred lunatics by the 1970s, and then to several thousand lunatics by the 1990s. It turned out that there was a bottomless supply of lunatics who wanted to throw themselves at the mountain, but because the Barr Trail was too narrow to allow a large field of runners, most of these would-be ascenders had to be turned away. Despite the difficulty of getting into the race, or perhaps because of it, enthusiasm for the event grew. The Pikes Peak Marathon had become an institution.

I wasn't aware of any of this history in 1998 when I mailed off my application to Colorado. I just wanted this race to be my thirty-seventh marathon. Lady Luck must have smiled on my application, though, because soon I received a confirmation of entry, along with a twenty-page information booklet. I was a bit mystified. Usually prerace instructions aren't longer than a page or two. But this booklet had twenty pages of instructions and warnings. *Twenty pages!* What had I gotten myself into?

I kicked off my shoes, threw myself onto my couch, and began to read. What surprised me about the race was the sheer volume of things to worry about. First, of course, was the climb. While most marathons have a significant hill or two, this one was nothing *but* hill; runners climb 7,815 feet up, and then race 7,815 feet down. The toll on the legs would be staggering, as muscles and joints would be tested in every possible way.

But that's not even the worst of it. The race *starts* at 6,295 feet above sea level, and climbs above the timberline where no tree can grow, into the thin air above 14,000 feet. At those heights, breathing becomes difficult, and running becomes almost unthinkable. The booklet recommended that participants train themselves in the technique of forced breathing, in which the diaphragm is repeatedly pushed to take in more air without exhausting the chest wall muscles.

But that wasn't even the worst of it. Apart from the climb and the altitude, there was the volatility of the summer weather on Pikes Peak to worry about. It was said to be utterly and dangerously unpredictable. "Pikes Peak can have rapid and extreme weather changes several times each day," the booklet warned. "Chilling rain, snow and sleet showers, high winds and dramatic temperature changes can occur [on race day] in August." The temperatures could drop by as much as fifty degrees from the starting line in Manitou Springs to the mountain peak. But that wasn't the real problem, the booklet insisted. The greatest danger to runners actually comes from sudden lightning storms above the tree line.

I put the booklet down and looked at the ceiling, pondering what I had just read. The contents of the booklet sounded frightening, and the chances for a flawless marathon looked slim. In fact, from the look of things, I would be lucky just to make it back alive and in one piece.

I smiled.

After conquering the challenge of simply getting into the race, I had to decide how to adjust my training to handle the unusual demands that the race would make on my body. The race organizers suggested arriving in Colorado two weeks before the event in order to begin acclimatizing to the altitude. Much as I would like to have done that, my boss, Uncle Sam, seemed to have other priorities, and I just couldn't take the time off. Other than constructing a hyperbaric tent over my bed to mimic high altitude—which I did consider for a hot second—my plan was just to fly out there the day before the race and hope for the best.

Training for the climb itself was also a matter of hope. I spent long hours laboring on the stepper machine and running hills, betting that would prepare me for the mountain. As for the dealing with the weather, I planned to bring enough gear to be prepared for any contingency. I packed layers and throwaway clothes—enough, really, for a week's worth of racing.

Finally, there was nothing left to do but rest and fly out to Colorado. I arrived in Manitou Springs in the early afternoon the day before the race, and spent some time walking around town before picking up my race packet. On the outskirts of town was the beautiful and aptly named Garden of the Gods, where a walking path snaked around pale red monoliths and rock outcrops. Manitou Springs itself looks like it had gracefully made the transition from mining town to tourist attraction, but without being infected with too much gaudiness. The streets were lined with small shops and restaurants nestled in century-old buildings. You had the feeling it wouldn't be all that unnatural to see a stagecoach rumble past. All this was interesting enough, but my thoughts were elsewhere. I wanted to get my race number and focus on the task at hand.

Usually, race organizers set up shop in a conference room of the host hotel, which is where you expect to go to pick up your race packet. Not so at Pikes Peak. Organizers set up their tables in a park, giving would-be racers a chance to look up at the Peak before they accepted their race number. Rather than filling runners with dread, however, the sight of the Peak seemed to inspire excitement in the race crowd. Newcomers and veterans alike seemed like so many greyhounds in the slip, waiting for the bell to ring. I tried to ignore it. I wanted to be calm, and save all my energy for the race.

The following morning I found myself shoulder to shoulder with other runners in Manitou Springs, near the park I had visited the day before. It was a cool morning, and I could see the breath of the runners around me as they stretched, pawed at the ground with their feet, and looked skyward toward our goal. This is the most difficult time for a runner—the twilight between preparing for a race and actually running.

There is nothing left to do but worry about things that had gone wrong in training, and there is not yet the reassurance that comes with actual racing, when the body tells you that everything will be okay. This is just the waiting, and it can seem endless.

That time passed, though, as it always does, and the blast of the starter's gun released us. We raced through town, past the storefronts and homes, seeking out the entrance to the Barr Trail. Soon we found it. We plunged into the woods and started to climb in earnest. Runners jock-eyed for position on the narrow trail, eager to spend their nervous energy. I held my position, but I didn't worry too much about skipping ahead. Passing people was not going to be my concern this day; I just wanted to make it up and back in one piece.

The air was clean and fresh, and the leaves around me were a vivid green as I settled into a smooth rhythm. The climbs were mixed with flat stretches, where our footfalls were muffled by soft dirt. Eventually, I realized that the forest was thinning, and that the soaring trees were shrinking. Soon, they gave way to large bushes, and then they, too, disap-peared, replaced by pale yellow and orange rock. We had reached the tree line, the point at which the forest had to turn back from the altitude and climate of the mountain. Now things would get interesting.

The sun shone brightly now as I made my way up the rocky incline. The gentleness of the forest floor had disappeared with the trees, and now I had to make my way over loose rock and sharp boulders. Looking up the distant cliff-side in front of me, I could see a line of tiny runners zig-zagging the switchbacks, looking like ants on a foraging mission. To my left stretched out the vastness of the southwest and an endless blue sky. It was a beautiful sight, but like the siren's call, it could lead me to disaster if gazing at it caused me to stumble and fall on the rocks underfoot. This was not the time for long, admiring gazes toward distant peaks.

I came across Barr Camp, a little oasis on the trail where volunteers waited with water and snacks. Their enthusiasm was infectious, and I threw myself back on the trail with renewed energy. Soon, though, my breathing became labored, and I realized that it wasn't caused just by the steady climb; the air was getting thinner. Everyone around me was moving slowly, and I joined them in walking the steepest sections of trail. My head started throbbing, and I leaned back on a boulder to rest. I tried to breathe down into my stomach, drawing as much precious air into my lungs as possible. From my rocky perch, I could see runners dotting the trail below me, forming a jagged seam on the mountainside. Wisps of clouds appeared overhead, and I wondered what the temperature was at the peak. I recalled that the race materials said that the typical time up to the half-way point at the top was the same as an entire flatland marathon, plus one half hour. I was starting to believe it.

I took another deep breath and pushed myself off the rock, reclaiming a spot in the line of runners inching their way to the top. I looked up, trying to gauge how much more there was to climb, but every spot I had been sure was the top instead turned out to be only a bend in the trail. I knew I was getting close, though, because the lead runners passed me on their way back down. I marveled at how fresh they looked; while I was struggling to walk, they flew downhill. I couldn't imagine having that kind of energy. For that matter, I could hardly imagine running the 13 miles back down to the finish line, but I refused to let myself think about that. I concentrated on simply putting one foot in front of the other, and blocked out all other thoughts.

The air became cooler, but there weren't any of the dramatic weather changes that we had been warned about. I moved mechanically, gulping air, wondering if there was actually a top to this mountain. And then suddenly, there it was. I had made it up to 14,110 feet, the top floor. There was a visitor center at the top, and plenty of spectators to cheer us on, but there was no time to celebrate. The top of the trail led us through a narrow defile through the rock, where volunteers unceremoniously spun us around and pointed us back downhill.

I pivoted and began to move forward, and then discovered an amazing thing: I could run! And more than that, I could run fast. It was as if I was being sucked into a vortex, and I felt better with every step. I slid on the gravel and hopped over rocks and boulders, spinning on the switchbacks like a car burning rubber on a wild turn. I couldn't believe how great I felt. It was nothing short of miraculous.

I had read that the difference between suffering altitude sickness and feeling fine can be as little as several dozen feet. I don't know if that's true, but I can tell you that each step down restored my strength and confidence. I was having fun. I ate up great chunks of trail with each stride, offering encouragement to the runners still moving toward the top. Like watching a movie in reverse, I saw the bits of brush appear between the orange and yellow rock, followed by small bushes and stunted trees. Soon, I was back in the woods again, below the tree line.

I was still flying, but my legs had started to protest. As much fun as downhill running can be, it's still hell on the quads, which have to work overtime to keep their fool owner from toppling forward and doing a face-plant. Not a problem, though: I had learned long ago how to ignore my screaming legs. I was more concerned about the footing. Downhill running on trail and broken rock is usually a recipe for disaster, but so far I had no problem handling the challenge.

No sooner had that thought entered my mind, hanging in the air like a thought balloon in a comic strip, than I found myself sprawled on the ground with my ankle screaming in pain. I pulled myself upright and took a tentative step. More screaming from below. I had twisted my ankle badly, that much was obvious. But standing alone in the woods, with runners off in the distance in front and behind me, and help—in the form of a rest stop—miles farther down the road, I had no choice but to keep moving. I took a few more easy steps. Not as bad as I first thought, really, once I got moving. I tried an easy jog. That seemed manageable. As I continued running, the pain subsided. Perhaps the adrenaline coursing through my body had blocked it out, or perhaps my body had responded by releasing a good dose of cortisol, a natural anti-inflammatory. Whatever it was, I was grateful for it, and promised to reward my body with a stop at the next aid station to have my ankle wrapped.

With the toughest part of the course behind me, I knew I wouldn't drop out unless I had no choice. I quickly constructed a cost-benefit test: how much of a layoff would I be willing to accept to complete the race? A week? Certainly. A month? Sure. Several months. Well ... I guess so. Permanent injury? No, of course not. But how could I tell which of these fates lay in my future if I kept running?

I decided to turn the question around: rather than worry about what might happen, I would look only for clues as to what would certainly happen. Unless permanent injury became obviously inevitable, I would keep running for as long as I could. At the next aid station a volunteer wrapped my ankle tightly, and I was off again, rolling downhill, betting on my ankle against the mountain.

The miles flew by, and soon I was reached the end of the trail. After so many hours of running on dirt and rock, it was strange to be on asphalt again. From there I only had a short piece of running through town to the finish line, and it was mostly downhill. Usually that would be welcome relief, but not now. My quads were screaming at me, and my toes jammed painfully into the front of my shoes with each step. I groaned out loud and rolled my eyes in agony; I didn't think I could stand much more. Finally, there was only one more corner to turn, and there it was: the finish line. The clock read 6 hours 58 minutes.

I collected my medal and sat down in a folding chair in the tent just past the finish line. I had been tested, but I had not broken. My ankle would recover, my toes would heal, and my legs would eventually forgive me, but this moment would never be forgotten.

Looking around me, though, I saw that my injuries paled in comparison to those sustained by other runners. The tent looked like an army triage center. There were bloody elbows and knees, as well as cut and bruised faces. There had obviously been a lot of falling up on the mountain. Despite all the blood and bruises, though, I didn't see any sad faces. We had all survived, and better still, had triumphed. The bloody bandage became a badge of honor, a sign of how close to the edge each of us had pushed ourselves.

Later that night, I laid my still-wrapped ankle on a pillow and slung a bag of ice over it. It was classic RICE therapy: Rest, Ice, Compression, and Elevation. I knew that was the proper way to treat a sprain, and I thought just this once I would play it by the book. I didn't have high expectations.

The next morning, I was surprised to find that the swelling of my ankle had gone down, and that the pain was mostly gone as well. This RICE thing actually worked. Who woulda thunk it? I was back running within just a few days, good as new. Better than new, actually, because I had conquered Pikes Peak, America's toughest marathon. I felt that victory in my 100-marathon quest was now assured. But if I thought that there would be no more challenges, I was greatly mistaken, as I would soon find out.

## Running Tip #5

### *Race Recovery*

- *Eat something 15–30 minutes after training or racing.* This will kick-start refueling of your muscles and repair of any cellular damage.
- *Take a cold bath, massage your legs, grab some couch time.* All of these will help move blood and waste products out of your legs.
- *Take the long view.* Plan on needing one day of rest or easy training for every hard mile you raced.
- *Get back to it slowly.* Run no longer than an hour at a time for the first few weeks after a hard marathon.
- *Beware the sniffles.* Your immune system takes a battering on race day, so get plenty of sleep, drink lots of fluids, eat well, wash your hands frequently, and avoid touching your eyes and nose.

The question would not go away. I would go days and weeks without thinking about it, but sooner or later I would figuratively reach into my pocket, pull it out, sit it on a table, and look at it. Why run the marathon? I couldn't seem to find a good, complete answer to that question.

In the years following my first marathon, I had pursued my growing passion for fitness and became a certified personal trainer and running coach, filling my early morning and evening hours with sessions in a local gym, and my weekends coaching charity fund-raising marathon teams. I became a fitness evangelist, preaching and living the healthy life. I did not want to induce any delusions of immortality, though. I told my clients at our first session that our goal was to improve where we could, maintain as best we're able, and extend the quality of our life; nothing less, but nothing more.

This sounded right to me, but it opened a door onto bigger questions. I thought about something I once read former New York Mets and Philadelphia Phillies relief pitcher Tug McGraw had said. After blowing a game, he would ponder something he called the Ice Ball Theory, which went something like this: some day, many millions of years from now, our sun will become a supernova, scorch the earth, and then flame out into nothingness. After that, our planet will wander eternity in a dark void, a giant ice ball hurtling through space. At that point, no one will be around to care that on a sunny afternoon Tug McGraw once served up a home run pitch to lose a baseball game. Tug found it much easier to sleep at night after running that scenario through his mind.

The problem with the Ice Ball Theory, as I soon realized, was that it proved too much. Instead of just showing how little any one mistake matters in the scheme of things, it showed how *nothing* really matters. Not a very comforting idea after all. The question for me, then, became not just why run the marathon, but instead, if all achievement and failure eventually fade into the void equally, why bother doing anything at all?

These philosophical musings suddenly took on an unexpected urgency. One of my new clients, Burt, told me that he was HIV positive, and that he was also undergoing chemotherapy. He seemed uncomfortable talking about his health, and I didn't press for details beyond what I needed to know as his trainer, but I did tell him that I was proud of him for taking control of his life and for trying to improve himself. It was the type of life-affirming act that brought me into training in the first place.

Burt had more body fat than he should have been carrying, and he wasn't as strong as he wanted to be. His self-esteem had also taken a battering from the disease. I knew that training him would be a challenge for both of us. We began slowly, getting him comfortable with the exercises, discovering his limits, and gently pushing them to new levels. As time went by, Burt was amazed to see his strength improving. Soon, he told me, his friends noticed as well, and commented on his changed appearance. Burt also experienced a change of attitude: instead of being the victim of his disease, he began to show confidence and a new enthusiasm for life. I was accustomed to helping people get results, but this was something new for me. Something special was happening.

One day I called Burt to set up another appointment. He sounded scared and very upset. He was feeling very ill, and he told me that a friend was about to take him to the hospital. I told him not to jump to any conclusions, since he had been feeling so good for so long. We would just keep an open mind and wait to hear what the doctors had to say. He promised to call me as soon as he felt up to it.

I was very busy at the time, and several weeks passed before I realized how long it had been since I'd spoken with him. I was filled with dread as I punched his phone number, made infinitely worse when I was patched through into another employee's voice mail. I left several messages at his home number that I hoped sounded calm and upbeat, but that urged him to call me.

Finally he called. It turned out that he had had a bad reaction to the various medications that he was taking. His doctors had given him a transfusion and kept him in the hospital for a week. He had lost a lot of weight and strength, but what was worse, he had also lost his confidence and sense of purpose, and was depressed about the big step backward that he had taken in his fitness program. He said that he doubted that he could get back to where he was before his illness. Not to worry, I told him. As my father used to say when my sisters or I had a setback, this was only a stumble, not a fall. I instructed him to use the weight machines for a week without worrying about how much weight he was lifting, just to get reacquainted with the movements. After that, I would put together another training program for him, and we would set about the task of rebuilding him.

Despite my confidence, Burt was still discouraged. He was sure that we couldn't possibly get back to where we had left off earlier. But I explained to him that as long as the laws of physics, chemistry, and anatomy still apply in our universe, we were sure to climb right back up the fitness ladder. It was just a matter of time. That's the wonder of the human body: give it a reasonable challenge, and it will rise to the occasion.

Burt took my advice, and we resumed our training. Soon, his strength and muscle mass started to return. It was only later that he told me how much my encouragement had helped him through his dark times. Instead of spiraling downward in free fall, he was able to once again take control of his life by having a plan to follow. Fitness wasn't just restoring his body; it was restoring his hope and his faith.

Burt continued to regain his strength, but his battle with his disease also continued. He moved to Boston to be closer to his family. We kept in touch, but then, suddenly, I stopped hearing from him. I found out that Burt had died from his illness. I'm usually very positive and upbeat about life, but I was suddenly filled with a sense of futility. What had it mattered that we had improved his strength 30 percent last year? What was the point of all that hard work?

I began then to think of my high school biochemistry lessons, about the energy bonds that held the electrons of our molecules in their orbits. The solidity of our bodies, of the entire physical world, really, was just an illusion; at the atomic level, there was more empty space than matter. I began to imagine my body—all of our bodies—not as whole organisms, but rather as collections of molecules bound together by only by these energy bonds. What if these molecules suddenly decided to disperse? What if the only thing keeping our atoms from flying apart was our own willpower, our stubborn refusal to cease to exist? How long could any of us be expected to hold these millions of molecules together before we tired and failed?

I began to think of the endless upkeep all of our bodies require to stay in proper trim. Every day, the body needs to be fed, to be trained, to be stretched and washed. The heart beats, the blood flows, and waste is eliminated. Sleep provides some respite, but then the cycle begins again, every day, until we cease to exist.

It was an exhausting thought. I began to imagine an escape from the tyranny of this routine, of a time and place without decay, where there is no struggle to improve and maintain one's collection of molecules. A place where there is no injury, no need to train, no need to run. A place where there is stillness.

I had reached the bottom, a place beyond the marathon, beyond running, beyond wondering about the active life. I had peered into a dark hole where existence itself is questioned. From the Big Bang through the thousands of millennia of existence, to the end of time and a return to the stillness from which it all was born, I saw that nothing truly endured but the stillness itself.

I shook off these dark thoughts, recoiling like a child touching a hot oven. Down that hole is a place where existence denies itself. A place without change is a place without the possibility of improvement, without challenge. Because it has neither success nor failure, it is a place without meaning. A place of such stillness is a place of death.

I decided to imagine my body differently. Instead of seeing it on the verge of pulling apart, I see my molecules spinning tightly in their orbits, strengthened and nourished by their numbers and their energy bonds. Every movement strengthens them further, and they shine brighter in the flexing and stretching of my muscles. I returned to solid ground, within the sphere of my experience. This was now familiar to me, because I knew the peaceful fatigue that I felt when I lived the active life; I knew that the joy of exertion conquers the stillness.

My body spoke in one voice, and made its choice. It chose movement, it chose running, it chose the marathon. It chose life. That was enough for now.

# To the End of the Earth

When January 1999 rang in, I had been racing for twelve years, and had run a total of 39 marathons. I had run up and down a mountain, and I had qualified for the Boston Marathon. In short, I felt that I was quite experienced. I had become something of a marathon connoisseur; while some people collected art or fine wine, I collected marathons. My collection had a serious flaw, however; I had yet to race away from American soil. That had to change. But I wanted my first race off American soil to be memorable. True to my nature, I wanted it to be *inspiring*. And I found it. After running my 40th marathon in Houston, I picked a jaw-dropping race for my 41st. In fact, I wasn't going to simply run a marathon; I was going to undertake an honest-to-goodness *expedition*. I had signed on for a race at the end of the world. I was going to run the Antarctica Marathon.

To be honest, the idea of running a marathon in Antarctica hadn't been burning in my thoughts. In fact, the idea never even occurred to me until I received a phone call from my friend Ginny Turner, a fellow marathoner who was also pursuing the fifty-state Holy Grail. I had met Ginny in South Bend, Indiana—at a marathon, of course. Standing inside Notre Dame's stadium after crossing the finish line, I explained to her the legendary "Touchdown Jesus," the image of Christ painted larger than life on the side of a building that can be seen from inside the stadium, beyond the goalposts. Some nameless smart-aleck many years ago had noticed how the figure's upraised arms resembled an umpire's signal for a score, and so a legend was born. Ginny and I became fast friends after that, and kept in touch over the following months, comparing marathon notes and schedules. So I wasn't at all surprised when she called me one day to tell me that she was planning to run another marathon. But I never expected to hear that it would be in Antarctica.

Ginny wanted me to join her on the expedition. I was interested, of course, but skeptical. I had been working as an attorney for a decade, but as a government employee, my salary was still low, and I was still saddled with massive student loans to repay. This would be an expensive adventure, and I just didn't think I could manage the cost. But as I opened my mouth to explain to Ginny why I couldn't go, she hit me with her final sales pitch: when she returned later and told me all about the journey, I would realize that I should have gone with her, and would forever regret not going. That stopped me cold. She was absolutely right. I found myself saying yes to her, even as my mind scrambled to figure out a way to pay for it. I got off the phone and signed up for the expedition that was to take place the following month.

Having committed to the race, I thought it would be a good idea to find out exactly what I'd gotten myself into. Once I received the race materials, I settled back for a nice read. The Antarctic Marathon—also called The Last Marathon, because that's the last place a sane person would think of running a race—is held in February, at the height of the austral summer. It was organized by a travel company that catered to marathoners, a reflection of the financial clout of the burgeoning marathon culture. Our group was comprised of over 160 runners from around the world, led by a team of naturalists who would handle technical matters and shore landings, and who would explain this vast wasteland to us.

My journey began with a 10½-hour overnight flight from New York's JFK airport to Buenos Aires. As if that wasn't challenging enough, I managed to arrive at the gate only 15 minutes before departure. This brand of reckless tardiness was, unfortunately, bred in my bones; the rest of my family treats deadlines no more respectfully than I do. Upon my arrival at the gate, the airline staff was both relieved and annoyed to see me, knowing that a member of a large group on the flight was unaccounted for just moments before the doors were to close. In their haste to get me on board, they assigned me to the first available seat they could find. It was in first class. Not really a good incentive for me to correct my errant behavior. Of course, this occurred in the years before the post-9/11 security clampdown, when such last-minute adventures were possible.

After arriving in Buenos Aires and meeting other members of the team, I joined a few of them for a little walk around the city, to shake off the kinks and to get the lay of the land. Getting around Buenos Aires turned out to be easy; it's really a walkers' city, crisscrossed with broad, beautiful boulevards, and filled with beautiful European architecture. Avenida 9 de Julio, at some 600 feet across, is one of the broadest thoroughfares in the world, while Florida and Lavale avenues are open pedestrian malls. We saw tango dancers whirling among street musicians, vendors in the flea market of San Telmo, and one of the copies of Rodin's *Thinker* pondering ceaselessly in front of the Congreso Nacional. Nearby was the beautiful opera house, the Teatro Colón, where Toscanini and Caruso had performed. And, of course, we made our pilgrimage to Eva Perón's tomb in the Recoleta cemetery. The site itself is unremarkable, but the cemetery as a whole is fascinating. It's a virtual city of the dead, filled entirely with mausoleums, each vying to be the most ostentatious.

Being a native New Yorker, however, I also insisted on descending belowground to check out the subway system. I discovered that the stations were like underground cities, containing dozens of small shops and eateries. The platforms were lined with beautiful ceramic murals, and the trains were wood-paneled antiques.

Making our way back to our hotel, we strolled along Puerto Madero, where a canal lined with fine restaurants opens into the Río de la Plata. Couples strolled the promenade, sharing ice cream cones and whispered conversations. When we finally made it back to our hotel room, I fell into my bed and, as my grandmother would have said, slept like the dead.

By the following morning, I was recovered and ready to run. I found the Parque Natural y Zonade Reserva Ecológica Costanera Sur, just east of Puerto Madero, where I did laps on a popular running and cycling circuit: an 8-kilometer hardpack dirt and gravel road that encircled the park. Later, I joined the full team and the travel company staff for a debriefing. In addition to other warnings, the hotel staff cautioned us about a tourist scam that involved one conspirator spraying mustard on an unsuspecting victim, while another conspirator suddenly appears and offers to help clean off the mustard. That's when bandits suddenly appear from nowhere to snatch bags and cameras from the distracted victim, and run off in different directions. This must be a joke, I said, but I was assured that it was true.

As if to prove the point, Ginny and I later got mustarded while wandering around near the Teatro Colon opera house. Although we didn't see who had surreptitiously sprayed us with mustard, we knew what to expect once we saw that we'd suffered a condiment attack, so we ignored offers of "help" from a nearby elderly woman, and quickly walked off before any bandits appeared. I was indignant; I didn't grow up on the streets of Manhattan to get mugged in Buenos Aires!

Finally, it was time to begin the next leg of our journey: a 4½-hour flight south to Patagonia, at the tip of South America. On the way down, strong winds buffeted our plane, and the pilot made an emergency landing to wait out the squalls. We stayed in our seats as the jet shuddered on the tarmac, silently exchanging worried glances among ourselves. Finally, the winds died down, and we returned to the air. As far as I was concerned, this is when the expedition officially began.

Eventually we arrived in a small but beautiful airport, topped with a latticework of timber and glass. We were in Ushuaia, in Argentinean Tierra del Fuego, the land of fire, named for the burning torches along the shore that were spotted by passing sailors. It was an apt name, because it was a dramatic place. The wind blew, the rain fell, clouds drifted in and out, and sometimes the sun even shone—often all within half an hour. The turbulence of the weather was echoed in the forbidding look of the cragged peaks surrounding the city. I had heard the place described as the City at the End of the World, and that seemed appropriate, too. Despite the human footprint on the land, it still appeared primordial.

Ushuaia is small, but it still offered some interesting sights, like the old prison, now open for nonconvict visitors. There was also a large nature preserve, and, most interesting to me, little houses mounted on sleds. As I learned, real estate ownership had been a loose concept at the tip of the world. When a dispute over land occurred, local residents traditionally solved the problem by simply moving their houses across the road. There weren't many of these sled-houses left, though; in Ushuaia, as in so many northern cities, open land was becoming a less and less readily available commodity.

With our time in Ushuaia concluded, our group met on the dock to board one of two chartered Russian research ships for the two-and-a-half day journey south through the treacherous Drake Passage. I had signed on with the smaller ship, which carried forty-six passengers. At this point we met our full expedition staff, led by Shane Evoy, a large, bearded, garrulous man who seemed perfectly suited to his work. The staff seemed to be a fun and enthusiastic bunch. One crew member confided to me that they had been looking forward to seeing us for weeks, since our ultra-fit group was a nice change from the often sedentary, elderly tourists that they usually escort to the Southern Continent.

Along with the expedition staff was the Russian crew who manned the vessel. Not many of them spoke English, but they proved themselves to be very hard-working, prompting me to learn at least one word of Russian: *spaciba*, meaning thank you. We were allowed to go up to the bridge and watch them in action, as long as we kept out of their way. The kitchen staff was equally good, providing three great meals a day, plus snacks. As a bachelor living alone back in the States, I found myself eating better aboard the ship than I did at home.

The ship itself was comfortable, but utilitarian. There was no lido deck or pool, but there was a bar—well-used on our trip—a lecture room, a small library, and even a sauna. Bathrooms and shower stalls were shared, with plenty of hot water available. The cabins were wood-paneled, each with two closets and a desk. Bunks had reading lights and curtains for privacy. Laundry service was available on the ship as well, though that seemed to be the kind of extra frill this group wouldn't go for. We thought ourselves hardier stock than that.

As part of the prerace package, I received an informational guidebook, which I devoured along with a score of other books on the history and environment of the White Continent. Once on the ship, I watched films and attended lectures offered by the expedition's naturalists. Surprisingly it wasn't hard to get a feel for the place. Antarctica, I learned, had no indigenous people, and was populated only by whales, penguins, seals, a few species of birds, and the shrimplike krill on which many of the other animals fed. Not much of anything, really.

Still, Antarctica proved fascinating in the way a simple, pure color on canvas can be captivating. But I couldn't help viewing all of the information I came across through the eyes of a runner, so when I read about air avalanches, called *katabatic winds*, I felt myself gritting my teeth. While most wind is caused by differences in air pressure, these winds are caused instead by gravity. Just as hot air rises, cold air can fall, and in Antarctica, cold air sometimes falls so rapidly that it can blow at 40 mph or more. I knew that if this occurred during my race, there wouldn't be much I could do about it other than lean in and fight like hell. As I read about those winds, I suddenly realized that nothing I had done before—including Pikes Peak—had really prepared me for what I might find down here on race day.

No Antarctic education is complete, of course, without learning the story of exploration. The tales of courage, suffering and vanity left me awestruck. Especially memorable was the Shackleton expedition. Ernest Shackleton set out in 1914 on the aptly named *Endurance* to become the first man to traverse the Antarctic continent, the South Pole having already been won. Before he even managed to reach land, however, his ship became ice-locked. All efforts to free the ship failed, and by late 1915, the shifting mass of ice had crushed his ship, leaving the crew to live on the ice with three lifeboats and whatever supplies they were able to salvage from the *Endurance* before it went under. Eventually, the ice broke up, and the crew took to the lifeboats and made their way through rough seas and freezing weather to a spit of rock called Elephant Island.

Their new home was well outside any established shipping lanes, and realizing that their chances for rescue were slim—and recognizing, too, that a steady diet of nothing but penguin meat was taking a terrible toll on his crew—Shackleton set out with a few handpicked men in one of the lifeboats to find help. In what has been hailed as one of the all-time greatest feats of seamanship, Shackleton managed to steer his 22-foot open boat 800 nautical miles through wild and freezing seas to King George Island, where there was a whaling station. But the currents had forced Shackleton to land on the far side of the island, and now he and his crew had to scale uncharted mountains to reach the station. Once again, Shackleton accomplished the impossible, and after they stumbled into town, the station's captain could scarcely believe the tale that the ragged, unshaven, exhausted band of men told him. By August 1916, Shackleton managed to secure a ship and rescue his crew. All hands made it back home alive.

Lying back in my warm and comfortable bunk, I could scarcely believe such a thing had ever happened. But there was a postscript to the story. When Shackleton returned to England, he expected to be hailed as a hero, but in his absence all of Europe had been embroiled in the bloodbath known as the Great War. Faced with the story of men who risked their lives for adventure and glory, and who lived to tell the tale, a weary and grief-stricken public gave a collective shrug. Shackleton's agonies paled in comparison to the tragedies *they* had endured.

Somehow, I felt an odd kinship with Shackleton. He set out to face suffering—perhaps not as much as he bargained for, but guaranteed suffering nonetheless—when it would have been just as easy and acceptable to stay home. Although his aim was clearly fame and fortune, I felt that there must have been something more to make the deprivation worthwhile: a desire, a need, to test his own limits. That much resonated with me. I knew that I, too, valued suffering for its own sake, though mostly just in 26.2-mile doses.

Our ship made its way from Ushuaia through the Beagle Channel into open water, escorted by Magellanic penguins swimming below, and albatross soaring above. After rounding Cape Horn, we entered the dreaded Drake Passage, where the Atlantic and the Pacific oceans converge to create the roughest seas on Earth. Waves routinely crest there at 25 to 30 feet, and often higher. For me, surviving the Drake was the biggest challenge of the trip. I never had what you would call a strong stomach, and I was well aware of the irony of my being on a ship on high seas after a lifetime of enduring queasiness on ferries and carnival rides.

I hadn't come unarmed. I'd prepared for the "Drake Shake" with every antinausea treatment known to science, and a few others besides. My doctor provided me with antinausea scopolamine patches, my pharmacist provided me with acupressure wristbands and old-fashioned Dramamine, and an herbalist sold me ginger candies to settle my stomach. I also knew that gazing at a stable point on the distant horizon while breathing deep gulps of fresh air would be helpful. With all these remedies in my bag of tricks, I felt as ready as I could possibly be.

I was surprised, then, and even a bit disappointed, to find that the seas were calm. Instead of the Drake Shake, we got the Drake Lake. All that worrying for nothing. With such calm waters, I was even able to get in a workout, ducking though portholes and sliding around the corners of the deck as I ran for 45 minutes. Several team members joined in, and we quickly dubbed our workout the Drake 5K. Much to our delight, we were told by the expedition staff that the Russian crew thought we were crazy.

After two-and-a-half days of listening to lectures, socializing at the bar, and gazing out at the horizon, we finally saw a few bits of sea ice. Then we had our first glimpse of land. We were out of the Drake Passage and were approaching the South Shetland Islands, just off the Antarctic Peninsula. It was summer in Antarctica, but the temperature was still in the 20s and low 30s, with gusting winds bringing it down into the teens. We all dug out our waterproof gear as the expedition staff prepared for our first landing. There weren't any docks or piers to welcome us, so all landings were wet. After scampering down a gangway, we climbed ten at a time into inflated, motorized boats called Zodiacs, which were driven as far up onto the rocky beach as possible. One by one, we swung our legs over the side and charged the surf like soldiers at Normandy. After experiencing this landing, I understood why we had each been required to acknowledge in writing that we were not guaranteed a marathon; if bad weather made a wet landing hazardous, there would be no race.[2]

When I first signed up for the expedition, the tour company director told me that although I was coming down to Antarctica for the marathon, it would slip into lesser significance when compared to everything else I would see down there. He was right. Our first stop was a visit to the Polish scientific base camp, followed by a landing at a penguin rookery, where thousands of Chinstrap and Gentoo penguins mingled about, molting and nesting. Following the staff's directions, we sat very still, and soon the cute, impossibly clumsy little guys came right up to us, climbing onto our laps and nibbling on our pant legs. I captured their cooing and braying on a micro tape recorder, which I thought would provide a perfect soundtrack for slide shows back home. All of this was wonderful, but one thing was not: the smell. These were wild animals, after all, and when they crowd together in one place by the thousands, there were bound to be repercussions.

Not so different from runners at a starting line, actually.

After making several other Zodiac landings, including one to the ruins of a former whaling station at Deception Island, we finally made our way to King George Island, where the staff laid out our marathon course. It was to be a double figure-8 loop, and it was every bit as difficult as we imagined it would be. The first loop of the figure 8 (which would also be the third loop as I made my way around the course for the second time), was a 1½-mile run across a rocky beach, up the side of a glacier, and back. We would then run along rough dirt roads and across a frigid stream past several scientific bases.

---

2 In fact, in the very next Antarctic Marathon expedition, held two years later, a landing was not possible. Nonetheless, in a feat that could be described as either monumentally determined or frighteningly compulsive, a marathon was held onboard the ship, consisting of 420 laps around the deck. Let's just say that I'm glad that I didn't have to consider that option.

This island, and indeed, this entire frozen continent, is governed by the Antarctic Treaty system, which provides that while no country may claim sovereignty over these lands or engage in commercial exploitation of its natural resources, countries may establish scientific bases to conduct research. A human presence is especially evident on King George Island, where seven nations built small villages. Our group was hosted by the Uruguayans, and their base would mark the start and finish of the race.

On race day, we awoke early and ate breakfast. The waters were calm, so we were able to land without incident. We were allowed into the small dining hall in the Uruguayan base to prepare ourselves for the race, but because their living space was modest, we weren't allowed to keep any of our bags inside the building. It was a small inconvenience, and no one seemed to mind. We also had to provide our own water bottles, which the staff placed out on the course for us.

As we lined up for the start of the race, I saw that several of the local residents had taken up the tour leader's offer to join us for the race. Most striking was an older, plump Russian woman who wore running shorts, a T-shirt, and oven mitts instead of the tights, long sleeve shirts, jackets and running gloves that the rest of us wore. Clearly, improvisation is a crucial skill down there.

The starting signal was given—a horn blare from a megaphone— and we dashed across the broken rock toward the glacier. I had expected that its surface would be a slippery sheet of ice, but instead I found it to more like an ice chip mountain. That made it not only more treacherous than I was expecting, but also prone to suddenly giving way, leaving a runner knee-deep in a previously hidden hole. Cracks in the ice only compounded the problem, making for very slow going.

After reaching the turnaround point on top of the glacier, and smiling for the official race cameraman, I carefully made my way back down past the Uruguayan base, and then continued along rough dirt roads, over steep hills, and past a small lake, toward the Chilean base and on to the Chinese and the Russian bases that lay beyond. I later learned that one member of our team stopped into the Chinese base, where he bartered for a watch and was treated to a warm drink.

Not being as creative, I just focused on the race. A spot of warm weather created mud fields for us to slog through, as curious penguins watched closely. There was something eerily magnetic about the penguins; I saw more than one runner veer off course toward them, as if hypnotized. A few shouts brought them back to their senses and to the racecourse. More perilous, though, were the skuas: big, darkly colored birds that were reported to be fiercely protective of their nests. If we wandered too close to one of their nests, we were told, a skua would swoop down and attack us. The problem, though, was that their nests weren't always in plain view. At one point on the course several of us apparently came too close, because a skua took wing and made repeated dives at us, which we warded off by wildly swinging our arms.

After more than five hours of sliding, mucking, hiking, and even running across the Antarctic tundra, I finally crossed the finish line. Marathon number 41 was in the books. I was neither the first nor the last runner to finish. Since the fancy new trail shoes I had brought had given me some nasty blisters, I was perfectly happy to have just made it through the whole way. We returned to our ship to clean up, nap, and fill our bellies, and then were transported to the larger ship for an onboard awards presentation.

The following day, we set off for another highlight: our dramatic landing on the Antarctic mainland itself. We boarded the Zodiac boats again, and made out way to a landing on the Antarctic Peninsula. It was similar to the other landings we had made, but somehow, it felt different. Gazing at the rock and ice around us, I think we all felt that we were finally, truly, at the bottom of the world, at one of the last unspoiled expanses left on Earth. I wondered whether our brand of ecotourism was helping to build political support to preserve it, or whether, despite our precautions and good intentions, we were the beginning of a flood of tourists who would unwittingly destroy it.[3] Our usually rambunctious group had fallen into silence; I supposed that they were all wondering the same thing.

And then it was back through the Drake. This time the seas were not so friendly, as the ship pitched and rolled through 35- and 40-foot waves. We were banned from the outside deck, as well as the bridge. Digging deep into my bag of tricks, I managed to keep my insides inside and my stomach quiet, provided that I stayed prone in my bed. Strangely enough, the same corkscrewing, rolling action that slammed me from wall to wall and turned my stomach when I tried walking felt comforting once I lay down. I decided not to fight it; I buried myself under my covers, and drifted off to sleep, rocked by the southern ocean like a baby in a crib.

Two days later we landed in Ushuaia, and few days after that I was standing in a terminal at JFK airport in New York City. It was snowing, and the temperature was near zero—colder, in fact, than it was just then in Antarctica. I stood for a few minutes off to the side of the arrival gate, trying to adjust to the sudden noise and bustle. I had never before felt so different from everyone else.

---

3 My fears were, unfortunately, well-founded. In November 2007, the cruise ship *MS Explorer* sank in Antarctica. While all 154 passengers and crew were rescued, the ship left behind a mile-long oil spill that could not be immediately cleaned up because of bad weather. As scientists worried about the effect of the spill on the 2,500 penguins who were about to pass that area, the Argentinean government announced that it was considering limiting the level of ecotourism to the area.

## Running Tip #6

### *Preparing for Antarctica*

- *Don't bother with speed work.* The Antarctic Marathon isn't for PRs, so instead, concentrate training on hills and trails.
- *Bring the right clothing.* Dress in layers: running tights, a long sleeve wicking top, and lightweight running gloves to keep warm, covered by wind pants, a lightweight water-resistant running jacket, and lightweight water-resistant gauntlet mittens over your gloves. Shed clothing cautiously, since the wind could suddenly pick up and the temperature drop.
- *Bring the right gear.* Use trail shoes, gaiters (short, protective ankle sleeves that help keep out dirt and water), and mini-crampons (rubber outsoles with short, plastic spikes for better traction on ice).
- *Bring a disposable, panoramic camera.* After all, this is a once-in-a-lifetime kind of race.

# Finally: Boston!

After returning home from Antarctica, I felt oddly depressed. For the first time as a runner, I felt unmotivated. I realized that Antarctica was to blame. I had harbored so much anticipation for the race that once it was over, I felt let down. The Boston Marathon was coming up in just two months, and I couldn't afford a training slump. To properly prepare for Boston, I needed another marathon to restore my motivation and keep me in prime condition. That's how I came to run the 1999 Los Angeles Marathon.

Signing up for the race was the easy part, but I was a bit sloppy on figuring out the logistics. I had traveled alone to run the race, and ended up staying in a hotel about 8 miles or so from the race start. I took a taxi to the race packet pick-up the day before the marathon, which was located near the race start, and was surprised to see how expensive the cab ride would be. Not wanting to blow my budget on transportation, I researched bus routes, and discovered that one bus would drop me off right next to the start. Perfect. The following morning I got up early and waited at the stop next to my hotel. I had given myself plenty of time—unusual for me, but I didn't want to take any chances. Finally, the bus came, and I settled back for a relaxing ride. Everything was under control.

And then, suddenly, there was chaos. The bus pulled over and the driver announced that this was as far as the bus would go, due to street closings caused by the marathon. How could I not have realized this would happen? Anger and frustration boiled up inside me, stoked by the realization that we were still about six miles from the race start, with precious little time to spare before the gun.

No need to panic, yet; I just had to hail a cab, and everything would be okay. I began walking down the street in search of a taxi. I quickly realized, though, that the streets were deserted due to the street closings. All I saw were traffic cones and occasional police cruisers. Checking my watch, I saw that there were just 5 minutes until the race start. It was time to panic. I broke into a run, scouring each street that I passed for signs of life. I picked up the pace, and went into top gear. I knew this wasn't the way to warm up for a marathon, but I had little choice.

Finally, I saw a cab, and was able to flag it down. I explained my situation to him, and he zipped off to the freeway, promising to get me to the race. We had just a few scant minutes, and six miles to go. I anxiously counted the passing seconds as we weaved through traffic. With my eyes glued to my watch, I saw the official starting time come and go. We were still on the highway. I was heartbroken. My driver reassured me that we were close, and as we neared the start downtown, I told him to just pull over. I threw money toward the front seat and leapt out of the cab, scrambled up the embankment, and hurtled over the guardrail. In front of me was the starting area, now bereft of all runners. The race was already 10 minutes old. People were milling about, and workers had started taking down the starting sign. This race was not turning out to be a good motivator for running Boston the following month!

"Runner coming through!" I yelled, dodging and weaving through the crowd. Up ahead, an electronic mat straddled the street, activated by a chip containing a transponder that each runner fixed to his or her shoe. Most big races use these to track runners and record each runner's finishing time. As I crossed the starting line, the very last person to do so in a field of more than 10,000 runners, I heard a reassuring beep. I was officially in the race.

Starting dead last has its benefits, as I soon learned. Usually the ranks of runners in a big race are shoulder to shoulder for the first mile or so, until they begin to spread out. It's only then that you can settle into your own target race pace. Not so for the last-place runner, however. From my vantage point, I could see that the field had already spread, and I was able to run as fast as I wanted from the very start. I began to wonder if this might not be a good way to intentionally start my races, but I quickly put that thought out of my head. Like a dog ordered to sit still while a juicy steak was inches from its nose, I knew that I wouldn't be able to fight off the urge to run once the gun goes off in a race and everyone surges forward. I was disciplined enough to run the marathon, but not disciplined enough to not run it, even for ten minutes.

I soon discovered another great benefit to starting in the back; you get to pass people. You get to pass *a lot* of them, and that's a good feeling. But more than that, you get to really see the race; I saw people who would usually be invisible to me, buried in sea of humanity far behind me. Among these faces in Los Angeles were several runners I knew from other races, people I didn't even know were planning to run L.A. If I hadn't started in the back of the pack, I never would have seen them, and never would have had a chance to say hello. It was a rare and welcome treat.

When all was said and done, I crossed the finish line in L.A. with a good time, and a story to boot. Marathon number 42 was history. And better still, I had restored my desire to race. I was like a lion pacing in a cage, and Boston was the meat laid in front of me.

Boston had always seemed like a dream to me, like a Camelot for runners, more myth than reality. I had run it once before as a charity fund-raiser, but that didn't feel right to me. Not to take anything away from all those dedicated and caring runners who race as fund-raisers—many of whom I coached myself—getting my Boston race number without running a qualifying time was hollow for me because I hadn't *earned it*. But in April 1999, I had earned my spot officially. From the barren waste-land of Antarctica to the famous starting line of the Boston Marathon in the outlying town of Hopkinton, I was on quite a roll.

From the moment I arrived in town, I couldn't help but get swept up in the excitement. While other cities sometimes ignore or tolerate their marathons, Boston is absolutely in love with theirs, and it showed. Banners and signs advertising the race were everywhere. Stores offered marathon merchandise—and not just the running stores—and seemingly everyone I met asked if I was running the race. Strangers smiled and wished me luck. Suddenly, marathoning wasn't a fringe sport, it was front-page news.

The runners themselves flooded the streets, shops, and restaurants like locusts. There was an audible buzz in the air, made up of dozens of simultaneous conversations about training, about the racecourse, and about qualifying races. The Boston Marathon began to feel like it was something more than a race; it began to feel like a mass movement.

And that, of course, is what it is. Any doubts were dispelled at packet pickup at the cavernous convention center, where thousands of people lined up to get their race numbers and to check out the expo. At most races, packet pickup is often little more than a quick, prerace chore, but here it's an *event*, a celebration of life and of running. Just making it into Boston is an achievement, and being part of the race said something about a person's work ethic and lifestyle.

Even the official Boston Marathon shirt made a statement. It was devoid of any splashy multi-color race emblem, and it lacked the tangle of corporate sponsor logos that covered most other race shirts. In Boston, you always get a long-sleeved shirt with a small Boston Athletic Association logo on the breast and *Boston Marathon* written down one arm. The color of the shirt varies from year to year, but the design never changes. It's quiet and dignified, and there's no other running shirt like it.

After picking up my race packet, I wandered around the expo. The energy was unbelievable. There was a palpable excitement in the air, heightened by the presence of so many of the world's greatest runners, past and present, signing autographs and talking with fans. In contrast to many professional athletes in other sports, these pros were friendly and accessible, swapping stories, training tips, and race strategies with anyone they met. I wondered whether this easy rapport stemmed from the fact that on race day, we would all face the same challenge. While even the most rabid Red Sox fan would likely never dig in at the plate at Fenway Park, any runner of any ability can go head-to-head against the best runners in the world by simply entering a race. Even Boston, with its qualifying times, provides a place where runners of modest ability can mix with the elite. And on race day, we have a shared experience: we all have to handle the weather, the course, and the challenge of covering the miles as fast as we can. It's a leveling experience.

Perhaps, too, the difference between running and other sports lies in the basis for excellence. While all top athletes train and practice, runners rely mostly on the relentless grind of their training, and not on any superior hand-eye coordination, as baseball and basketball players do. Elite runners are genetically gifted, sure, but without intense training, those gifts are wasted. Their training creates a strong work ethic that leaves humility in its wake. There are no short cuts in marathoning, so anyone who is a marathoner has worked hard. It's a lesson no one forgets.

After a few hours, I had had enough of the expo, and staggered out with a bag of promos, giveaways, premiums, and samples. I ate an early prerace meal, and spent the next few hours lying sleeplessly in bed. Finally, it was race day. Not Sunday morning, though, as it would be with most races, but Monday, the state holiday known as Patriot's Day. In Boston, that means a day off, a Red Sox game, and the Marathon.

Getting to the marathon was an adventure in itself. The Boston Marathon, like marathons in New York City, Las Vegas, and numerous other places, uses a point-to-point course. This turns the marathon into a true journey, as runners pass from town to town, along country roads, over train tracks, into the heart of the city. The problem, though, is that unlike loop or out-and-back courses, runners don't return to where they started. This creates a logistical challenge: thousands of runners have to be transported from downtown Boston out to the start line, where water, shelter, and bathrooms are provided for them as they wait several hours for the last of the participants to arrive. I'm sure race morning is a mad scramble for the race staff, but for the runners, it's an exercise in rushing to do nothing, and it can be quite frustrating.

Most point-to-point races require a predawn lineup for bus transport. In Boston, the race doesn't begin until noon, and the wait at the high school in Hopkinton—transformed into the Athletes' Village on race day—can be three hours or more.[4] This is my least favorite part of the marathon experience. I've learned to deal with it, and I've even found some ways to make the process a bit more tolerable. At the New York City Marathon one year, instead of waiting on line with other runners for the bus to starting area in Staten Island, some friends of mine and I rented a limo to drop us off at the starting line. It felt decadent, but split between us, it really wasn't too expensive at all, and not only did we avoid the predawn bus lines and were able to sleep a little bit later, but we were able to enjoy the envious and curious stares from other runners as we emerged from our ride.

In Boston, though, I wasn't so lucky or creative. I waited on one of the many long lines at Boston Commons as the fleet of yellow school

---

4  In 2007, years of tradition were abandoned as the race was moved up to 10 A.M. to avoid the worst of the midday heat that had plagued runners in the preceding few years.

buses made their circuit to the race start and back. Eventually, I boarded one of the buses, and settled into a window seat. As the bus droned and rocked, I fell into a drowsy stupor. Finally we arrived at our base camp. Rows of Porta-Jons and several big tents had been set up on the school grounds, along with a stage where various speakers and musicians provided information, advice, and entertainment. My drowsiness quickly disappeared, both from a sudden adrenaline rush and from the shock of cold air. April is a tricky time in Massachusetts; it could be scorching hot or icy cold, but no matter which it is, the chances are that at some point you'll be uncomfortable on race day. That year, it was cold, which made waiting for the race to begin an awful ordeal.

Well, not entirely awful. There was one special marathon tradition that I witnessed and would never forget: the moment marathon legend Johnny Kelley took the stage. Kelley first ran the Boston Marathon in 1928, and won the race in 1935 and 1945. He finished in second place seven times, and was in the top ten eighteen times. He also competed in the 1936 Olympic Games, but he was perhaps more famous for holding the record for the number of times he'd entered the Boston Marathon (sixty-one), and the number of times he finished it (fifty-eight). He was also immortalized in the 1936 race, when eventual winner Tarzan Brown (and how's that for a name!) passed him on the last of three brutal hills in the town of Newton, a moment, the press reported, that broke Kelley's heart. That hill would forevermore be known as Heartbreak Hill, and would eventually be the site of a statue depicting a young Johnny Kelley running hand in hand with an older version of himself.

As I stood before the stage in Hopkinton that morning, Kelley looked thin and frail, a vestige of the great athlete that he once was. Then he spoke. He told us to enjoy the day, to be careful on the course, and to enjoy ourselves. Finding a reserve of strength, as he must have done all those times on Heartbreak Hill, Kelley asked if we'd like him to sing for us. We all clapped and cheered, and Kelley broke into his signature song,

"Young At Heart." The crowd went crazy, laughing and applauding, as cameras clicked all around me. Everyone seemed to recognize that this was one of those special moments, one we would carry with us and share with others for many years to come.[5]

After several hours, we were called away from the school and out onto the street, where corrals had been roped off to separate runners according to their expected finishing times. Standing around for hours drinking water, coffee, and sports drink—as nasty a combination as I could think of—had taken its toll on many of the runners, but the good folks of Hopkinton didn't seem very sympathetic to our plight. Many homeowners patrolled their bushes like guard dogs, shouting away any runners who tried to take care of business surreptitiously. Rather unfriendly, I thought, but what did I know? I lived in a condo, and knew zilch about gardening. For all I knew, the cumulative effects of 18,000 or so overly hydrated, nervous runners could lead to permanent deforestation, so I tried to be sensitive to the concerns of the local community.

The excitement grew as noon approached. Then finally, after years of dreaming, months of planning, hours of waiting, we were off. The Boston Marathon had begun!

The cheering at the starting line was incredible, as the runners passed through a gauntlet of spectators and tried to settle down into their pace. The Boston Marathon is really a tour through a series of towns, which the marathon fanatics can recite in order: *Hopkinton—Ashland—Natick—Wellesley—Newton—Brookline—Boston.* Strategically, this presents some interesting possibilities. Most people focus on the big hills of Newton, stacked one after another between miles 17 and 21, where runners have just started feeling deep fatigue and doubt. What most people don't really consider, however, is that the Boston Marathon is actually a

---

5 Johnny Kelley last ran the Boston Marathon in 1992, when he was eighty-four. He died on October 6, 2004, at the age of ninety-seven.

very fast course, dropping 413 feet over the first 17 miles. Over the next 4 miles, in Newton, runners must climb back up 187 feet, but then the course drops another 127 feet from Newton to the finish line. Apart from those difficult hills in Newton, then, the Boston Marathon is mostly a downhill course.

So, what to do? Conventional wisdom is to run the first 17 downhill miles conservatively and save energy for Newton. Once those big hills are conquered, it would be time to turn on the gas and fly through the final 5 miles to the finish. That was the way Boston was supposed to be run.

Naturally, I decided to do something different. My problem with the conventional wisdom was that the miles before Newton represented two-thirds of the whole race. If I ran that part conservatively, then even if I felt great in the last 5 miles and ran that section hard, I wouldn't be able to make up for all those mediocre early miles, and I would wind up with a mediocre finishing time. On the other hand, if I ran those first 17 miles hard, and struggled through the hills of Newton, I would have only 5 miles between myself and the finish line. I would no doubt be dog tired at that point, but if I could just muster up a little more courage and manage to hold onto my pace, I could wind up with a great finishing time.

Or, I could blow up, and find my body in full revolt in Newton, leaving me sprawled on the grass on the side of the road, exhausted and broken.

Those were basically my options as I saw them. Dare greatly and risk dropping out, or run conservative toward a good, if not glorious, finish.

I thought back to the words of the late Steve Prefontaine, probably the greatest middle-distance runner the United States has ever produced. Pre would often flout conventional wisdom by running out front instead of biding his time for a strong finish. In the 1972 Olympic Games, he pushed the pace in the 5K, running a courageous race but ultimately finishing fourth. "A lot of people run a race to see who's the fastest," he said. "I run to see who has the most guts." That's how I wanted to run. I couldn't win in Boston, of course, but I would run as courageously as anyone there.

With that settled, I streaked through Hopkinton, weaving my way through the runners and enjoying the loud encouragement of the fans packing the roadsides. My legs felt fresh and strong, with lots of pop. In the words of the old Irish toast—appropriate in Boston—it felt as though the road were rising up to greet me. I recognized Darryl, a fellow runner from my track group in D.C. I shouted hello as I flew past. I was running well, and enjoying myself.

The sights of the marathon came and went. I flew past the clock tower in Ashland, the old train station in Framingham, and approached Wellesley. I had heard other runners joking about the enthusiastic co-eds there, but I wasn't prepared for the sheer bedlam of it all. Row upon row of women screamed out to us, offering us encouragement along with offers of kisses. Some guys grinningly took them up on their offers and received a peck, but I was too shy even for that. And, of course, I still had my race to run.

Next up was fabled Newton, and I knew this was where my race would truly begin. If I could make it through the three hills of Newton without breaking, I would have a chance at a great finish.

I hit the first hill, and rode it as the course turned onto broad Commonwealth Avenue. The climb was over a mile long, but I kept my legs churning, and finally I crested the top. The next mile was a gentle downhill, giving all of us a chance to recover our strength and determination for the next challenge ahead. The runners around me were silent, their faces held tight. They seemed like fishermen sailing into a squall, determined not to break. We rode the next hill the same way.

And then Heartbreak Hill was upon us like a storm. Runners swung their arms and fought to hold their pace, grunting and breathing heavily. The crowds were thick along the street and in the broad, grassy median, screaming and waving banners and signs. They knew that this was the most dramatic part of the race, because it was here that the race was usually won and lost; the finish was only for the coronation. And it was here, too, that the humanity and courage of the runners was most evident. We spoke to each another, offering encouragement, trying to share our energy, hoping that together we could bring everyone to the top. A stranger looked over at me and said, "Run with me. We can do this. Run with me."

I pushed to keep up with him, repeating the mantra, "We're almost there, we're almost there, we're almost there." I saw the hilltop just up ahead, and I lowered my eyes. It was so far away, and the road was so steep. I counted off ten seconds before I looked up again. The top of the hill still seemed so distant. I looked back down. Finally, I was there, at the top. I had conquered Heartbreak Hill. I had slowed, but not by very much, and now I just had to pick up the pace and race to the finish in Copley Square.

But did I have anything left in my legs?

I took a moment's breather, and then tried to accelerate. There was that moment's gap, that briefest moment between the command my mind gave, and the response of my legs. I lived a lifetime in that moment, fearful that my legs would refuse to answer my call. But they did. They had not abandoned me. I streaked down the back side of the hill, with renewed strength and hope.

Soon, the excitement of Newton faded behind me, and with it, the adrenaline rush that conquering the hills had given me. There were still 5 miles left to go, and that was a very long way to run on tired legs. I tried to focus only on the patch of road in front of me, and concentrated on maintaining my pace.

I streaked down Commonwealth Avenue, along the train line, and looked up for the massive neon Citgo gas sign in Kenmore Square that would tell me that the finish line was only a mile away. Seeing the sign would be like spotting a lighthouse in a storm at sea; it was the promise of safety, of release from pain and fatigue.

Suddenly, someone jumped in from the crowd and began to match me, stride for stride. It was Lynn, a teammate from my Antarctica adventure. We had kept in touch, and since she lived nearby, she said she'd come to Boston and try to run me in to the finish line. Now there she was, when I needed her most. She didn't have to say much as she ran with me, but I drew energy from her, taking strength from her companionship. I ran like a machine now, thinking only about keeping my legs moving, pushing, pushing, pushing, concentrating on nothing but running.

Finally, the course veered away from Commonwealth Avenue and turned right onto Hereford Street for a couple of blocks, and then left onto Boylston Street. The finish line was just up ahead now. I could see it. It was just a few blocks away. I only had a minute of running left, I told myself. After all these hours, just one single minute. I told myself that I could endure any kind of pain for just one minute. I pushed as hard as I could, sprinting toward the finish line. Lynn matched me, and then drifted away as I flew through the finish line.

I had run the Boston Marathon in 3 hours, 9 minutes, just a single heartbeat slower than my personal best. In the process, I also requalified to run the Boston Marathon the following year. Most importantly, though, I had run courageously, and I felt like I truly belonged at Boston. In this, my 43rd marathon, near the halfway point to reaching my 100-marathon quest, I finally felt like a marathoner.

There was another thing about Boston that was auspicious. I hadn't kept in touch with too many of my old high school friends, but I'd heard through the grapevine, such as it was, that one of our classmates, Stephanie Kay, was teaching art at Boston University. Stephanie and I had been friends in school. We were not very close friends, but I always thought that we got along well. I liked her, but I thought that she was perhaps a little out of my league. She was very pretty, and being an artist, she hung out with the cool crowd. But we were adults now, and I was curious about what she looked like and how she was doing. I left her a message through her office, just letting her know that I was coming into town for the race and would love to catch up with her. I didn't hear back. Well, that was all right. It had been well over a decade since we'd last seen each other, and my message had come out of the blue, so I couldn't blame her for tossing it aside. I guessed that she just wasn't interested.

It would be a while until I found out how wrong I was.

## Running Tip #7

### *Massage*

Nonrunners assume that it's better to run downhill than up, but that's not always true. Downhill is *faster*, but it's far more brutal than uphill. After crossing the finish line in Boston, my joints stiffened and my muscles began to ache from all the pounding my body had absorbed. The quadriceps muscles on the front of my legs, which had kept me from falling right on my face, were totally shot. A few days' rest didn't bring much relief. I needed help. I was ready for a massage.

Hard training and racing causes micro-tears and the accumulation of waste products in muscle cells. Adhesions also can occur, in which muscles cells stick together, limiting flexibility and healing. Massage forces waste out of the muscle tissue and breaks up adhesions, resulting in reduced recovery time, improved range of motion, and a lower occurrence of injury.

It can take a while for the benefits of massage to become fully apparent, although the results could sometimes be very dramatic. Once, a massage therapist was working deeply (and painfully!) on a spot in my upper back where I'd been feeling pain, when I suddenly broke out in a drenching sweat. The therapist said it was common for stressed bodies to release their tension that way, and it really did feel as though a clenched fist had suddenly opened up. I felt better immediately.

But don't get massage only when you're injured; aim to get a massage monthly, or even biweekly or weekly if you can afford it. Or try self-massage: knead and rub your target muscles deeply, stroking toward your heart, using massage oil to reduce friction. There are also products available to facilitate self-massage, such as a rolling-pin like device that works especially well on hamstrings and quads.

# Across the Pond and Around
# the World

After conquering Antarctica, traveling abroad for a marathon didn't seem to be such a far-fetched idea. Following Boston, I ran the Salt Lake City Marathon in Utah. Even though I had raced to the top of Pikes Peak, I had never run an entire race at altitude before, and it seemed to have an effect on me that I hadn't anticipated: I suddenly developed an endless need to pull over to the bushes. I had never experienced anything like it before, and I don't know why it happened, but the result was that I was alternately passing and getting passed by the same handful of runners. Finally, one of them had had enough, and as I emerged from the woods for what must have been the tenth time, he yelled out "stop passing me!" All I could do was sheepishly apologize.

Next was an uneventful marathon in Tupelo, Mississippi—uneventful for me, though not for Dave, who joined me for that race. While I flew down for the race, Dave opted to minimize costs by taking an overnight bus down. At one rest stop, he lost track of time, and watched in alarm as his bus pulled out without him on board, but with all his racing gear sitting neatly on his window seat. He hopped the next bus and gave chase. Luckily, this new bus was an express, and he overtook his gear at the next major stop. After all that, running the race was easy for him. Once the race was over, Dave and I decided to go have lunch and celebrate with a few beers. The lunch was easy to find, but not the beer; we couldn't find any place to serve us alcohol on a Sunday. Tough lesson for a city boy like me to learn!

Following Mississippi, I set my sights on Berlin for marathon number 46. Berlin was a city in transition, ground zero for the collapse of communism and the birth of a new Europe. I read about how the city was rebuilding itself and was bristling with energy and excitement. The racecourse was supposed to be a very flat and fast course—several marathon world records had been set there. It seemed like the perfect marathon adventure.

I managed to talk two of my running friends into going with me. Our flights went smoothly, and we checked into our hotel without a problem. We also made it to the packet pickup easily enough; the Berlin Marathon is a huge race, with 20,000 or so participants, so all we had to do was get close to the race headquarters and look for people in running shoes toting their race packets and the goodie bags. We made our way to the great hall and collected our paperwork, only to discover that the race instructions were written only in German.

It's my conceit as an American that no matter where I go, I expect the locals to speak English, and that all instructions will be translated for my convenience. Apparently, the Germans had different ideas on the subject. I scanned the runner instructions. Some of the words bore a passing resemblance to English, but others were just a maze of letters. I was baffled by the German propensity to take lots of small words and mash them together into mammoth tongue twisters. Luckily, the materials had a similar layout to American race instructions, so we were able to more or less figure things out.

However odd and unsettling packet pickup had felt, race morning seemed as familiar and comfortable as an old shirt. Runners gathered at the starting line and did what runners everywhere do; they ate energy bars, drank water, stretched, napped, talked, paced, worried, and relaxed. Eventually, they huddled close together behind the starting line, and then exploded forward en masse at the blast of the starting gun. I found myself part of a teeming, sweating mass pouring through the Brandenburg Gate. It was unforgettable. I was surprised, though, to see mile markers popping up more often than I expected. I checked my last split time—the pace in which I'd run my last mile. My watch read 3:44. That would put me right about at the world record for the mile. *That can't be right,* I thought. Then it dawned on me. *Kilometers.* Those markers measure *kilometers,* not miles. The world record was safe, and worse yet, I would have to pass another 41 of those markers before I was through.

I immediately understood the downside of measuring a marathon course in kilometers—when I see a sign that reads "26," my body knows, like one of Pavlov's dogs, that it has only another minute and a half or so of running, and then it's quitting time. Not so in a European marathon. Marker 26 only tells me that I have another 16 kilometers to go. It's a definite downer.

On the other hand, kilometer markers fly past quicker than mile markers, which gives the feeling of progress being made. It's also an ego boost to pass numbers that get so staggeringly high: 35, 36, 37! On a practical level, having such a profusion of markers also provides runners with more opportunities to check their pace and make any necessary adjustments.

I also discovered anew that a marathon is a splendid way to tour a city. Anyone can lay out a 5K or 10K race course to avoid the seamier sides of a city, but a marathon exposes all there really is to see, the warts along with the beauty. In Berlin, we snaked our way over to the former East Germany, and what I saw there startled me. I had grown up during the Cold War, and had imagined East Germany as the formidable industrial muscle of the Soviet bloc, churning out weapons and superior athletes.

What I saw was no mighty enemy; the buildings all seemed shoddy and in disrepair. If ever this had been a place bustling with energy, that time had long since passed. I felt like I had peeked behind the curtain looking for the Wizard of Oz, only to find a little tired old man.

There *was* bustling energy in Berlin while we were there, but it was coming from the West. As we ran, we could see dozens of construction cranes dominating the city skyline like mythic giants. Berlin was a city in transition, and as I ran the course, I thought it would be interesting to come back and race the city again in a few years to see what it would grow to be.

Everything about the Berlin Marathon was as I expected it to be, but after crossing the finish line, I encountered one of the oddest sights I'd yet seen at a race: race volunteers carrying large bundles of cash for on-the-spot deposit refunds for race chips. I couldn't imagine anyone flashing wads of cash like that in Central Park in New York City, not even on marathon day with mounted police nearby. Fuhgeddaboutit.

After Berlin, I ran the Marine Corps and New York marathons again—a personal tradition at this point—and then ended 1999 by adding Washington State and Florida to my list of completed states. That made it eleven marathons in 1999, which was a new record for me, and I had reached marathon number fifty, the halfway point in my quest. But I didn't stop to ponder it, because I was busy running marathons in South Carolina, Maryland, Boston again, and Maine. Next up: joining a running group to head to Beijing for marathon number 55.

Beijing, like Berlin, was another city in transition. Its biggest changes would not come until years later, when it began building up in earnest for 2008 Olympic Games, but even in October 2000 there were signs of the coming transformation. There were more cars than I expected to see, and the clothes and bicycles of the younger Chinese were flashier and more colorful than the dour, drab designs sported by their elders.

Our tour guide helped minimize communication problems, but there was still opportunity for misadventure. One day, with no group activity scheduled, another team member and I climbed into a taxi, aiming to visit a local temple. We showed a photo of our intended destination to the driver, then sat back in the cab. Before long, the driver turned onto a highway, and as the miles and minutes ticked by, my friend and I exchanged nervous glances. After a 45-minute odyssey, the cab pulled up in front of a marketplace. We had no idea where we were, but we knew one thing: if we let that cab drive away, we might never find our way back. Having had the foresight to bring a book of matches from our hotel, we showed it to the driver and pointed at the address. He shrugged, and set off to return us to where we started. We never did make it to that temple, but things could have turned out much worse.

On race day, my traveling companions and I gathered with the other runners in Tiananmen Square. As we waited for the start, I looked around and tried to imagine the confrontation a decade earlier between government troops and the mass of protesters who had camped there. Our group had talked about it, but it was a topic that none of the local Chinese seemed willing or able to discuss with us. On race day, there was no dissent visible among those gathered; we were all runners. Crossing the cultural divide, I bartered my American running jacket for a Chinese Olympic team jacket, a deal consummated wordlessly with a Chinese runner, using rough pantomime to transcend our language barrier. It's a marathon treasure that's as meaningful to me as many of the medals I've earned.

Finally, we all gathered at the start line, and the familiar crack of the starter's gun sent us out on a loop of the square, under the larger-than-life gaze of Chairman Mao. His stern image was everywhere—not only on official posters but also on clock faces, shirts, mugs, and souvenir trinkets. He seemed to be making a transition himself, from revered leader to high camp. Ironic comeuppance for a despot.

After exiting Tiananmen Square and racing through the city, we were herded out onto one of the city's surrounding highways, where we tallied most of the miles in our race. The few spectators we passed stood in hushed observance, offering support with only an occasional clap or shout. After the spectacular start, the rest of the race was, to be honest, a very boring slog.

We finished our race on the highway, an appropriate end to a mostly disappointing race. I was still glad to have to have made the journey, though, especially after visiting an unrestored section of the Great Wall in an area well outside of Beijing. Still, the race itself seemed like a missed opportunity for the Chinese. A marathon should be used as a forum to showcase a city, to give visitors a glimpse into its natural and architectural beauty, its history, and its culture. Beijing had so much to offer, and yet the race did so little with it.

In addition to running on foreign soil, I undertook another challenge that year; in addition to my regular job, I became a marathon coach for a charity fundraising team in my spare time. I had jumped from being a marathoner to being a marathon evangelist. In 2000, I signed on with the Arthritis Foundation's Joints in Motion program, and the following year also signed up to coach the American Diabetes Association's Team Diabetes. Coaching forced me to articulate many of my beliefs about marathoning, and also to reconsider the elements of my training regimen. It was a great way to share my passion for marathoning, and I grew to love it. Also, as the old Navy recruiting posters used to say, it was a great way to see the world. I traveled with these teams to Dublin, Rome, Athens, and Amsterdam, and in each of these places, I ran along with them. I was as happy as an obsessed runner could be; I was helping charities and sharing my love for the marathon as I experienced races all around the world.

The trade-off, however, was my commitment to never running a marathon all-out if I was with a team. I didn't want to be in a position where I might be unavailable to help my team, whether from injury or mental and physical fatigue. I wanted to be able to not only finish the marathon with the runners I was pacing, but to also run back and see after our other, slower participants.

Still, it was an enormously rewarding experience. Many of our team members had never considered themselves athletes, and by the end of our time together, they had discovered a strength and resolve they never knew they possessed. This realization was a powerful thing, and I was thrilled to be part of it for so many people.

My first trip abroad with a charity team was for the Dublin Marathon, in October 2000, just two weeks after Beijing. Conditions in Ireland were brutal that year, as race day greeted us with driving rain and high winds. During the race, I tried ducking behind larger runners to lessen the impact of the wind, like a cyclist drafting another rider. Nothing helped, though. It was just one of those days.

The Irish fans seemed undisturbed by bad weather, however. They lined the roads and shouted "Well done, lads!" to the runners flying past. One spectator in particular remains in my memory: at mile 11, a golden-haired girl, no more than seven or eight years old, looked up hopefully as we ran past and squealed, "Give us a smile!" Those of us within earshot of this little sprite couldn't help but comply.

One unexpected feature of the race was that rather than hand out cups of water like they do in the States, the race volunteers in Dublin handed out full bottles. Not a bad idea, except that few runners drank the entire bottle, or even carried it for very long. The result: for the block or two after each water stop, half-filled water bottles flew through the air like hand grenades.

At the finish line, exhausted, shivering runners were treated to coffee and chocolate—not the bananas and bagels found at most races, but still very welcome. It had been a grueling day. I felt worst for the first-time runners, who perhaps didn't know that a marathon didn't have to be this hard. They had conquered more than the usual marathon challenge, and I tried to help them realize that. They were finally convinced by the front page of *The Irish Times* the following morning, which ran the headline "Runners Defy Wind and Rain in Marathon of Suffering." I kept that page, and have it somewhere still, buried in a stack of race memorabilia.

One month later, I found myself flying out to Hawaii with a different charity team for the Honolulu Marathon. Although we were still technically in the United States, Hawaii felt exotic. Perhaps that was because Hawaii is the only state with an historic palace, and because so many Japanese runners had entered the marathon. At one store, I actually wondered for a moment if they accepted dollars, proving true the old saying, better to be silent and thought a fool, rather than speak and remove all doubt.

In most marathons, my plan is to start out comfortably and slowly ease into my goal race pace, saving enough energy in reserve for a fast finish. But in Honolulu, with the threat of a hot sun weighing heavily on me, I decided to flip my strategy; I would start out fast and try to get as many miles as possible under my belt before the heat set in. It was a risky strategy, especially since I was committed to keeping some energy in reserve to use helping my team afterward, but I felt sure the best strategy would be to do what I could to avoid running more than necessary in the hot tropical sun.

We were in the Christmas holiday season, but the weather was warm as we lined up with 20,000 other runners in the predawn darkness in Waikiki, awaiting the traditional fireworks show that accompanied the race start. After looping Waikiki, we were sent out for two loops around Diamondhead, the volcano that dominated the Honolulu waterfront skyline. Despite my attempts to avoid spending too much time in the sun, I still found myself feeling dehydrated and depleted by the time

I made it to the finish line in Kapiolani Park 3 hours and 25 minutes after having started the race. Luckily, I recovered quickly, and was able to head out back on the course to run with my team and make sure they were all having the experience they had trained so faithfully for. And as for me, marathon number 57 was in the books, and Hawaii was on my list of states.

## Running Tip #8

### *Avoid Dehydration*

Your body uses water, in the form of sweat, to shed heat. This water comes mostly from blood plasma, and unless you replace it, your heart won't be able to pump the resulting sludge to your working muscles. As little as a 2 percent loss in body fluid can seriously affect exercise performance. Loss of blood plasma also makes it harder for your heart to send blood to the skin to cool off your core. When this happens, you risk heat exhaustion, and even heat stroke, which can be fatal.[6]

*Signs of dehydration*

- *Dry skin*
- *Cold or clammy skin*
- *Nausea*
- *Disorientation*

---

6 There's been some research, especially by Dr. Timothy Noakes of the University of Cape Town—who himself has run more than seventy marathons and ultramarathons—suggesting that dehydration isn't really dangerous at all. Instead, he argues, it actually helped early man hunt game across the open plains by reducing his body weight. Rising core temperatures and reduced speed are not caused by dehydration, he says, but instead by overexertion. While these are certainly intriguing ideas, and might very well be true, I'd recommend caution here, and stick for the time being with the conservative viewpoint until more research is done in this area.

*Your plan of attack*

- *Drink regularly.* Water is the old standby, but a sports drink also replaces essential minerals and provides some simple sugars for fuel. Drinking is the key; what you drink is up to you.
- *Weigh yourself.* Comparing your weight before and after exercise will tell you how much fluid you need to replace under various conditions.
- *If in doubt, act.* Slow down and take in more fluids. Slurp water from a garden hose, or knock on someone's door and explain your problem. Pour cool water on your wrists, arms and head. Sit down in a shady area. If you don't feel better quickly, call 911. Don't be brave; this is a potentially dangerous situation.

# Island Running

As the jet descended toward the runway, it wasn't hard for me to remember why I had decided to come to Bermuda. Looking out the window, I saw palm trees. It was the middle of January, 2001, and here I was, looking at *palm trees.* Back home in Washington, D.C., I wouldn't see green outdoors for another two months or so. The temperature, as promised in the Department of Tourism brochures, was in the mid-60s, with cloudy skies. A little warm for running, perhaps, but I knew what to do about that, right?

Often thought of as one of the Caribbean islands, Bermuda actually lies far to the north, some 570 miles east of the North Carolina coast. Although it's commonly considered a single island, it is actually a collection of some 150 separate islands, many of them no more than a speck of rock peeking above the bright blue waters. They are the tips of long-dormant volcanoes, together forming a long, fishhook-shaped archipelago, inhabited by some 61,000 people. Because these islands are swept by the friendly Gulf Stream winds, the temperature in Bermuda stays moderate all year long, with temperatures ranging from a low in the upper 60 degrees Fahrenheit, to a high in the mid-to-upper 70 degrees Fahrenheit.

In the middle of this fishhook is the city of Hamilton, established in 1790 as a convenient meeting place for all of Bermuda's scattered residents. Now the capital of Bermuda, its streets are filled with pubs, restaurants, and little shops. The main thoroughfare here is Front Street, which runs parallel to the harbor, and which features a roofed sentry box affectionately called "the birdcage," from which a police officer directs traffic.

Near the birdcage on Front Street is the Number 1 Passenger Terminal, site of the race packet pick-up. When I arrived to get my number, I found that the field would be, well, an *intimate* gathering of runners. There were only 392 runners registered for the full marathon, and 313 registered for the half. This was a far cry from the huge crowds at the marathons in New York, Boston, and Chicago, but small races do have their charm.

I spent the rest of the day doing a little sightseeing and a little eating, but mostly just resting and waiting. Rain was predicted, and sure enough, I heard the tapping of rain splashing against the window in the middle of the night. By the time I got up and went out the door, though, the rain had tapered off, leaving a cool, overcast morning. Perfect.

By 8 A.M., I was back on Front Street for the start of the race. The course is a double loop, with the half-marathoners pulling over to the side in Hamilton as the marathoners forge ahead for another lap.

I always have mixed feeling about that kind of format. It's nice to muster the entire running crowd together for as long as possible, especially in small races, but it's also quite a letdown to head toward the half-marathoner finish line with a pack of runners, and emerge alone on the other side.

As the starter's gun went off and we surged up Front Street, I thought about The Hill. When I first began to consider running the Bermuda Marathon, my first question was, where's the hill? In a marathon, there's almost *always* a hill. Sure enough, it's there: a nearly 40-meter climb at 3½ miles called McGall's Hill, revisited at 16½ miles.

The first mile flashed by in a blur of storefronts and adrenaline, and then we slipped out of the city center, onto a beautiful country road heading east. The road wasn't crowded, but neither was it empty; there were runners everywhere. We rolled over a few small rises, and then we were upon The Hill. It looked impressive, but it was early in the race, and we collectively ate it up.

Green. I'd noticed it upon arriving, but now I saw it everywhere. Lush green, bright green. The island doesn't have a soil base deep and rich enough to support large-scale agriculture, but its native plants thrive tenaciously, lining the marathon course with color. And there were other colors as well: houses splashed with blues and yellows and pinks, with bright white rooftops, kept clean so rainwater falling from their sides may be captured in underground cisterns for later use.

I noticed something else, too. Something that was *not* there. Garbage. I didn't see any trash along the streets, not in Hamilton, not on the country roads, not anywhere. So far, it was a runners' paradise.

We turned north onto the wonderfully-named Devil's Hole Road, and soon, at mile five, we were treated to a spectacular view of Harrington Sound. From there we turned toward Flatts Village, a former smugglers' haven that served as the site for the execution of witches in the mid-1600s. Today, the village is a benign and friendly haven for sailboats and fishermen, and true to its name, it was flat. The crowds had been sparse so far, but now there were several small groups of spectators. They seemed interested and supportive, though more reserved than the usual marathon crowd. That didn't surprise me. Bermuda, as a British possession, retains some Old World mannerisms that were brought across the Pond, including a tradition of high tea. Bermudans don't scream and yell along the course, but they are quick to return a polite "hello" or "good morning."

After Flatts Village, we turned onto North Shore Road. It was here, at mile 8, that I was rewarded with the first ocean view of the race, and it was breathtaking. Jagged dark volcanic rock met glorious blue water in a spray of white foam. It was almost enough to make me stop to enjoy the moment, but I knew I'd be back to see it again on my second loop.

The road settled into a pattern of rolling hills, and I noticed that the porous limestone, used widely as a building material, left structures appearing weathered and ancient. A stone archway overhead looked absolutely medieval. I also noticed the salty breeze blowing in off the ocean—another welcome distraction. On the left were signs for the Railway Trail, a running path made up of segments from Bermuda's old narrow gauge railway line, completed in 1931 and abandoned in 1947. It looked full of beauty and adventure, carved through rock and draped in foliage. I fought the urge to veer off and explore it. At mile 11 we turned south, back toward Hamilton. An old man sitting in a folding chair by the side of the road called out, "Once you pass me, it's easy to the finish!" I called back, "See you again soon!" I hoped I would.

The last 2 miles into Hamilton were downhill and fast. The sun fought its way through the clouds and scattered them, and the foliage retreated. The temperature climbed as the halfway point loomed ahead and the half-marathoners put on a burst of speed. I joined them and flew through the finish line, but my race was only half over, and my legs suddenly seemed to lose their bounce. McGall's Hill, redux, was just 3 miles away. As I tried to regain my focus and marshal my reserves, a man on a scooter passed by and offered me a candy. "I'll be with you guys all the way!" he promised as he sped ahead to the next runner. An older Japanese man passed me and called out "I'm faster than last year!" "Good for you!" I yelled back, and felt energized by his enthusiasm. I threw an invisible lasso around him, and let him pull me along for a few miles. Before long, I found my stride again, and settled into a groove.

And just in time, too. McGall's Hill loomed ahead, and it seemed to have grown since I'd last seen it. That leaden feeling crept back into my legs, and I concentrated on just moving ahead, putting one foot in front of the next. Looking off to my left I saw rolling green fields. Sitting there on the hillside was a woman with long brown hair, with her dog by her side. She smiled and waved, and I waved back.

And then I was at the top of the hill. This time, I noticed that there was a church on the hilltop, and, to its right, a cemetery. I was glad I didn't notice it earlier; it would have seemed too ominous. But not now; McGall's Hill was history.

Now I relaxed, remembering the flat miles that lay ahead. The heat was taking its toll, however, and I worried that soon I would start slowing down. As I re-entered Flatts Village, I tried to put a confident face on my running, for myself as well as for the spectators. I heard someone call out "You're seventeenth!" Me? Really? I've never had someone yell out my place during a race before. One more benefit of a small race field. It was enough to give me a boost over the next few miles.

I realized that the crowds, sparse though they were, were as determined as the runners to see the race through. They remembered me from my first lap, and called out as I passed by. The children waved and the women smiled. "You're looking good!" the old women said. "You too!" I replied, and they laughed and laughed. The old man I saw on the first loop, still sitting in his chair, waved to me like he's known me for years, and up ahead I saw Runner Number 16. It seemed that he wasn't that far ahead.

The street signs read "4 kilometers to Hamilton," and I tried to accelerate. The scooter-man pulled alongside again. No thanks, no candy for me, but thank you, thank you. More people lined the path now, and I started counting down the minutes I thought I had left to run. Mile 25 was downhill, and I wondered whether the extra speed I gained from the descent was worth the pain in my legs and lungs. But there was Mr. 16, and I was near to him, very near, then next to him. He smiled and said hello. I smiled back, and surged onward. Up ahead was Front Street again, and the finish line, meant for me this time. I crossed it, relieved and grateful for having completed another marathon, to have another medal. I turned around, and there was Mr. 16th, though now he was 17th. We smiled, less competitors now than comrades-in-arms.

I stepped inside the terminal, and went upstairs where there was the promise of food and drink. I took in fluids during the race, but it was so hot, and now I was so thirsty. Race Secretary Pam Shailer told me that it actually *hailed* during race weekend the previous year, and I was happy to have been spared any rain or ice. There were pastries, fruit, hot chocolate, and soup laid out for us, and soon I felt revived. Downstairs, there were two massage therapists ministering to the runners, and I got in line. When it was my turn, the therapist introduced himself—his name was John Ford, and he seemed to know just about everyone there. More importantly, his fingers were magic, and brought welcome relief to my tired body.

Marathon number 58 was in the books.

## Running Tip #9

### *Avoid Hyponatremia*

Hyponatremia is the opposite of dehydration; it's a dilution of sodium and other electrolytes caused by drinking too much water, which is most common among athletes who are on the marathon course for more than 4½ hours. It can be deadlier than dehydration, and in extreme cases, can lead to coma or even death.

Because its symptoms are similar to those of dehydration, hyponatremia is often misdiagnosed. The first question to ask a runner in distress is how much water have they been drinking? That will tell you what their problem likely is.

Over-the-counter nonsteroidal anti-inflammatory drugs ("NSAIDs"), such as aspirin, naproxen sodium (Aleve), and ibuprofen (Advil and Motrin), seem to increase the risk, perhaps because they inhibit the body's ability to excrete water. Women might also be at higher risk because they're smaller than men and can more easily overload on water.

*Symptoms*

- *fatigue*
- *cramping*
- *dizziness, nausea and vomiting*
- *bloating and puffiness in the face and fingers*
- *headache, confusion, and fainting*

*Prevention*

- *Use sports drinks that contain sodium.*

- *Add salt to your food in hot weather, unless you're on a salt-restricted diet.*

- *If you feel symptoms of hyponatremia while running, eat some salty food, like pretzels.*

- *Don't take any NSAIDs immediately before or during your race; if you must take a pain reliever, take acetaminophen (Tylenol).*

# Running Here, Running There, Running Everywhere!

In March 2001, I traveled with an American Diabetes Association fund-raising team to Italy for the Rome Marathon. With the ancient Coliseum as a backdrop, the race start was as impressive a sight as one could ever hope to find. As I stood shoulder to shoulder with the mass of other runners, I realized that I'd never before encountered such a stink from a race crowd, particularly before the event even started. Did no one here ever use deodorant?

Self-preservation led me to work my way out of the crush in search of fresh air. I wriggled to the outside, and wandered forward, where the elite runners waited in secure corrals. I saw the Africans, loose and smiling and confident. And there was an Italian team, laughing, standing around ... and smoking. I blinked in disbelief. Yep, there they were, sneaking in a last butt before the gun went off. *Only in Italy*, I thought.

With the race start just minutes away, I gulped in a lungful of fresh air and dove back into the crowd. Suddenly the mass surged forward. I assumed that the race staff had opened up the corrals, and that the crowd was pressing forward toward the starting line. I expected that our advance would soon grind to a halt, but somehow the crowd kept pressing forward. Soon there was enough room for us to break into an easy run. I couldn't understand what was going on.

Slowly it dawned on me that the race had begun. There had been no announcement, no starting gun, and no countdown. The race utilized an electronic chip system, to track each runner, but still, it was a very unsettling way to start a race. A friend with more European racing experience than I had later told me that this was typical of races abroad; if the runners get impatient, the officials just send them, like a mother telling her whining kids, *Fine, you want to go out and play so badly, well, go!*

Organization continued to be a problem after the race was under way. The first water stop wasn't ready for us by the time we came streaking by. Since Rome, like many European marathons, provide water and sports drinks every 5 kilometers—3.1 miles to us Americans—rather than the traditional mile or two in the United States, that meant that many runners went without any water for the first 6 miles of the race. It was already shaping up to be a hot, sunny day, so I knew that dehydration would be a problem. I began forcing down extra fluids as soon as drinks were available, and I told the runners I was pacing to do the same.

Not everyone was thinking ahead, though. I spotted a runner from the Canadian Diabetes Association, who was wearing an outrageous sunburst team singlet, in contrast to the solid red shirt that my Team Diabetes runners wore. I introduced myself. His name was Geoff, and he was running his first marathon. I was pacing several of my teammates already, and we all decided to run together. Geoff was running very well, but he hadn't been taking in enough fluids, and as the miles wore on he began to cramp. My teammates and I made sure he drank more, helped him stretch, and even rubbed his aching calves. Geoff urged us to go on, but I told him that if I surged ahead to the finish line, this would be just another race for me, neither the best nor the worst of my finishing times. But if I stayed with him and made sure he finished, it would make the race much more meaningful. The other runners in our little group agreed, and we decided to finish the race together.

We continued past the Vatican and the Circus Maximus, down cobblestone streets and narrow alleys. The cobblestones turned out to be more foe than friend, as they robbed our legs of their bounce and left them sore and aching. Spectators yelled out *forza!* (strength). At one point I overheard a spectator yell out *bocca al lupo!* as we passed, to which one of my runners yelled back *crepi il lupo!* I asked the runner what all that ruckus was about.

"Ah," he said, "that's just something people say in Italy during races. He yelled, 'you're in the mouth of the wolf!' and I called back the traditional response, 'may the wolf die!' It's how they wish you good luck." Like almost everything Italian, it was more dramatic than how things are done back home.

As we ran, we picked up a few more Team Diabetes runners who were happy to share in the team spirit. Finally, the Coliseum, and the finish line, loomed up ahead. We crossed the finish line and celebrated like it was New Year's Eve. It was as happy a finish as I've ever seen, and Geoff thanked me by giving me his team singlet—more appreciated once I'd laundered it!—as well as buying me several beers at our team get-together that evening. The friendship we forged proved to be lasting; Geoff and I kept in touch after we returned home, updating each other on our lives and running, keeping alive the hope that we'll be able to meet up for another marathon someday.

After returning from Rome, I ran Boston again—I was becoming a regular, though I never took it for granted—and then I met up with Dave in Austria for the Vienna Marathon in May. He was there for work, and the timing seemed too good to pass up. We raced along the Danube, passing beautiful parks and buildings, as the Viennese called out "*Hopp hopp!*" meaning, "jump faster!" I felt like I was where I was supposed to be, doing what I was supposed to be doing. I was flying around the world, meeting wonderful people, running marathons, and also feeling like I was making a difference in people's lives. It all felt like an amazing dream. Everything was perfect.

It was May of 2001. It was the last season of our national innocence, before everything would change forever.

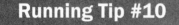

## Running Tip #10

# *Travel Like a Runner*

*Before you go*

- *Be willing to go it alone.* It's more fun to travel with friends, but you can make new friends easily during a race.
- *Clip your toenails before you leave home.* That's one less thing to worry about, and one less piece of equipment to risk getting confiscated by security.
- *Bring only carry-on baggage.* You'll be able to safeguard your racing gear, and you can more easily switch flights if there are any delays, or take advantage of requests for volunteers to give up their seats in exchange for free-flight vouchers.
- *Make a list of the essentials, and pack before the day of departure.* But don't panic if you forget something; unless you're traveling to a remote locale, you can still buy what you need when you arrive.

*Be prepared for the flight*

- *Drink plenty of water and bring your own healthy snacks.* Bring your own bottle and ask flight attendants to fill it.
- *Flex your legs or move around often.* The risk of developing potentially life-threatening blood clots during a long flight is higher among runners, perhaps because of our lower heart rate and blood pressure. Wearing compression socks might also help.

*Have a plan*

- *Deal with time zone changes.* Plan on one day of adjustment for every hour you lost or gained, although sometimes not adjusting works better if you're traveling east to west and you have a very early race start.
- *Scout around.* Become familiar with the course and the city. If you're racing in a high altitude, arrive in town a week early, or add 30 seconds per mile to your expected race pace.

# Speed Dreams

It was a conundrum. I loved marathons so much that I wanted to run them as often as possible, yet the more I ran them, the harder it would be for me to reach my potential as a marathoner. Running a marathon just about every month relieved me of the need to do long training runs, since my races *were* my long training runs. But I sacrificed intense training between races, since I was usually either recovering from one race or tapering for the next. I knew that I was also preventing my body from fully recovering from each of my marathon efforts. This hadn't resulted in injury, but I wasn't priming my body for one supreme effort, the one that would get me to my next goal in running: a sub-three hour marathon.

Finally, in the summer of 2001, I decided to take up the challenge. I had run six marathons in the first half of the year, but I committed to making my next one—number 64—"The One." I took a month off from hard running to let my body fully rest, then picked the Steamtown Marathon in Scranton, Pennsylvania, in October as my target race. My work colleague and running buddy Jim was planning on doing it, and had been talking up its virtues. It was known as a fast race, mostly downhill, with a net drop of 955 feet. Eventually I was won over, and signed up, hoping that as long as I could keep my feet moving, I could count on gravity to bring me home in record time

That summer, Jim and I trained ferociously. Although I had done speed work with my running friends and run marathons with them, I had never before focused on a single race with any of them. Jim and I developed a unique camaraderie, stopping by each other's office with updates on our workouts and pace calculations. Our lunchtime tempo sessions, run faster than race pace, were epic. I loved them, and began to keep a journal to record my thoughts.

*It's Thursday afternoon, and Jim is waiting for me. Today is our tempo run, a 10-mile loop that is supposed to leave us breathless and exhilarated. Last week Jim ran strong, and opened a half-block lead over me with two miles left. I forced my leaden legs to give just a little bit more, and Jim slowed just a bit to let me pull even. Afterward, I was exhausted. And now Jim is waiting for me again.*

*We start out easy, weaving through crowds and traffic. The D.C. parks insinuate themselves through the city like vines wrapping around a tree. Our loop takes us from the downtown business district to Georgetown, and from there onto a 3-mile wooded trail. We would emerge at the northern edge of the city and run down Connecticut Avenue, back to our starting point. It's a beautiful route, about 10 miles long, but it's also our proving ground. These weekly runs are an important part of my plan to build speed for Steamtown. If I can just keep up with Jim.*

*We work our way through Georgetown, and enter the woods. We're running well, but shorter on breath than either of us would like. Our conversation dwindles down to a few short words, and then just the sound of our heavy breathing. As we jump logs and hop over streambeds, I imagine that I'm an early settler, chasing game for the family dinner. Or perhaps an escaped convict, with the howl of bloodhounds getting ever louder behind me. Leaves brush past my face, and I feel a surge of energy. I pick up the pace.*

*We leave the woods, and I glance down at my watch. We're ahead of our usual pace, but the toughest part lies ahead. The downhill must be run hard if it is to be run honestly. It's a 4-mile stretch that should leave my lungs burning and my thoughts muddled. Less effort than that makes it just another easy run, and puts Jim a half block ahead of me.*

*We sweep down the avenue and overtake a bus picking up passengers. I consider the traffic lights ahead, and the scheduled stops the bus has to make. We'll run along the bus route for the next three miles, and if we run hard, I think to myself, we can beat it. Again, I pick up the pace.*

*Now we're flying, our bodies moving smoothly, feet barely touching the ground. We've raced the bus a full mile, and it still hasn't gotten the better of us. It pulls close, flirts with us, but then brakes to pick up passengers, or is halted by a red light. I become accustomed to the ebb and flow of its loud, droning engine. And then the National Zoo appears, its entrance gate enveloped by a swarm of tourists. We step out toward the street, and collect the open-mouthed stares of children. I pick up the pace.*

*Ahead is the bridge over Rock Creek Park. This is where I watched Jim surge ahead last week and was unable to match his strength. Today, my lungs are burning, but I feel strong. Jim falls a few strides behind, surges to make up lost ground, then falls back and surges again. He will not gain a half block on me today. The bus is behind us now for good, vanquished. We have less than two miles to go. I pick up the pace.*

*Now we make a left onto broad Massachusetts Avenue for the last few blocks of our run. We are running without thinking, like machines, just trying to hold on. "Almost there, just a little bit more," I intone, as much for myself as for Jim. And then we are just one block away. I am tired, but I am in love with the effort, and I tell Jim I will sprint the last block. He joins me, and we tear down the street, mad for speed and adrenaline.*

*And then the workout is over. We shuffle, letting our heartbeats slow and our breathing return to normal. I look at my watch. Six minutes faster than last week. "Great run," Jim says breathlessly. "Great run. My best 10-miler ever." I smile and nod, happy and alive.*

*We take turns, Jim and I, pulling and pushing each other through our training runs, tearing through the woods and racing buses, chasing after our marathon dreams. We are athletes in the greatest, craziest, most competitive, most supportive, most elegant, most brutal sport in the world. And next week, with any luck, Jim will be waiting for me again, ready to hit the trails.*

That was my summer: sweat and effort and dirty running clothes. The days shortened, and a chill crept into the air, and summer faded behind us.

It was September, 2001.

When I was growing up, my parents and my older relatives would sometimes recall exactly where they were and what they were doing when President Kennedy had been shot. It seemed so odd to me for so many people to have such a personal memory of such a famous moment.

Not any more.

I recall exactly where I was and what I was doing on the morning of September 11th. I was in a neighborhood local gym where I trained, making my way through a cardio session on some of the cross-training machines. I distracted myself by looking up at the overhead TVs, catching the morning news. Little by little, reports came in about an errant plane that had struck one of the World Trade Center towers. Like everyone else, I thought it must have been an accident, similar to when a plane struck the Empire State Building decades before. But of course, it was nothing like that, and as the events of that morning unfolded, I stayed glued to my LifeCycle, extending my workout from one hour, to two, to three. I couldn't leave my seat, and almost compulsively, maniacally, I kept pedaling.

Reports of the second plane hitting a tower came in, and the footage was horrible and mesmerizing. At one point, as the commentators talked on about what was happening in Manhattan, I realized the footage of a smoking building being shown on TV wasn't the World Trade Center; it was the Pentagon, right here in my city's backyard. Obviously, something had happened there as well, but hadn't yet been reported. I climbed down from the exercise bike. Everything seemed unreal as I made my way downstairs. By the time I got there, a staff member at the front desk told me that one of the towers had collapsed. The second one followed shortly after.

I called my office and spoke to one of my friends there. He told me that everyone who was there was preparing to leave, and that I shouldn't bother coming in. I cleaned up and went over to visit a friend who lived on the top floor of an apartment building. He had a beautiful view of the city, facing south to the Potomac River. Toward the Pentagon.

When I arrived there, I found that several others had come as well. We stared at the horizon, where a smoke cloud hung in the air. It was the first tangible proof that something terrible had happened. We sat most of the day with our eyes glued to the television, taking in the reports and trying to make sense of it all.

The next meeting of my charity marathon training group was somber. Instead of being upbeat and boisterous as usual, they were quiet and apprehensive. We had been training for a return trip to the Dublin Marathon, but with our departure only a month and a half away, there was little chance that we would see a return to normalcy before we were scheduled to depart. This was what we had to deal with.

We started off by talking about the toll that the recent events had taken on all of us. I said that I planned to continue training the group and would go to Dublin, as I hoped all of them would also do. Some people said that they no longer felt comfortable leaving the country. I wanted to tell them that everything would be okay and that they should still go, but how could anyone be sure?

Most of the runners opted to continue with the program. We would continue training, and go to Dublin. I hoped that I had not just put all of their lives at risk.

Meanwhile, Jim and I made it through our own training program, and drove out to Scranton on October 6, the day before the Steamtown Marathon. Scranton is an old locomotive town, and though its glory years are long gone, it honors its past with a museum and, of course, the race. I had calculated that I needed to run at a 6:51-per-mile pace to get my sub-3-hour time. 6:51. Just thinking about those numbers made me nervous.

On race day I felt good. The skies were clear, and there was a slight chill in the air. I did a light warm-up, and waited for the starter's gun, shaking my legs, looking for clues as to how they felt. Did they feel strong? Did they have pop? Was I hungry? Stuffed? Thirsty? Bloated? I considered it all, and decided everything was right. I was ready to go.

The race started, and we ran through the city streets, immediately lurching downhill. I was breathing cleanly, strongly. We twisted and turned on the city streets, and soon left them behind, heading out toward quieter roads. I felt great. I pulled ahead of Jim and weaved through the small crowd, feeling like I was hardly touching the ground. As we ran past tall trees bathed in green leaves, I struck up a conversation with a man next to me, and then passed him behind. I had never felt so good before so early in a race. I pitied all the other animals in nature for their slowness. I looked down at my watch. I was running 20–30 seconds faster than my goal pace. I should have been worried; energy is like a bank account, and if you spend it in one place, particularly early in a race, it won't be there later when you really need it. I was blowing my reserves with wild abandon, but I felt confident that I was fine. I had trained hard, and this was the pace that felt comfortable. Perhaps my energy account had accrued interest, I thought. I would not slow down. I would run hard and hold on to the finish line. It would be like Boston, but better.

It wouldn't take long for me to realize how wrong I was. I had carefully drawn up a training plan and spent months following it, but then I threw all that hard work away on race day. It was a rookie mistake, and there's a price to be paid for such recklessness. By mile 16, I knew that I would have to ante up. I hadn't yet slowed, but that intoxicating energy was ebbing, and I realized that I wouldn't be able to sustain the pace I had set. If I could just keep running well, though, I told myself, I still could make my sub-3-hour goal.

Over the next few miles, I slowly began to accept the reality of my situation. The hard downhill running had taken a toll on my quadriceps. I began to consider fallback goals as my sub-3-hour dream began to slip away. By mile 20 I was running on a beautiful bicycle path through the woods, but I couldn't enjoy it. I was in trouble, and like a beaten fighter looking for a place to fall down, I began to consider when I would start walking.

Walk breaks are an accepted part of racing for many people, especially first-time marathoners, and I recommend them to my teams. When you take a walk break, you give your running muscles a moment's rest, and you also give your mind a manageable goal to work with: just run reasonably hard for another mile, and then you can have another walk break. Breaking the race up into segments like that makes it seem much easier to handle. As I've told my teams, the marathon is just too big to swallow in one gulp.

In Steamtown, though, my walk breaks during the last 6 miles of the race were not strategic. They were acts of desperation. My legs ached with fatigue, and they demanded that I stop running. As soon as I started walking, the race I had trained for was effectively over. I managed to talk my legs into running again for a few minutes at a time over the final few miles, but as the minutes ticked by, I saw even my various fallback goals slip away. First, my dream of a sub-3 hour finish vanished, followed shortly by my hopes for a new personal record. Eventually, I realized that I would not even achieve a Boston qualifying time. Finally, I reached the last stop on my descent: I just wanted to finish the race. When it was finally, mercifully, over, my official time was 3:20:14. Not bad, really: it was the eighth best time of the sixty-four marathons I had run, but that was a deceiving statistic. The Steamtown Marathon had broken me.

As I gathered myself and waited for Jim, I thought about a story a childhood friend recently told me. Supposedly, a new guy had recently walked into a gym back in New York where we used to train and started boasting about how much he could lift. "It's all mind over matter," he said. "If I can believe it, my body can achieve it." With that, he loaded 300 pounds onto the bench press, laid down on the bench, lifted the bar off the support, and … crashed it down onto his face, knocking out three teeth.

The lesson, of course, is that mind over matter works *as long as you're in the ballpark.* I could believe with all my heart and soul that I could fly, but if I jump out of a top floor window, I'm still going to go splat on the sidewalk.

That's how I felt about my performance in Steamtown. I went splat. There was nothing in my training to justify the early pace I had set for myself. My training hadn't put me in the ballpark for the race I was running. It was a difficult lesson to learn, especially at this late date, when I already had a dozen years of marathoning experience behind me and should have known better. As much as I tried to put on a happy face, it was hard for me to hide my sadness and anger. I had wasted a good opportunity to achieve something special.

Once, long ago, I swore to myself that if ever I crossed a marathon finish line and was disappointed, I would hang up my running shoes. Was it now time for me to quit? I thought things over during the long drive home. By the time I reached my apartment, I had reconciled myself to what had happened. I decided that whatever my original goal had been, finishing the race was still a wonderful achievement, especially given how badly I felt during those last few miles. I could have quit, but didn't, and that was still something to be proud of.

I wasn't ready to hang up those shoes just yet.

## Running Tip #11

### *Training Food*

People exercising for 90 minutes should take in 4 calories per minute to maintain performance—that's up to 240 calories per hour. Not an easy task.

That's where sports gels come in. Basically, they are just sugary syrups, often caffeinated, that are easily digested for a quick mid-run energy boost.

- *Take with water.* They need water to break down, so take with 6–8 ounces of water. Sports drinks won't do the trick, since those extra carbs may be more than the stomach could absorb.
- *Experiment with the different flavors.*
- *Aim to take one every 45 minutes to an hour.*
- *Consider alternatives.* If you can't tolerate sports gels, experiment with other low-fat, easily-digested foods, like energy bars. There are even chewy bite-sized blocks and jelly beans especially for athletes.

# Back to Where It All Began

I was glad to have worked my way through my disappointment with Steamtown so quickly, because my charity teams were making their final preparations for their own races. It wouldn't have helped them much to have a despondent coach.

First up was a return trip to Dublin. I was thrilled to be back; Dublin had become one of my favorite cities, and this time I knew exactly where I wanted to go and what I wanted to do. There was my favorite fish and chips stand next to the Jury's Hotel, and a pub in the Temple Bar district that had the best traditional Irish music. I also wanted to visit a great sweater shop I discovered on the previous trip, and revisit the beautiful Book of Kells at Trinity College.

And then, of course, there was also the race. This time we got lucky with the weather; skies were gray, but there was none of the rain and wind that had vexed us all the year before. All team members crossed the finish line without any significant problems, making me a happy coach indeed.

After the race was over, I set out with a woman I was dating and a few other people for a side trip to western Ireland, to visit Galway and the surrounding areas. The Irish countryside is starkly beautiful, with a checkerboard of stone fencing surrounding small, romantically weathered castles. We visited the Cliffs of Mohr, with its sudden and dramatic 700-foot drop. I was brave and cocky until we neared the cliff's edge, and then I chickened out like all the other visitors and got down on my belly and crawled to the edge to peer over the side.

I also learned the origin of the intricate piping patterns on the traditional Irish sweaters that I had bought. Traditionally, each clan was known by a particular pattern knit into their sweaters, much like a heraldic coat of arms. But instead of just being for show or vanity, these patterns served a grim purpose—they enabled the quick identification of drowned fisherman when their bodies were recovered. This was a harsh reminder that for all the beauty of the land, this could be a difficult and unforgiving place to live.

My Ireland trip drew to a close, but I wasn't ready to go home. I was about to meet up with another of my charity teams for a different adventure. We were going to visit the roots of the marathon, to retrace the steps taken by the ancients. We were going to Greece to run the Athens Marathon.

The racecourse would roughly follow the original route Phidippides supposedly traveled, from the still open and wind swept plains of Marathon, around the burial mound underneath which lay the remains of soldiers who fought that battle so long ago. From there, the route passed through the Greek countryside from town to town, until it reached its finish in the heart of Athens. It felt like a homecoming of sorts to me, though I'd never been there before. It was a race that I'd known for a long time that I would have to run.

Although cloaked in myth and legend, this event was still an actual race, and organizers would have to overcome the usual logistical problems. For years, the knock against the Athens Marathon was that it failed to provide enough water on the course. In 2001, the organizers finally solved that problem, placing drinks every 5 kilometers, and adding a few more water stops for good measure.

But we also had some unexpected water; the torrential downpour we missed in Ireland caught up with us in Greece. Most runners sought shelter in a nearby stadium construction site. Eventually, with clenched teeth and muttered curses, we all made our way through the downpour to the starting line. The race I had dreamed about for years was about to begin.

Running in the rain is not really such a bad experience. Even if it wasn't raining, we would all be soaked eventually by our own sweat. Our concern was really for our feet. When socks get wet, there's a greater chance of getting blisters, and a bad blister could ruin the most well-prepared athlete.

That day, things were not looking so good for our feet. Several sections of road were flooded under several feet of water. Some runners tried to cope by using garbage bags as waders, but discovered that the bags quickly tore and let water in. Others charged through, and either soaked their shoes or had them sucked off their feet by the thick mud below. Most of us just circled as wide as possible around these little lakes, climbing around grass and bushes. In the end, it didn't matter what each of us did; we were all going to get drenched by race's end. I was as soaked as I'd ever been, and that includes swimming.

The race presented other surprises as well. Athens is famous for its pack of wild, though mostly friendly, dogs. I had seen them and been trailed by them throughout the city, but I didn't expect to see them on race day. But there they were on the course, eyeing us curiously. Several of them decided to run alongside us for several kilometers. I was leery at first—even a friendly dog may be tempted to bite a runner—but they were as amiable and uncomplaining as any companion I've ever run with, and I was a bit sad when they decided not to go all the way with me to the finish line. They made a much better impression than the famous cats of Rome, who were nowhere to be found on race day.

Finally, the rain tailed off as we neared the outskirts of Athens. The traffic thickened, and stores and stop lights appeared. Near the 18-mile mark, we hit the big hill—there's always a big hill, remember?—and then we descended into the city for one of the most glorious finishes in marathoning: a loop on the track in the 1896 marble stadium that hosted the first modern Olympic Games. As the stadium came into view, my pulse quickened, and I picked up the pace for a strong finish. The course brought us closer to the stadium, and then … led us past it. We had to run a little farther down the street and double back to the stadium. I felt like one of my canine companions might feel if a juicy steak waved in front of his nose, only to have it yanked away at the last second. It was a deflating moment, but when I finally did enter the stadium minutes later, my loop on that historic track made up for all the difficulties I'd had to overcome that day. It was my 66th marathon finish, and it was as sweet a moment as I'd ever had in road racing.

## Running Tip #12

### *Running Etiquette*

- *Stay to the right.* It's the rule with cars, and it should be the rule with people, too. Let faster runners and cyclists pass.
- *Don't run more than two people across.* If you hog the road, you're asking for trouble.
- *If you need to slow down or stop, step to the side.*
- *Be responsible for your own needs.* If you see someone else's cache of water or goodies sitting by the side of the road, don't touch it. They'll be counting on it being there when they need it. Choose training routes that pass by water fountains or convenience stores, or plant your own provisions by the side of road.
- *Be an honest racer.* If you're not a 5:30 mile, don't line up in the front of the pack before a race; you'll only get in the way of the faster runners. Plus, it's no fun getting passed.
- *Go the extra mile.* We're all part of a fitness community, and we should act like it. Wave and say hi to other runners, and offer extra water or goodies if you have them handy and someone looks like they could really use it. But be respectful of others; friendliness in the running community is not an invitation to distract or harass other runners.

# Why Run the Marathon? Third Lap

As my marathon tally rose, I never gave up trying to understand my passion for the marathon. I knew instinctively that my running was meaningful in a way that I hadn't yet been able to explain, but now that I was recruiting and training team participants for my charity fund-raising teams, I knew that I had to find a way to articulate my reason for running 26.2 miles.

Information meetings usually began in the evening, after I had left my regular day job and my work as a lawyer. I began with the easy stuff, speaking about the joy of experiencing your body moving easily and powerfully, of the need to break through assumed or self-imposed limitations to discover the true potential hidden within all of us. I spoke of the satisfaction found in accomplishing the seemingly impossible, of proving wrong all those people who doubted not that it could be done, but that *they* could do it. I told them of my belief that everyone ought to have something they do that causes them to lose track of time, whether it's music or art or reading. For me, it's running. I rely on that quiet time to balance out the other demands on my life. I told them it might be the same for them as well.

Warmed up, I then spoke of the rewards to be found in accomplishing a difficult task. In a high school mythology class, we had been assigned Joseph Campbell's *The Hero with a Thousand Faces*, which explains the common threads of humankind's hero legends. The hero, Campbell explained, always sets out on a quest, separating himself from the ordinary routines of everyday life, and ventures to a land of danger. He confronts a great challenge, and after emerging triumphant, he returns home with a boon for mankind, whether fire, the Golden Fleece, defeat of the Minotaur, or great wisdom.

That is the hero's tale, I told my audience, and that is the tale of the marathoner, because the marathon is a heroic journey. Setting ourselves apart from our neighbors through our months-long ritual of training and sacrifice, we face the challenge of race day, when we test our resolve and preparation over miles of arduous roads, emerging, we hope, at the finish line, having gained wisdom about ourselves. Upon crossing that line, we are all of us transformed, having sensed our own power and determination, capable now of being masters of our fate rather than passive spectators.

I told them how running seems to bring out the best in all of us. I told them about Grete Waitz, the nine-time winner of the New York City Marathon. In 1993, Grete was in New York just as a friend of the race, and to support her husband, who was running. While she was there, she met Zoe Koplowitz, a marathoner who suffers from multiple sclerosis, and who competes while using crutches. It usually takes Zoe about 24 hours to finish a marathon, by which time there is hardly anyone at the finish line. Grete promised Zoe that she would wait for her at the finish line.

In the early hours of the morning following the race, Grete ran out to the finish line to see if Zoe was there yet; Zoe was close, but hadn't yet come into view. Then Grete discovered that there weren't any more finishers' medals left. Horrified and embarrassed, she ran back to her hotel room and grabbed her husband's medal, telling him "you don't really need another one," and made it back to the finish line in time to put it around Zoe's neck when she crossed it.

I told them that I often think of that story, about the caring of an elite runner for all the other brave people who attempt the marathon, and of the courage of a challenged runner like Zoe Koplowitz, whose achievement makes me thankful for simply having the opportunity to train and race. I don't know if running attracts good people, or if running makes people good, but there is a shared sense of understanding and respect among marathoners, a camaraderie forged by sweat and effort and sacrifice.

This is the marathon experience, I told them, and it is wondrous. I recalled for them the running of the 100th Boston Marathon in 1996, when defending champion Uta Pippig faded back behind young and strong Tegla Loroupe. It soon became apparent that Uta's difficulties were caused by the onset of menstruation and related intestinal problems, but Uta would not give in to the pain and discomfort. She gritted her teeth and flew past Tegla in the last few miles, en route to another first-place finish. That was as heroic an achievement as I've ever seen. When once asked why she runs the marathon, though, Uta simply answered, "I make the marathon beautiful for myself and for others. That's why I'm here."

I repeated that word, "beautiful," and looked out on the puzzled faces in my audience. Pain itself isn't beautiful, I said, but there is a beauty to effort, to perseverance, that marks it as special, as near as we may come to perfection.

I told them, too, of my own marathoning history. This is always a tricky business because I wanted to inspire them, not intimidate them. Many people find it easy to draw a distinction between what I've done and what they can do, saying that I must have some special gifts that enable me to accomplish these running feats. I told them that if I have any special gift, it's just stubbornness. There's nothing special about me that enables me to run so many races. My body might be a bit more durable than others, but there's really no reason why most of them couldn't run the same races that I do. All they need, I told them, is the determination to try. And despite my own experience, most people find that one marathon is plenty!

Some people nodded their heads, and some seem moved. Others sat politely in mute attention. Many of them joined our teams, and many did not. I always came away from these meetings with mixed emotions, feeling that I touched on something important, but that I'd circled rather than pierced the bulls-eye. I didn't manage to get to the heart of it; I couldn't fully explain what I felt. It was a frustrating, tiring business.

One moment crystallized my thinking. I had returned to Rome in 2002, and I had just finished pacing a group of my Team Diabetes runners to the finish line—marathon number 68 for me. Their day was over, but mine continued, as I ran back and forth on the course to cheer on the rest of my team and all the other race participants. I awaited two young women in particular: members of my team who were pushing against the clock. The race director, I knew, would shut off a section of the course at an appointed hour in order to let the city reclaim its streets, and the remaining runners on the course would have no choice but to cut the race short. It was a bum deal for those who had worked so hard and been struggling for so many hours, but there was no possibility for appeal. As I waited, I realized that my last two team members had not made the cutoff. They would cross the finish line, but they would not have completed 26.2 miles.

After the race, all of our teams from across the country returned to our host hotels, freshened up, and then gathered in the evening for a celebration dinner. There were smiles by the hundreds, and stories of obstacles overcome, random moments of hilarity, and new friendships forged. Above all, there was the electricity of accomplishment and pride. Whatever else may ever be said of them, they were now and forever marathoners.

But my two young women were not there. They were still upstairs in their shared room, and would not join us. Their marathon had been one of sacrifice and persistence without reward. They felt that they had nothing to celebrate. When I realized that they hadn't come down, I went up to talk with them.

I knocked on their door, and they let me in. I sat down, and asked how they were doing. Their words tumbled out in a flood, mixed with tears of frustration and anger. They spoke of their bitter disappointment, of the months of hard work they had poured into their dream, of their confidence in their ability to realize that dream if only it had *not been stolen from them*, of their dread of having to explain their failure to friends and family when they returned home. I sat and listened and tried to think of a way that I could tell them that there was nothing to be upset about, but I could not. It would be a lie.

But I did have something to say. I told them of the history of the race, of Phidippides's 25-mile journey, of the modern Olympic Games and the 1.2-mile accommodation to the British Royal family. I explained that the modern marathon is an exact distance, but that there is nothing sacred or immutable about the number 26.2. By itself it is without meaning; we alone give it meaning.

I spoke about time. I explained that my best time in a marathon is not the race in which I ranked highest; on that grand day in Detroit, I finished far behind the lead pack of runners, but I have never run faster. In other races, such as in Bermuda, I ran slower, but I finished higher in the final tally because my competitors were slower still. On which day, I asked them, was I the better runner? Of which day should I be proudest? I told them of my race in Pittsburgh, where I fought through heat and dehydration to finish over an hour slower I expected to. Rather than being despondent, though, I was thrilled with my performance that day, because I felt that I had shown courage.

So, I asked them, if distance doesn't matter, and time doesn't matter, what is the marathon about? What remains? In the end, what matters?

I spoke more about Detroit and Pittsburgh. Anyone can run well on a day when everything is in magical alignment, when your training has peaked, when injuries have been held at bay, when the course and the weather are perfect. Then performance is easy. In Detroit, I simply ran, like a machine. But in Pittsburgh, on the day when things were most difficult, when it would have been easiest to quit, that was the day when I asked more of myself than I thought I was able to give. It is in that kind of moment that glory can be found.

But in Rome, these two women had been denied their moment of glory. I told them that I knew that their victory had been stolen from them. But they had not given up. They had struggled, and had not turned away, even when they knew that they would ultimately not make the cutoff time, and would be rerouted on the course. There was no shame in what they had done, and their accomplishment was not lessened by the race director's decision. I told them that they had not completed a marathon; that was a simple fact that none of us could ignore. But they had not quit. They had transcended distance and time, and found something greater than just crossing a finish line; they had discovered the depth of their own power and determination. There would be other finish lines if they wanted them, as there were for me after my first disastrous marathon attempt, but they were already heroes, because they had journeyed and sacrificed and brought back the wisdom of self-knowledge.

We sat a while longer, and finally I stood up to leave. They thanked me earnestly, perhaps more for recognizing and validating their pain than for any other solace I tried to give them. As I walked away, I thought about what I had said, and tried to hold onto those thoughts the way you try to hold on to a dream upon waking. I felt that I had touched on something. This time, I had not become lost in a fog of words. This time, perhaps, I had moved just a step closer to finding the answer to my question.

In the meantime, I kept racing. Having tasted racing on foreign soil, it was all I really wanted to do. In March 2002, I raced Rome again, and then in April, I flew to Paris. I was certain that there was no better way to see a city than by running through it, and if there was one city that was big enough and beautiful enough to amaze runners over 26.2 miles, I was sure it would be Paris. But on race day, as I joined the 20,000 other runners gathered in the shadow of the Arc de Triomphe, I wondered whether it was fair of me to hold this race to such a high standard. It was a living city, not a museum showpiece, and this was a race, not a luxury tour. I tried to temper my expectations. There would be good parts and bad parts, I reminded myself, and all that I could be certain of was that eventually, if I kept moving forward, I would reach the finish line.

I needn't have worried. The City of Light turned out to be as glorious as I'd imagined it would be. After racing down the Champs-Élysées, we toured the parks and streets of the city, and then raced along the Seine. The Eiffel Tower loomed in the distance. It was breathtaking. Along the way I saw couples running in wedding attire, and heard shouts of *"Bon courage,"* and *"Allez! Allez!"* meaning, "Go! Go!" I later read in the *New York Times*[7] that spectators had taunted runners by shouting "Only 500 kilometers left!" and "Run faster! They're about to open the street up to cars!" According to the *Times*, the French appreciate track and field stars, but feel an ambivalence bordering on disdain for middle-of-the-pack runners. But I didn't hear any of those catcalls. Or maybe it was just that I don't speak French. For me, at least, marathon number 69 was perfect.

After returning from Paris, I settled into the morass of heat and humidity that is D.C. in the summertime. With temperatures climbing up into the 80s and 90s, there wasn't much for a marathoner to do; it was too hot for race organizers to safely hold any long distance events in all but the most northern of cities, or in chilly San Francisco, which is no surprise to anyone who's been there in July. So summer usually stretches out into a long season of training and catching up with running friends. And of making plans for the smorgasbord of fall races.

My grandmother used to have a saying: you make plans and God laughs. She was about to be proven right.

---

7 April 14, 2002, p.10.

# Running and Romance

I have to admit it: my love for running marathons required a certain amount of understanding from the women I dated. We marathoners are a tough group for nonrunners to understand. We train our bodies for our own health and vanity, and then race to prove to ourselves how tough we are. Every day's activities are planned around the run. Friends and families sometimes take a back seat. Like most marathoners, I didn't really see anything wrong with this. I thought it was fair for me to have a space in my life that was all my own. As long as I didn't ignore any responsibilities, I didn't see anything wrong with doing what I wanted to do.

Unless, of course, I wanted to share my life with someone else. Most women who at first were attracted to my passion for running soon tired of my priorities. My getting up at 5 A.M. to run or meet with personal training clients, and fading by 9 or 10 at night, didn't help either. Eventually, they all asked why I couldn't just sit down and relax.

On occasion I dated another runner. It seemed like the natural thing to do: find someone who shared my passion and interest. All of my friends expected this of me; what could be more natural than for a marathoner to be involved with another marathoner?

As it turned out, it wasn't really that simple. Learning to date and train with someone as active as myself raised new issues. We all define ourselves in many different ways. For me, being a marathon runner is a big part of who I am. The athletic women I dated felt the same way, but sometimes their emotional lives were more complex. One woman in particular that I dated had always been the athletic alpha partner, faster and fitter than her dates. In this important arena, success defined her as a person. Things were different when I came along. Suddenly, she wasn't the one who could run or bike farther and faster, and she wasn't used to that. Whether we realized it or not, we weren't just romantically involved, we were competitors. Even as she tried to hide it, resentment and anger grew, and spilled out in small ways, and I didn't know how to handle it. After all, *I* didn't feel the need to compete with *her*. But it was easy for me to feel this way, since I wasn't the one having my self-image challenged. Would I feel comfortable if she was a better runner than I was? I'd like to think so, but I don't know for sure.

Ultimately, that relationship didn't work out, and not just for that reason, but it did play a part. I knew that things didn't have to be like that in every dual-athlete relationship; there were plenty of successful running couples out there. It just wasn't happening for me. But that was okay. I didn't feel the urgent need to settle down anyway.

But I did want a special person in my life someday, and to have a home and family: the whole nine yards. Suddenly, that person entered my life. Or rather, re-entered. It was Stephanie Kay, the former high school classmate from Boston whom I had tried to contact years before. Our class was now about to mark its twentieth graduation anniversary. Some class members had set up a Web site, and e-mails were flying in all directions. I thought I'd give it one more shot, so I sent her an e-mail. She wrote back. I answered, and then so did she. She told me that she had gotten my message years earlier, and had wanted to call me back, but that my message had been lost at her office. We now exchanged phone numbers, and had hours-long conversations about running and art and anything we could think of. One night, as we spoke on the phone, we hit a natural stopping point. There was just nothing else that came to mind to say. I expected her to wrap things up, but instead she waited on the phone for wherever our conversation would go next. It hit me right then: she liked me.

It was a long time coming, actually. I first met her back in 1976, when we both entered junior high school together in New York City. I was just twelve, and was immediately smitten, but at that tender age I was too shy and inexperienced to know what to do about it. So I did nothing.

The years passed, and although I never managed to ask Stephanie out, I did manage to become friends with her. Finally, we were in twelfth grade—seniors at last! Our senior trip was a ski weekend, and one night, as several of us were relaxing after a long day of skiing, I managed to finally ask her for a date. Sort of. I asked if she'd like to take a walk in the woods with me. With hindsight I can see how this could have seemed a little too bold. Stephanie must have thought so, because she politely declined. Later, she wrote some nice things in my yearbook, but signed it "wuv." Sadly, the replacement of that "L" with a "W" told me all that I needed to know about her feelings for me.

And now, all these years later, we were talking, and then making plans to meet up in New York. Then she visited me in D.C., and I visited her in Boston. By the time the reunion came around we were a couple. Little by little her "W" turned into an "L."

I had come to think of D.C. as my home, but the more time I spent with Stephanie in Boston, the more I grew to love it there. Which is not to say that every visit was like a fairy tale come true. For example, that summer I went up to visit her for the July 4th weekend. We avoided the throngs of people mobbed along the Charles River to watch the fireworks and hear the Boston Pops, but the next morning was clear and beautiful; a perfect day for an easy 8-mile run along the river. Evidence of the previous evening's celebration was everywhere, although cleanup crews were already hard at work emptying overstuffed trash cans and picking up litter, oblivious to the runners and cyclists flying past them.

Along the bicycle trail sat row upon row of portable toilets, put in place over the previous several days to handle the crush of revelers. Now, like cannons left on a battlefield, they sat silent, but apparently still usable. I don't usually have access to such conveniences except on race day; my training runs are often marked by moments of brilliant improvisation in dealing with bathroom issues. But now, faced with such opulence, I decided to use one of the silent soldiers.

I swung open the door on the nearest Porta-Jon. Just as I was getting comfortable, I heard the sound of a truck nearby. Very nearby. Suddenly I felt the stall move. I jumped to my feet and grabbed at the door, but it was pinned shut by the long metal arms of the truck's hydraulic lift. I was trapped!

I wasn't sure whether to laugh or scream. I opted for shouting, and after several tense moments of yelling and peering out of the mesh screen at the top of the stall, I finally caught the driver's attention. He motioned to me to stay put—where would I possibly go?—and he moved the truck so that I could free myself from my little prison. As I resumed my run under the bemused gaze of the driver, I wondered whether anyone would believe what had just happened to me. What if I couldn't get the driver's attention? Is there a secret Porta-John burial ground? Would it be more than a days' run from where I was staying in Boston? Would Stephanie recognize me if I even made it back to her? Would she want to?

But luckily, I made it back to Stephanie safe and sound, and we continued our courtship.

And that's how I found myself one afternoon at the top of Old Rag Mountain in the Shenandoahs, about to get down on one knee. It was a beautiful, sunny day, with a nice crispness in the air. I had packed a lunch, including chocolates with strawberries, and a bottle of wine. And a diamond ring. My plan was to find just the right spot; someplace sheltered from the wind, but bathed in sunshine, with a sweeping view of the valley below. And I found it. Everything was perfect. I began to set out our lunch.

Just then a young woman and a few men passed by. We exchanged hellos, and then I heard a loud thud. The woman had fallen heavily while jumping from one rock to another, and had twisted her ankle badly. Right next to our spot. I suddenly had a vision of all my carefully laid plans going up in smoke. I reached into my bag for an ace bandage.

"Would you like to wrap your ankle, so you can *get going*?"

"No," she said. "But it hurts so much, I'm feeling nauseous."

Nauseous. Right next to our perfect spot. I waited twenty years for this moment, and now this woman is going to throw up on us.

"Would you like some water, so you can *get going*?"

"Ugh," she said. "I'm seeing spots."

Spots. I couldn't believe it.

"That must be the altitude," I told her. Look, I know the Shenandoahs are not the Himalayas, but I was improvising. "You need to be at a lower altitude. You really should *get going*."

Finally, I realized that this woman wasn't going to be able to move anytime soon. Her friends were helping her, so I wasn't needed, but I would have to change my plan. Luckily, Stephanie and I were able to find another suitable spot, and this time there were no interruptions when, all these years after I had asked her to walk in the woods with me, I asked her my second bold question.

And this time she said "yes."

## Running Tip #13

### *Strength Training*

There are runners who believe fervently in strength training, while others argue just as strongly against it. I'm a believer; strength training helps maintain good bone density, and running efficiency, and keeps injuries at a minimum.

- *Invest in some expert advice.* Paying a personal trainer to show you the right way to do your exercises is money well spent.
- *Always change your routine.* This keeps you and your body from getting bored, and provides the best stimulus to your body for adaptation, so alternate between free weights, cables, machines, and body-weight movements.
- *Work the core.* Any exercise that forces you to balance will work muscles crucial to your running, including your abdominals, lower back, glutes, and hip stabilizers.
- *Do complex movements.* The more joints you get involved, the more muscles you'll be training. So forget bicep curls; do some squats and push-ups.
- *Don't rest; alternate body parts.* You've got the endurance for this, so use it, and get your workout over in lightning speed.

# A Race Like No Other

My fall 2002 racing campaign began with a solid run in the Toronto Marathon in September, followed by the Portland Marathon in early October, which enabled me to add Oregon to my list of states completed. Portland's race was as scenic and well-organized as any of the other dozens of marathons I'd run, but what stood out in my mind was a short, brutal climb up and over a short suspension bridge, and the tiny redwood saplings the volunteers handed out to finishers at the end of the race. The rest of the country had not yet added "carbon footprint" to their lingo, but Portland was way ahead of them.

Two weeks after crossing the finish line in Portland, I flew out to Amsterdam with a small team of Arthritis Foundation charity fundraisers. Little by little, I was working my way to Europe's greatest cities, and each one was proving to be more astonishing than the last. I loved Amsterdam for its streets and canals and museums, and yes, even its red-light district and marijuana-selling coffee shops, though I was too shy and conservative to do more than quickly walk past either. More to my liking was the wonderful Van Gogh Museum. There was also the famous Rijksmuseum to stroll through, as well as a somber visit to the house of

Anne Frank, the young victim of the Holocaust whose memoirs touched the world.

But I had other things on my mind as well. I was especially looking forward to the race; Amsterdam's marathon course had once held the marathon world record, and was reputed to be as beautiful as it was flat and fast. But the day before the marathon I fell ill with a bad cold, and on race day I felt miserable. Still, after traveling all that way to be with my team and run the race, I wasn't about to let a cold stop me.

The cold had other ideas. By the halfway point, I knew that I wouldn't be able to run the entire race, and that I'd be lucky to even finish as a walker. Still, I pressed on, running as much as I could, and walking the rest. As I stumbled on, I tried to appreciate the beauty of the course. It had meandered through the downtown area, then wandered to the out-skirts of town, passing along a river and old windmills. It's often difficult to be objective about a racecourse when you've had a rough day; it's too tempting to think badly of a race in which you performed badly. But in Amsterdam, it was easy to see that despite my own difficulties, it was a wonderful race. I only regretted that I wasn't able to make the most of it.

Even in my depleted condition, however, I found myself trying to push as hard as I could. Seeing other walkers brought out my competitive juices, and I silently took aim at each one directly in front of me, quickening my pace to catch and pass them. It might sound compulsive, but this helped me feel like I was still part of a race, even as my expected finishing time soared higher than I ever thought it could be. When at long last I crossed the finish line, though, I wasn't concerned about my time; I was just thrilled that I had managed to go on when it would have been so easy to quit. It was a lesson I had learned before, but which was worth learning again: some of my best moments aren't my fastest moments.

Marathon number 72 was in the books.

Two weeks after running Amsterdam, I ran the New York City Marathon again. I had beaten my cold, and was ready for a real race.

But even with all I had experienced in fifteen years of racing, there were still some things to learn. For example, I had believed it to be impossible to urinate while running. To the extent that I had ever thought about it—and I know that by thinking about it at all I am among 1/100th of 1 percent of people on the planet—I had thought it was like keeping your eyes open while sneezing: theoretically possible, but not likely to be seen in my lifetime.

As it turned out, I was wrong. The race had just started, and all of us in our tens of thousands were huffing our way up the Verrazano Bridge, when I noticed some runners to my right who were transfixed with something just ahead of us. They seemed amazed. I saw why: a woman wearing nylon shorts was letting go as she ran. Besides being inconsiderate of those of us behind her—and was there ever a better incentive to pick up the pace and pass someone?—I couldn't imagine running 25 more miles on a crisp November morning in those soaked shorts. But maybe she had once had a bad Porta-Jon experience, too.

But that wasn't my problem. In fact I had few problems at all that day, and I was rewarded with a finishing time almost an hour faster than I had just posted in the Netherlands.

And then two weeks after that, I ran a local race in Maryland. It was a cold, wet day, and when I crossed the finish line, I was relieved to see that the race organizers had put out soup and pizza to revive us. I was famished, and stacked three slices of pizza one atop the other, downing them all at once like a big hoagie. I'm glad the race photographers didn't capture that moment.

Two weeks after *that* race, I returned to Hawaii with another charity team to run the Honolulu Marathon. On the flight home, I thought about how, after fifteen years of marathoning, my body seemed to need less and less recovery time. I didn't know exactly how this had happened, but my body had obviously adapted on a very fundamental level.

The marathons kept coming. Number 76: Miami; number 77: Boston, number 78: Kona, Hawaii.

Ah, Kona. A race obviously dreamed up by a sadist who knew nothing about running. It was held on the Big Island of Hawaii, which sounds like a tropical paradise to anyone who hasn't been there. To those in the know, however, most of the island is a hot, barren lava field. A friend of mine had run it the year before and had lost eight of her toenails due to swelling of her feet during the race. I had already weathered plenty of hot-weather racing, so I knew what to expect and how to handle it, but for the uninitiated—that is, for the virgin marathoners on my charity team—it was a brutal awakening. I tired to help them understand what they were up against, but no amount of talking was going to fully prepare them for the broiling moonscape on which they found themselves. I stayed on the course helping our runners—and anyone else I saw in difficulty—until our very last participant crossed the finish line. As much as I love the marathon, I think the best that could be said of this one is that we all managed to get through it.

After Kona, I believed that I had pretty much figured out the marathon. The scenery might change from race to race, the temperatures and elevation might vary, and the crowds might differ in size and enthusiasm, but the overall experience would usually be the same. There would be an adrenaline rush at the blast of the starting gun. There would be early optimism, shouts of support, and periodic aid stations. There would be eventual fatigue, and perhaps blisters. There would inevitably be a moment of truth, accompanied by a wave of determination, and then perseverance, culminating with euphoria at the finish line. This is the beauty of the marathon—its predictability, and its simplicity. You just run 26.2 miles as fast as you can, and if you do it right, there are usually precious few shocks along the way.

Or so I thought. Then I read about a marathon that is different from all the others, the name of which brings a smile to the face of those who are in the know: the Marathon des Châteaux du Médoc, or as it is more commonly and simply called, Médoc. If the marathon is the serious-minded older sibling of running, then Médoc is the wild child, looking for the nearest party. In a sport defined by discipline, Médoc is the Dionysian exception: a race that is more revelry than competition.

Created in 1985 as a tour for a group of athletic wine connoisseurs, the race is a September jaunt along roads and trails, past fifty-nine vineyards in Pauillac, in the Bordeaux region of southern France, by the shores of the river Gironde. To say that it is just a race through wine country, though, is like saying that Mardi Gras is just a celebration of Fat Tuesday, because the organizers have turned the marathon into a uniquely local creation; a celebration of the senses. It has become famous for wine, food and music stations along the course, and for the outlandish costumes worn by its participants. Even the race materials caution you to think of it as more of a tour than a competition. It is truly what Ernest Hemingway named Paris: a moveable feast.

I first learned about Médoc in the mid-90s in a newspaper article that took a "look what those crazy foreigners are up to now" approach to reporting on the race. The race was described as being more notable for the quantities of wine and oysters consumed than for fast times produced. While most marathons are a 26-mile adventure, Médoc sounded more like it needed a twelve-step program, but I was more intrigued than dismayed. I knew that some day I would have to experience it for myself.

Several obstacles became immediately apparent, starting with simply getting into the race. Like most chronic marathoners, I had become accustomed to having to compete with other applicants to get a number in the most popular races. Over the years, the Marine Corps Marathon began to fill up more and more quickly, and soon would close out within days of being open, while New York required split second timing just to get a race application considered. Still, these races offered enough slots to give most runners hope: 18,000, 25,000, or 35,000. Not so with Médoc. The narrow lanes along which the course meanders makes a huge field of marathoners impossible, so the race is limited to only 8,000 participants. It is also an immensely popular race, and registration closes out quickly. To race Médoc, you have to commit early and keep your fingers crossed.

In April 2002, when I traveled to Paris, I thought I had managed a particularly good coup at the marathon expo: I convinced a race official at the Médoc Marathon information booth to let me reserve a block of one dozen slots for my running friends and myself. I thought it would be an easy sell back home. The race official put his initials on an application and told me to send it in with payment for the reserved slots as soon as possible. I was so pleased with my good fortune that I sent in the money while I was still in France. But when I got back to the States, a voice mail message was waiting for me that said, in a thick French accent, that there was a problem with my race application. Not trusting phone contact, I sent an e-mail explaining the arrangement I had worked out with the race official. All settled, I thought. Then I received an e-mail in return telling me that my demand to talk to the race director was refused. I was confused. Obviously, this was going to be more complicated than I thought, especially since I didn't speak French.

As I tried to sort out the application process, I also began to consider the logistics. There weren't any direct flights from the United States to Bordeaux. The best that I could arrange was to fly direct to Paris, and then either take a connecting flight or a bullet train to Bordeaux. And on arrival, the difficulties don't end; Pauillac is far from the Bordeaux city center, and lodging there is very limited. The only workable option seemed to be to stay in the city and arrange for a driver to take me for the nearly hour and a half long ride to the race start.

Ultimately, my plans to run Médoc collapsed that year like a house of cards. Still, I had caught the scent, and I would not give up hope. And then suddenly, in 2003, the opportunity arose: Jenice Cunningham, a coach and team coordinator for the Arthritis Foundation based in Atlanta, was putting together a team. I knew Jenice from the Honolulu, Dublin, and Amsterdam marathons. Jenice had worked out all the details, and she had called me to find out if I wanted to come along. I answered yes before she was even finished asking the question.

With the logistics all taken care of, I settled into deciding on a training plan. Knowing that Médoc is no ordinary marathon, I wondered if I needed to alter my usual routine. Speed work is usually a part of my regular marathon preparation, and speed can pay off handsomely in Médoc, where I had heard rumors that the winner in each age category receives his or her weight in wine. I'm not an elite runner, though, so a fast marathon would leave me without the winner's prize and also without full enjoyment of the race's amenities. Even if I could somehow miraculously take first place, I didn't think I would be able to survive the reward, even with the help of my friends. I decided on a more leisurely approach to the race. I crossed speed work off my to-do list. So far, so good.

The next issue was thornier. How does one prepare to drink wine during a race? I considered adding alcohol to my training regimen, but I was unable to find any advice on how to do this. Should I slowly increase my intake week to week, along with my mileage? Would it matter what kind of wine I trained with? I scrapped the whole idea; I just would build up a solid running base and let the race-day drinking take care of itself.

Although I couldn't find any information on training for Médoc, I did find plenty of advice on how to actually run the race. The first suggestion I came across was to skip wine altogether for the first half of the race, on the theory that if I should then encounter any ill effects from wine tasting, I would be close enough to the end to successfully make it across the finish line. The second tip was to not actually swallow the wine. Instead, I was told to just swirl the wine in my mouth like a professional taster, and then spit it out. This would theoretically give me the pleasure of experiencing the wine without actually getting drunk, the reasoning being, I presume, that being drunk diminishes the chances of crossing the finish line. A third idea was to simply run the race in a straightforward, no-funny-business manner—no wine, no food, no partying. Then, after coming across the finish line, I could make my way back on to the course to eat and drink to my heart's content.

These all seemed like very well-reasoned strategies. Naturally, I ignored them all. I had decided against running Médoc carefully and strategically; that just didn't seem to be true to the spirit of the race. Spitting out wine must be a kind of heresy in France, and as for backtracking the course, when my legs cross a finish line, they know the race is over, and they don't like to run after that. I decided to experience the race fully and let the chips fall where they may.

There was, however, one more issue I would have to consider before making my way to the starting line: what to wear. Usually this is a simple matter: shorts and singlet in warm weather, graduating through different combinations until I came to tights, gloves and a hat, with a long-sleeved top and jacket, in the coldest weather. Médoc, of course, demanded a different approach. The race materials not only mentioned that most participants wear a costume, but also promised an extra prize for all participants who did so.

What's that old phrase? In for a penny, in for a pound. Everyone in my group—myself included—decided that we would go the extra mile, so to speak, and wear a costume. But whatever we chose would have to be not only eye-catching, but practical as well. After all, this wasn't just some Halloween bash or a Thanksgiving Turkey Trot; we would have to wear this costume for 26.2 miles. With that in mind, Jenice's group agreed on the perfect outfit: grass skirts and leis over our running duds. I daringly cut the skirt down to make it more suitable for running— almost a grass miniskirt, really. I smiled at the incongruity of seeing it lying next to my usual race gear, but I began to relax. All the big issues were now decided.

Finally, September rolled around, and I found myself boarding a jet for a red-eye flight to Paris. I arrived almost too tired to appreciate the gleaming glass and steel of Charles de Gaulle airport as I made my way to my connecting flight. In the months since I committed to the race, international events had stormed onto the front pages as we moved closer toward war with Iraq. I wondered whether the rift between the U.S. and French governments would affect my travel and race plans, and whether Americans would no longer find themselves welcome in Bordeaux. I've long believed in the spiritual healing power of a marathon, but this was a tall order. Could wine, food, and running bring us together? I'd soon find out.

My flight landed in Bordeaux without incident, and if I had any doubts about where I was, they were quickly dispelled as giant bottles of cabernet sauvignon stared down at us from atop the baggage carousels. After a short ride to our hotel and a quick check-in, several of us went out for a walkabout.

Bordeaux seemed to be in the early stages of a renaissance, with ongoing restoration and construction projects throughout the city center. Its old-world charm was still evident, though, as cafes, restaurants, and shops lined the streets in centuries-old stone buildings, all leading down to the wide Gironde River. The streets looked impossibly narrow, and the traffic was choking, but to us, it was a beautiful place. We were even able to find a place that served pizza—or, at least, a version of it. And better still, we located a nearby supermarket for loading up on water and fresh fruit.

The following morning we piled into our chartered bus for the hour-long drive out to Pauillac for the race expo and number pickup. After entering the athletic center that served as race headquarters, we encountered a small sample of what to expect the next day, as an older gentleman in full American Indian costume stared us down at the entryway, and made folks jump by periodically letting out a short war whoop. Being a city boy, I admit to only a sketchy knowledge of Native Americans, but even I knew this was very odd. It would prove to be only the first of many such moments.

We proceeded to get our numbers, shirts, and race timing chips. Having a chip in a race like this seemed out of place; it was one of the few telltale signs that this was an actual competition at all. We then made our way to the modest Médoc Marathon expo. A few other races, including the Chicago Marathon, were represented, and among the race memorabilia that was available for purchase were bottles of wine with the race logo emblazoned on the label. There was also another uniquely Médoc concession tucked in among the stalls: a costume seller catering to those who hadn't yet settled on a race day outfit. As I looked over the racks of Viking, maiden, and clown costumes, I realized that my team's Hawaiian ensemble would probably seem very conservative compared to what we would see the next day.

I mulled that over as we went back to Bordeaux and spent the day lounging around waiting for our pasta feed. The race organizers put on their own prerace dinner—complete with copious amount of *le vin*, of course—but we opted to be closer to our hotel and an early bedtime. Though the race was scheduled to start at 9:30 A.M., the long drive necessary to get there required a predawn departure. Far from being annoyed, I was almost soothed by this return to a slice of my usual prerace regimen.

The next morning I scarfed down a light, high-carb breakfast, then boarded the bus and settled into a doze as the sun rose over the French countryside. The air was crisp and just a bit cool, with temperatures nudging into the 60s.

Stepping out of the bus in Pauillac, I couldn't help but think of the colorful world into which Dorothy's house fell in *The Wizard of Oz*. All around me were odd characters in running shoes; mimes, devils, cavemen, bunnies, pirates, prisoners sporting a helium ball and chain, cats and mice, and all manner of cartoon characters. There was face paint galore, and even teams of runners pulling theme carts, like mini floats in a Thanksgiving Day parade.

I had read that 70 percent of the participants were costumed, but on race day it felt like a much higher percentage; it seemed not just like many people had a costume, but rather that virtually everyone had one. Dressing in a plain running outfit suddenly seemed like a mortal sin, and I was glad that my team had at least made an effort, humble as it was. As I walked past a row of portable toilets, though, I wondered how all these odd and otherworldly people would manage the details and necessities of running a race. No matter; we were a colorful group, and we were having a good time.

In fact, we were the most self-aware race group I'd ever seen. In the minutes before most races, runners seem lost in their own thoughts, full of nervous energy about the challenge they would soon face. In Médoc, though, the prerace mood was festive; it was all about people-watching, preening, and enjoying yourself. There were dancers gyrating on platforms above the crowd, and everybody was posing and snapping photos of those around them. A Japanese group, dressed as samurai, even had their own camera crew following them around the starting line to record their encounters with other outlandish runners. It all reminded me of the crowd I'd seen at Grateful Dead shows years ago, which was so happy to just be there that watching the band almost seemed like an afterthought. Watching us laugh and point at one another at the starting line, it was almost easy to forget that we would soon be running a marathon.

But there was indeed a race, and suddenly we were off. We wound our way out of town, past scenic storefronts and booths offering food and wine-tasting, and past cheering supporters. We made our way toward the vineyards, and soon came upon the first official aid stop, just a few kilometers into the race. It was amply supplied with water, cake, cookies, raisins, dried apricots, and even prunes—prunes, for heaven's sake!—but no wine. In fact, there was no wine at any of the early aid stops. I wondered whether the race directors thought it best to protect us from ourselves. As the sun poked its way though and the temperature began to climb, I began to think this might not have been a bad decision.

Kilometer 9 brought our first wine-tasting opportunity. I was treated to the unusual sight of tables lined up with glass after glass of dark red Bordeaux. Never has being a runner seemed so rewarding! I slowed to a walk and lifted a glass. As I savored the first sip, I knew that I wouldn't remember the taste of the wine or even the vineyard, but I'd certainly remember the sensation. I tossed the glass in a receptacle and resumed running.

As we made or way past the châteaux and back into the fields, I saw a number of runners split from the pack and head out between the rows of grapes. It took me a moment to realize that they were taking bathroom breaks. A runner would not be surprised at such behavior, but I bet that wine connoisseurs would certainly be shocked.

We continued through the French countryside, passing the occasional stone châteaux and cyclists on holiday. We ran on paved roads, but more frequently on dirt paths alongside the vines, the pounding of our feet kicking up the soft, powdery dirt into low clouds. We didn't come across another wine-tasting stop until kilometer 16, but there were plenty of aid stations along the way offering refreshments and cool, wet sponges. The sun was shining brightly by this time, and I was starting to wonder about how the heat would affect our ragtag group. As if on command, some dark clouds rolled in, bringing along a welcome sprinkle of drizzle that cooled us off and quieted the billowing dust around our feet. The drizzle continued, however, and grew in strength, and soon became rain. Usually a cause for disgruntlement, the rain instead became a cause for more drinking.

At some point along this part of the marathon I had the most unusual sensation; I thought I saw flowers blowing around me, as if a herald were scattering petals in my path. Perhaps I was having a bad reaction to the wine. But no. Slowly recognition creased my bewildered brain—my lei had broken, and was quickly dispersing itself. I gathered up the loose ends and tied them together tightly. Just as my grass skirt had been shortened, my lei was now a streamlined version of its former self.

We also began to come across bands along the course offering up some musical distractions. Oddly enough, when I passed a couple of them, they were playing old American country and rockabilly tunes, like "Blue Moon of Kentucky." Not exactly what you'd expect to hear a band playing in France, but sometimes it's better to just appreciate a moment than to ask why and how.

After the second wine stop, the tastings came more frequently, and I stuck with my promise to taste each and every wine that they put in our path. Soon I lost count, but I knew that in all, there would be twenty-one wine-tasting stations. I've never been a math whiz, but even I could figure out that with there being only two wine stops in the first half of the race, there would be quite a bit of catching up to do. I mustered my best bit of marathoner's determination for the task that lay ahead.

As I continued on my way, I also realized something else about the course: its sheer beauty. I knew that it wasn't just the alcohol talking as I wondered whether this might not be the most beautiful marathon course I've ever run. It wasn't just that there were breathtaking sights along the way, although there were plenty of those. It was the absence of something; the inevitable marathon dead zone, the dry spot to be found in all races, where we labor though industrial parks, past train tracks and factories and parking lots, with no supporters to cheer us on, and no eye candy to distract us from our boredom and suffering. Boston has such a zone, lined by railroad tracks. So does the New York Marathon, in Queens, before hitting the Queensboro Bridge. And so do countless other races. But in Médoc, I realized, there was nothing but row after row of grapevines, full with their dark fruit, and beautiful châteaux lording over their fields.

The beauty of the course and the glory of the wine couldn't stave off the realities of running a marathon, however, and despite my leisurely early pace, I began to slow in the second part of the race. I won't blame it all on the wine, not when there were also some other obstacles I could point my finger at, like the food. At one station I took a bit of unidentified food and shoved it into my mouth. After all, no one would put out food on a marathon course that would be bad for us, right? Wrong, I realized too late. Wrong, wrong, wrong. Of all the foods in the world, the only one that I truly hate was liver. What I had now in my mouth was some type of liver-based lunchmeat. Yuck. The memory of it still haunts me, and has led me to instituting a new racing rule: put nothing in your mouth that you can't identify. My mother later insisted that she taught me that rule years ago, though I'm not so sure about that.

The race continued onward, past kilometers 25, 30, and 35. Then, at kilometer number 38, with just four kilometers to go, the race let loose, like a child that's been quiet too long and needs to scream. First came the oysters, piled ostentatiously on serving tables. A teammate of mine later told me of a writer's observation: "Oh, the courage of the first brave soul to slurp an oyster!" On that day in Bordeaux, I can tell you, there were plenty of brave men and women, and I struggled to be among the bravest.

Next up was a steak station, where bits of grilled beef on sticks were served up to runners. I took just a small piece to taste, then moved on to the next station just down the road, the cheese tables! And after that, more wine! I gulped and chewed and gulped some more, and then, as I slowly fell back into an easy running pace, a little voice somewhere deep inside began telling me that my gluttony wasn't such a great idea. I slowed down a little more as the oysters began to talk to me, and I reminded myself that I only had a little over 1 kilometer to go. I also said a little prayer of thanks to the race directors for not putting the oysters in the first half of the race.

One last unexpected race amenity awaited runners who made it this far: face paint. For those who had been too shy to wear a costume, or who had somehow lost it along the way, there was a chance for last-minute redemption. A couple of volunteers were quickly dabbing color onto runners on request. I opted for some black and red stripes down my nose and across my cheeks. All I can say is that it seemed like a good idea at the time.

And finally, the finish line was just up ahead. As I crossed through, I was given a backpack with the race logo on it, and a bottle of wine to put in it. For my costume-wearing efforts, I was also given a fanny pack bearing the race logo. And last but not least, I was pointed toward the finisher's tent, where wine and beer were being freely doled out. Perhaps not surprisingly, I had had enough by this point, and as appreciative as I was of the postrace offerings, I decided to head to the bus instead. And probably not in a straight line, either, despite my best efforts.

The afternoon was spent recovering from the race, followed later by more wine and food. The next day, we all decided to partake of the vineyard walk offered to race participants, featuring—you guessed it— more wine and food. A highlight was the lunch tent set up at the end of the tour, where oysters and other fare were doled out as a French chanteuse belted out old American tunes and various national anthems. Somehow, I wasn't at all surprised. By this time, I had learned to expect the unexpected.

After the race, we took a train back to Paris—still drinking along the way, of course. We then spent a few days drying out and sightseeing. As I gazed at the now-familiar Eiffel Tower and wandered the Latin Quarter, I tried to put the race in perspective. It seemed to fit into no readily available category. It belonged in a category all its own.

The winners of the marathon, incidentally, posted times of 2:32:52 for the men and 2:56:27 for the women; entirely respectable finishing times that seemed incongruous with my own experience. My finishing time was just about the slowest I've ever had—let's just say it was between four and five hours. Still, it was good enough to put me first in my little group; this was probably more of a reflection of the party instinct of my group than my own speed. But my slow time seemed to show the truth behind the race's motto: below an image of an apparently snookered runner weaving from pillar to post is the phrase "Médoc, Le Marathon Le Plus Long Du Monde," "Médoc, the Longest Marathon in the World." While it might have felt like an ultramarathon, I knew that Médoc is not really a race to be measured in time, or perhaps even by distance. It really was like no other race in the world.

As much fun as racing in Bordeaux proved to be, it wasn't the only excitement I had running that September. There was Hurricane Isabel to consider. It started as a small updraft as water evaporated over warm south Atlantic waters. The updraft gathered strength and grew into a tropical storm, and then flexed its muscles and grew into a Category 5 hurricane, with winds raging at 160 miles per hour. Inexorably, it moved toward the Carolina coast, and up toward Washington, D.C. Naturally, I took that as a sign to lace up my training shoes for the run of a lifetime.

As the storm drew near, batteries and bottled water were cleaned off store shelves, and schools, as well as federal and local government agencies, announced that they would be closed. Thursday—hurricane day—started out gray and windy, and I felt a sense of expectation among those out on the streets, rushing through last-minute preparations. As the day ebbed into evening, the winds picked up to a howl, and rain swept through in waves. The storm was drawing near, and it was almost time for me to go.

It was 9:30 P.M. when I finally ventured outside. The first thing I noticed was how very warm it was. It must have been in the upper

80s, and I immediately regretted bringing a light jacket. The rain had let up, and the winds had died down a bit as I ran southwest toward the Potomac River. If there were a front-row seat to the storm, it would be on one of the city's bridges, where wind can whip over the open water like race cars at Daytona.

As I ran down the city streets, I passed shuttered and boarded businesses, but also some open bars and restaurants, catering to the adventurous, the bored, or the addicted. There were already a few trees down, and debris littered the road. A handful of taxis roamed the streets, and there were a few police cruisers out, but little else. I ran down the center of M Street in the Georgetown district, one of the busiest thoroughfares in the city, and I was all alone. It was the first time I'd ever been able to do that. I felt giddy with power; this storm was not as bad as I thought it would be. Clearly, Isabel had lost a great deal of her punch as she made her way inland. Just then, a branch swatted me across the back of my head, as if to remind me that the storm had not yet lost all of its teeth.

I turned onto Key Bridge and looked across the Potomac River toward Virginia. I was about a third of the way across when the big winds hit. I was blown from side to side of the walkway like a pinball, despite my best efforts to run a straight line. As wind whipped my face, I found it difficult to breathe. It was exhilarating, but also terrifying, and it occurred that it wouldn't take very much more wind to send me hurtling over the railing for a hundred-foot plunge into the river below. I made it to the other side, then turned to head back home. My ambitious 12-mile course had been cut to a short 5-miler, but that was enough of a taste of the hurricane for me.

As I neared my apartment, the storm picked up in intensity, as if to say that it had only been toying with me so far, and that it was now ready to really play. Rain began to pour down again, and the wind increased. I raced toward my building and burst through the doors like it was the tape in a 5K race, then stood there, dripping and panting as the storm raged on the other side of the glass door like a lion in a cage. By that time, Stephanie had moved down to D.C. and was living with me. She just handed me a towel and shook her head.

By morning, the storm was all but spent. I ran different trails during the following days to assess the damage. Fallen trees across one of my favorite bike paths made for a unique climbing-running duathlon. Friends in the suburbs reported that their power was out, and would be for at least another week, from what they'd been told. Still, the city had been lucky to escape with relatively little damage; it has been far luckier than many other coastal towns. And I was lucky to have unwittingly found a relatively gentle hour during the storm to squeeze in my hurricane run.

## Running Tip #14

## *The Bathroom Break*

One thing that sets runners apart is the utilitarian view we take of our bodies. We see them as machines, built through training for high performance. Our need to relieve ourselves before a race is usually no more embarrassing to us than a need to check the oil in our car. This might put us at odds with the rest of the civilized world, but we're okay with that. Still, there are basic guidelines to follow to avoid any problems in this area.

- *Deal with bodily needs before the race begins.* All major marathons provide hundreds of Porta-Jons at their race starts, but before a race, the lines to get in one are usually very long. Minimize your need for them by cutting off the fluid intake a full hour before the race start. Wait until just 5 minutes before the race is to begin, then gulp down 6–8 ounces of water or sports drink.
- *Don't be too shy during the race.* Marathoners tend to act with unspoken cooperation during a race; we keep an eye out for places other runners choose to use. But sometimes, a race course simply doesn't provide any secluded spots to take care of business. Like Superman without a phone booth, I've sometimes found myself looking in horror at fields without trees and city streets without dark alleys, and those are somehow also the spots where the crowds of spectators seems most dense. In such situations, do what you must. Remember: during a marathon, the regular rules of proper public behavior don't apply.

→

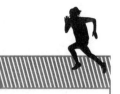

## Running Tip #14

If you doubt me, think of marathon world record–holder Paula Radcliffe, who, en route to winning the London Marathon in April 2004, crouched down on the course to relieve herself. She apologized afterward, but runners knew no apology was necessary. We understood.

# A Bit of Hardware

By 2004, I had run eighty-four marathons, and my collection of medals was something to see. My first medal was earned in the Marine Corps Marathon in 1987, and though I was fiercely proud of it at the time, I can now admit that it was a cheap little thing. It was fashioned to resemble a dog tag, but looked like it had been pulled from a cereal box. As the race matured over the years, though, and received corporate sponsorship, its medals improved, and now they're smart, gleaming works of running art.

Twelve years later, when I crossed the finish line in Antarctica, I didn't get a finisher's medal at all. I wasn't concerned, though, because all of the runners were told that medals would be mailed to our homes later. Sure enough, it showed up in my mailbox a few weeks after I'd returned home. It was the biggest, heaviest, and gaudiest medal I had ever seen. I was thrilled; it was a tangible reminder of where I had been and what I had accomplished. But receiving a medal was not a surprise; most marathoners—even many elite runners—work so hard with so little tangible reward that we have come to expect, even demand, that we be given a finisher's medal upon completing the course. And in commenting on a race, a description of the medal is often right up there with reviews of the course and the race support. And woe to the race director who fails to deliver; he will not be spared the wrath of the runners.

There have been several races where I crossed the finish line and did not get my expected award: in the Northern Central Trails Marathon in Maryland I was given a cheap glass mug, which was also the reward handed out one year at the Houston Marathon. The race director in Virginia Beach was even stingier; there, I was only given a finisher's certificate. Although I never uttered a word about it—at least, not to race officials—someone clearly did, because most of these races now offer finisher's medals. In fact, race directors now go above and beyond the call of duty, offering finisher's medals that are getting ever bigger, shinier, and gaudier. Proof once more that it's possible to have too much of a good thing.

Medals have now become so popular that many races of less than marathon distance award them to their participants. Nestled in my collection are medals from the World's Best 10K in San Blas, Puerto Rico, the Amish Country Half-Marathon, the New York City Road Runners New Year's Eve Midnight 5K run, and the Virginia Beach Rock 'N Roll Half-Marathon. I had run each of these races as hard as I could, and felt that I had earned each medal, and yet something was not quite right about receiving that hardware. Perhaps I had become a snob, but I felt that only races of marathon distance or more ought to award medals.

Eventually, the question came up of what to do with them. Originally, an ordinary nail in the wall was good enough to hang them on. I graduated to a bigger nail, and then a hanging display rack I picked up in a yard sale, designed to hold baseball caps. Finally, I just dumped them all into a cabinet drawer.

Packing them away, I found myself rating them. My Boston Marathon medals were my favorite, each one a symbol of high achievement. They knew their value too; no shiny gilded affairs, these. The

Boston Athletic Association opts for pewter, with its emblem, a unicorn, in relief on the front. It's the marathoning equivalent of a pinstripe suit.

In contrast was the playfulness of the Disneyworld Marathon medal. It was an oval with two smaller ovals affixed at the top, giving an approximation of that famous mouse's head. On the face of the medal was a likeness of Mickey himself, tearing down the road in singlet, shorts, and running shoes. The Las Vegas Marathon medal is in the shape of a roulette wheel, appropriately enough. I've also got a ceramic medal, and even an embroidered one.

The ribbons on which the medals were attached reflect each race's personality as well. Their colors range from black to purple, white, green, red, and orange, and in combinations from traditional red, white, and blue to all the colors of the rainbow. The ribbon for the Marine Corps Marathon medals are red and gold, the colors of the Corps, while the Honolulu Marathon medal came on a string of puka shells, and the New Orleans Marathon medal hangs from a string of Mardi Gras beads.

And then there were the shirts. For some reason, most races have traditionally distributed T-shirts bearing a race logo to all race participants. Early on, they were all cotton, but now most races provide technical racing shirts instead. It might be a good way to tell the world that you had done something extraordinary, and it's certainly a good way for a race and its sponsors to get some cheap promotion, but at some point, enough is enough. Every year or so I've had to cull less desirable shirts from the herd, setting them aside for donation to a local homeless shelter.

But there is another kind of memento that I covet, the ultimate kind of racing hardware: an actual award. After I had finished my first marathon, my father was very proud of me. By the time I finished my second one, though, he asked when I would win one. Win? Not likely, I told him. I was a good runner, and usually finished in the top 10 percent of most race fields, but the difference between being good and being elite is huge. As I explained, if I was rested and warmed up at mile 25 and jumped into the race with the members of the elite pack, who had already been running for 2 hours or so, they would easily blow right past me and leave me in the dust. I hated to disappoint Dad, but I told him that I would *never* win a marathon. Simple as that. Just finishing was an accomplishment in itself, and running as hard as I could every time was my victory.

Of course, that didn't mean I couldn't dream a little. I didn't expect to win any races outright, but just placing in my age group would be nice. I achieved a little recognition in a race at Dewey Beach, Delaware one year. It was a 10-mile race with an interesting side competition called the Pump 'n Run. Race volunteers weighed participants, and then loaded up a bench press—full body weight for men, two-thirds of body weight for women—and participants benched this amount as many times as they could shortly before running the race. One minute was then deducted from their finishing time for every repetition they were able to do on the bench.

I signed up for the Pump 'n Run, and bench-pressed my body weight twenty-one times. I then went out and ran a strong race. When it was all over, I discovered that I had won my age group. It was my first award, and even though all I received was a commemorative T-shirt—another T-shirt, for cryin' out loud!—I enjoyed hearing my name being announced, and taking those few but glorious steps forward to claim my prize.

I wasn't completely surprised by my little victory, though. Back in high school I had enjoyed lifting weights with my friends, and I had never given that up, even as I took up running. I might not have been the fastest runner or the strongest lifter, but I can run very fast for a weight lifter, and I am very strong for a runner. The Pump 'n Run rewarded this kind of balanced fitness, and I appreciated that.

But still, I had not won an award for being the fastest runner on race day. My trophy cabinet was still bare.

Then came the Hog Eye Marathon in Fayetteville, Arkansas. Marathon number 85. The night before the race, my friends and I went to a famous local steak joint, Doe's. Supposedly it had been a favorite eating spot for the press corps who followed Bill Clinton on his campaign tours.

They serve two kinds of steak in Doe's: one-pound and two-pound. I showed restraint and ordered the one-pound. It was as good as word of mouth had said it would be. I knew that come race time, the steak would still be with me, like bag of wet cement in my gut. But I wanted to enjoy this time and place with my friends, and one never knows when such a moment may come around again. After eighty-four marathons, I bet that my body would find a way to handle it.

The next morning, though, I worried less about that steak than about the driving rain and wind outside. At the sound of the starter's gun, I set out with several hundred other runners on a very hilly out-and-back course. There is something about truly horrible conditions that focuses the mind, and soon I found myself enjoying the challenge in a crazy kind of way. I wouldn't be out running a marathon in the first place if I didn't like a challenge, and the weather was just one more obstacle to conquer. I gritted my teeth and ran on.

Eventually, the course led us back to town square and the finish line. I collected my medal and then lingered indoors to warm up and have something to eat. When the race results were posted on the wall, I went to check my official time and discovered that I had finished second in my age group. I was going to win an award!

I'm embarrassed to say how excited I was. Dad passed away in 1989, but if he were still alive, I know that he would be thrilled that I had finally won something, even if it took me 85 marathons to do it. My award was a hand-made ceramic plaque, with the race name and logo drawn into it. Aesthetically, it's not much, but to me, it's beautiful.

Looking at all my racing hardware, I'm reminded not only of my years of marathon running, but also of one of my great fears for the future: that some day, all of these medals—and my few awards—will be in a box at a yard sale somewhere, three for a dollar. As I handled some of my medals, I noticed that some of them had already started to corrode. I realized that I didn't have to worry about that far-off yard sale; apparently, my medals wouldn't even last long enough to make it there. What if they all disintegrated little by little? Or what if they were lost in a fire? What was I without my medals?

I knew that if all my medals disappeared, I would feel the loss of the tangible proof that I had led a runner's life. But I realized, too, that they didn't really matter that much. With or without them, I knew what I had achieved. Truth be told, I hardly ever look at any of them anyway; they are to me like the gold in Fort Knox, more of an idea than a physical presence in my day-to-day life. I ran the marathon to discover the depths of my own determination and perseverance. I didn't need a medal to tell me who I was.

Meanwhile, I had other things on my mind that summer. It was June 2004, and Stephanie and I were about to be wed. Even we were surprised at how quickly our relationship had moved along, but though we had dated a little more than one year, we had known each other since we were twelve, so we really felt like we had known each other all our lives, which was more or less true. It was as if we were each getting to know someone we were already very well acquainted with. We had shared history, yet separate lives; wonderful and varied life experiences, yet the same background. As we liked to say to each other, it just made sense.

On the morning of our wedding I woke up early and went for a run—no better way to burn off some of the jitters I felt. I showered and dressed, and drove down from our hotel to the site we had picked: a castle nestled in the Hudson Valley in upstate New York. I marveled that so far, things were going perfectly. Just as that thought went through my mind—hanging there, like a thought balloon in a comic strip—someone asked me if I had the rings on me. I froze. They were still back in my hotel room. Oh, crap. Crap, crap, crap. Un-freakin'-believable.

I jumped in my car and raced the five miles back to the hotel, cruising through stop signs and red lights, almost hoping that a cop would stop me so that I could explain my dilemma and get a police escort. That didn't happen, but I did make it back to the chapel in time, and the ceremony went off without a hitch. After the reception, husband and wife made it back to the hotel room, exhausted but very happy. We celebrated by opening a bottle of '93 Château Lafite Rothschild I had brought back from Médoc. Despite the shaky start, it turned out to be a wonderful day.

The first thing people now want to know about Stephanie was whether she was a marathoner. The answer is no. At first, Stephanie was concerned that I might pressure her into running a marathon, but I told her I could care less whether she ever ran one, and I meant it. Sure, it would be great fun for me to run a marathon next to my wife, but I didn't marry her in order to fulfill that dream; I married her because I love her for who she is, not for what she might become.

Still, Stephanie is very fit. She's a bit of a gym rat, really, which is important to me because I want to be with someone healthy, someone who I can grow old with, someone who can still see life as a great adventure well into our senior years. But run a marathon? Nah. There's plenty of stuff I have no interest in doing. Bungee jumping, for example. I have absolutely zero interest in that.

If Stephanie were to tell me that she didn't think she *could* do it, though, that would be different. Running has taught me to not automatically accept limitations, whether imagined or imposed by others. I don't believe anyone should automatically expect and accept failure, especially not in regard to the marathon. Finishing a marathon is within the reach of anyone with the determination and courage to *just try*.

When we first started dating, Stephanie actually did show some interest in trying to run. Her plan was to run as far as she could and see how that felt. I saved her the suspense and gave her an immediate answer: if she ran for as long as she could, she would only guarantee that she would be tired and miserable when she finally stopped.

Over the years, I've seen the same pattern among people who hate running: when they gave it a shot, they almost always went too far or too fast. The trick, I told her, it to not run until you're exhausted—leave that for the marathons! Instead, I told her to run until she felt fatigued but comfortable at the end. If she didn't want to hate running, she'd need to keep it manageable.

And that's what she did. She began with some walking and easy running on the treadmill, and little by little she worked her way up to running for a half hour straight. In time, she stretched it to an hour.

In November 2003, we took our vacation in New Zealand, which we found to be a magical, wonderful place, filled with beaches, gorges, smoldering thermal springs, and breathtaking mountain ranges. The Kiwis don't take any of this for granted; I'd read that if there's a danger-ous, difficult, thrilling way of getting from one point to another, they do it. Naturally, I thought, there must be a marathon. Sure enough, there was, right in the capital city of Auckland, along with a 10K race. I signed up for the marathon, and with my encouragement, Stephanie signed up for the 10K. It was the first race she'd ever entered.

On race morning, I set out before dawn to get to the ferry that brought the marathoners across the harbor to the starting line. It was a beautiful course: almost pretty enough to keep me from cursing the bru-tal headwind I ran against over the last few miles of the race. As I neared the finish line, I wondered how Stephanie had done.

The race finished in a park, and it didn't take me long to spot her across the open field. As I waved to her, I ticked off items on my mental triage checklist: she was upright, she was walking, and she was smiling. When I got to her, I gave her a big kiss and asked how it went.

"Great," she said. "I finished in just under an hour."

"That's a great time," I told her. "You should be proud."

"Yeah, I am," she told me. "But around mile four, I thought, *Well, wouldn't a cup of coffee and a newspaper be nice right now?*"

So, there might be no marathon run together for us. Or maybe there will be. Either way, it's okay; Stephanie had proven—as much to herself as to me—that she could run one if she wanted to. But running isn't her passion, it's mine. Her passion is for art, both as a painter and a teacher. I love that she has such strong opinions, dedication, knowledge, and talent for it. That kind of passion is, to me, the fullest embodiment of what is best in our nature. Our appreciation for each other's passion is more important to us than being able to fully share in the object of each other's joy. We each feel deeply about something, and are willing to risk something of ourselves for it. That alone makes us kindred spirits.

We do actually run together sometimes. I think of these runs not just as workouts; they're couple-time, when we share stories or ideas, or just enjoy a break from the rest of the world. Instead of being in competition with our relationship, running has, I think, strengthened it.

After all these years, I think I finally got it right.

## Running Tip #15

### *How to Do the Thing You Love with the One You Love*

Training with your romantic partner is not impossible, but if you want to make it work, it's a good idea to follow some basic guidelines.

- *Put the relationship first.* Running with a mate can be tricky. The key is to not do anything to demean or demoralize your partner. So forget your training schedule. If you push too hard, he or she will get very cranky. The point is to demonstrate what you already know: that running can be fun. Do your hard workout earlier or later in the day, or on another day altogether.
- *Make your run together your entire workout.* Don't use your run together as a portion of a longer workout. That implies that the run was inadequate, which could undermine your mate's confidence. So start and finish together.
- *Make sure your partner has the proper gear.* Chances are your nonrunning mate will show up for your first run together wearing cross-training shoes, a cotton T-shirt, and sweatpants. In other words, all the wrong things. If you think missing your anniversary led to a big fight, see what happens when running with you causes your mate to have chafing and blisters. So go shopping together for proper clothing and good running shoes.

→

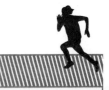

- *Figure out what works for your partner.* It's your job to show your partner a fun time; if he or she enjoys the run, he or she will be back for more.

- *Don't be the boss.* After years of running and racing, it's easy to think we know everything about running. But if you tell your partner what to do, you reduce him or her to an underling. So don't order; create a dialogue instead. He or she will probably follow your advice anyway, but that will be his or her decision. It makes a difference.

- *Don't forget these rules on race day.* When your partner is ready to try a first race, be supportive. Offer to run a race with her or him, at her or his pace. But remember: this is your mate's race, not yours; you're just support crew with a number. If your partner would rather run without you, decide together where you'll meet afterward, and ask what you should bring for after the race.

# Good Things Come in Small Packages

My next marathon was only a few weeks after I got married. I met up with Dave in Calgary, Canada, to run a marathon. The race was held in conjunction with the annual Stampede Rodeo—not really a sport that I could identify with. But stranger to me than the idea of roping cattle was the gold band that I fingered on my left hand during the race. I quickly got used to it, though, which I took to be a good sign, and when I crossed the finish line, I received a large western-style belt buckle on a ribbon as a medal, which seemed a fitting memento for that particular race.

That was marathon number 88. When people heard that I'd run that many races, they'd usually ask me which one was my favorite. I didn't know what to say. There were obvious contenders, like New York, Boston, and Paris. I did love them all. But like a child in a candy shop, I just couldn't decide. Finally, I came upon an answer that was honest: my favorite marathon is ... the next one. People smiled, but it was really a dodge, and we all knew it.

Little by little, I started to narrow the field, if not to a particular marathon, then at least to a category. The big races were the ones that people were most familiar with. These behemoths were cities unto themselves, and they were like huge running festivals. They were *events*. But with the bright lights and press coverage came the uglier side. These races were demanding, high maintenance mistresses, requiring one to fight for entry, to battle for hotels and flights, and to wake up early to rush to the starting line to wait with tens of thousands of other runners for the start, and then pick one's way through the crowds at the finish for family and friends, all lost in a sea of sweaty bodies. These races were memorable, but they often seemed like so much *work*.

That said, big-city marathons should not to be missed, and I returned to them again and again. But were they my favorite races? Not necessarily. There was something more important than the flash of the big-city races; I learned to love the allure of the small-town marathon. Modest, unassuming, more friendly and personal, these were the races I truly enjoyed. Still, people didn't seem to completely believe that. I could see it in their eyes. Sure, they seemed to say, that sounds nice, but you'd never turn down the New York Marathon for a race in, say, Idaho, would you?

Wouldn't I? I decided to put it to the test. I needed to add Idaho to my list of states anyway, so Idaho it would be for marathon number 89. The Mesa Falls Marathon in Ashton, to be exact.

First, I had to get there. Whoever said that it's the journey that matters, not the destination, never spent a lot of time waiting around in an airport. As soon as I went online to book my flights for the race, I realized that things would not be as simple as I expected. There weren't any direct flights from D.C. to Ashton, and among the circuitous routes that were available, there were precious few options.

But that was okay; I hadn't expected booking my flights to be a run in the park. Ultimately, the ones I chose would land me in Idaho well past sunset on the day before the race. No problem. I could handle that, too. There was no commercial airport in Ashton, which meant that I would have to rent a car in Idaho Falls and drive an hour to get to my destination. Still not a problem; I've had to do that before in other big-city races. I would miss the prerace pasta dinner and all the camaraderie that's usually found there, but that wasn't the end of the world, since there would be plenty of time to meet people on the course during the race.

After spending nearly the entire day outbound waiting for flights and making connections, I finally arrived in Idaho Falls. It was a tiny airport, but that was a good thing, since there was no need to take a shuttle to an off-site baggage claim area: I could just step down onto the tarmac, walk into the terminal, get my rental car and go. Except that despite having made a reservation, no one was available at the off-site office to set me up with a car. Quicker than I could say "grrrrrrrr," though, I rented another car from a friendly young woman at a competitor's sales desk, and was soon on my way to Ashton. Still, none of these transportation problems would have happened in Boston, Chicago, or New York. Advantage: big-city marathon.

An hour later, I was driving down ID-47 in Ashton, Idaho, also known more simply as Main Street. I was glad for the sign postings, because I easily could have missed it. With a population of 1,129, there wasn't going to be a lot of street life anyway, especially not around midnight, which is when I arrived. The marathon Web site had listed available lodging, and I opted for the Four Seasons Motel, which was said to be near where the runners were to line up for transport to the starting line on race morning. When booking the room a few weeks earlier over the phone, the clerk told me almost apologetically that the price would be $45 per night. I magnanimously told him that would be perfectly fine. As I edged down Main Street in the quiet darkness, I discovered it on my right, one of those wayside-type inns with parking spots in front of each room. There was a note affixed to the front door of the office addressed to me, letting me know which room was mine, and that it had been left open for me. This would NEVER happen in New York. Not on marathon weekend, not ever. Not even anywhere within 100 miles of

New York. I smiled with relief; at this hour, every moment was precious, and the sooner I could lay my head on a pillow, the better.

I ambled over to my room, swung the door open and found . . . pretty much just a room. It was nothing fancy, but it was certainly serviceable. A clean bed, a TV, and hot and cold running water. Gazing out the door, I realized that the local high school's parking lot, where we would board buses for transport to the race start, was literally right across the street. At least I could sleep to the very last moment, and needed only to make sure I had all my running gear on as I stumbled out the door.

The alarm woke me from a deep slumber, and I looked out the window. Still dark outside. Nothing unusual, since many races have a predawn starting time. There were already two school buses idling in the parking lot, with a handful of runners milling about. Only eleven racers participated in the race's inaugural running in 1997, and the field ballooned to forty the following year.

From what I could see while peering out that window, it hadn't grown very much since then. There were only a few hundred runners, apparently no media representatives whatsoever, and precious few spectators. Still, I don't think I'd ever before had such a comforting prerace moment. I'd had some close calls in the past getting to the starting line in time, but this would not be one of those days.

Fifteen minutes later, while identifying constellations in the clear sky, I walked up to the folding table that served as headquarters for race-day packet pickup. The temperature was in the upper 30s, although warmer weather was predicted for later in the day. Race Director Dave Jacobson checked my name off the list and handed me my packet and a smart-looking polo shirt with an embroidered race logo. "You," Dave told me, "are the first person from Washington, D.C., to run the Mesa Falls Marathon." That meant I would hold the course record for a D.C. marathoner just by crossing the finish line. I began imagining my press release as I trotted back across the street to my motel room to drop off my shirt and goody bag.

Climbing aboard one of the buses minutes later, I peered toward the back for the one thing worth its weight in gold to a runner before a race: a bathroom. There it was, tucked away in the corner. Breathing a sigh of relief, I settled into one of the plush seats, felt the warmth flowing upward from the bus's heaters, and unwrapped my personal "breakfast of champions": two energy bars and a sports drink.

The bus was buzzing with conversation, and soon I met all the runners seated around me. There was a father-daughter team, and quite a few out-of-town runners. As it turned out, though, no one had traveled as far as I did. More than one person wore confused expressions when they found out where I was from; they seemed to find it hard to believe that anyone would come so far for such a small race.

As I sat talking with my new neighbors, I realized that very few of them were first-time marathoners. In fact, several of the runners had already completed over 100, and one runner had completed over 200. Apparently, I was no longer the craziest person in the room. This highlighted a characteristic of smaller races that I soon came to appreciate; the average depth of experience among the participants in small marathons seemed to be vastly greater than that of the people to be found in the typical big city marathon. This meant that I'd be able to tap into the collective running wisdom of this group throughout the day about various other marathons, and, more importantly, get valuable information about the marathon course from people who had run this race before. As the bus pulled out of the parking lot for the 45-minute ride to the race start, I fell into a light sleep.

The bus groaned through a turn, and my eyes fluttered open. The sky was slowly beginning to brighten, and the bus, having left the highway, was coming to a stop next to, well, next to nothing, really. We were in the middle of nowhere. There was no building or man-made structure to be seen anywhere, apart from the road we drove in on. I didn't know it at the time, but we were in Targhee National Forest, by the Island Park caldera. We were at an altitude of 6,142 feet, roughly one mile above sea level.

The air felt crisp and clean as I left the bus and moved toward the impromptu starting line along with the rest of the runners. In New York, sheer luck gets you close to the front of the pack; in Boston, it's proven speed. In the Mesa Falls Marathon, however, all you need to do is step forward and pick your spot.

I chose to stand behind some of the faster-looking runners; close enough to feel the excitement of seeing open road ahead when the race begins, but not so close as to give myself illusions of being an elite racer. Dave Jacobson led us through the traditional prerace remarks, and then, without fanfare, sent us off.

This small phalanx of runners moved briskly along the asphalt as snippets of conversation broke out here and there among us. At that altitude, I knew I would be laboring to maintain my usual pace, so I tried to rein in my legs, which were feeling particularly springy. The course would eventually bring us down to an elevation of 5,260 feet, for a net drop of 882 feet, so I wasn't worried about a slow start; I would have plenty of opportunity to pick up the pace later on.

I followed the pack through a left turn, and found myself on a wide dirt road, heading deeper into the wilderness. Full daybreak was upon us now, revealing rolling hills on both sides of the road, covered in brush and short trees. Up ahead, I was told, there would be wonderful views of the Grand Teton mountain range. One thing I knew not to expect, though, were spectators cheering us on in the coming miles, but with all of the great scenery around me, I was starting to think that they might not be missed.

It was at that moment that I realized we were not quite as alone as I thought. Strange noises echoed from distance. There were wild animals out there howling at us. Another runner then told me that he had seen a moose in the first mile of the race. Despite its great size, the beast disappeared soundlessly into the brush. These other animals, however, did not seem quite as shy. A volunteer at mile 8 told me that coyotes and wolves had given him the eye as he set up our refreshments earlier in the morning. I felt an instinctual moment of panic, but then I realized that these animals were probably more afraid of us than we were of them. As long as I didn't drift so far back of the pack that I'd seem separated from the herd, I knew I'd be safe. Just as I relaxed, the howling subsided, as if on cue.

Just then the Tetons came into view, bathed in bright morning sunlight. They were indeed magnificent, even if we were too far away to fully appreciate their sculpted beauty. Then the fickle road turned us away from this sight and plunged us into the woods. We were led onto a bike path, which emptied onto a small scenic overlook. Hundreds of feet below us and perhaps a half-mile away, the Snake River plunged off what appeared to be a wide, stone tabletop. It was the race's namesake, the Lower Mesa Falls. I paused a moment to fully take in the beautiful view. Reluctantly, I turned away and followed the race path back into the woods.

It was about this time that I fell into a conversation with Matt, whose race turned out to be a family effort. Matt's sisters and cousins were providing vehicular support—"support" in the sense of screaming and yelling from an open van door during a slow drive-by.

"Know those folks?" I joked.

"Yeah," he admitted sheepishly. "My brother and cousin are out here also somewhere, running their first marathon."

Matt already had a little marathon experience, having run the Roxbury (Idaho) Marathon. "Now *that's* a small race," he told me. "Just twenty-two runners." I guess he entered the Mesa Falls Marathon to see what it would be like to do a big race.

At mile 13 we came to a short stretch of paved road that led us to Bear Claw Junction, which was the starting point for the half-marathoners. Some marathon runners don't like having fresh legs suddenly thrown in alongside them at a race's mid-point, since it can throw off their pacing. As for me, on that day at least, I was glad to have a little more company as we descended into the brush and found ourselves once again on a dirt trail.

The path on which we were now running was narrower than the road on which we had started, but it soon revealed itself as one of the most scenic stretches of any marathon I've ever run—four beautiful miles along Idaho's Warm River. Our trail was halfway up the side of a valley, providing commanding views of the river below and the valley around us. The weather had warmed, the sun was shining, the trees and bushes were lush and green, and the river was an inviting blue. Matt told me that there was no truth to the river's name, however; the Warm River was frigid this time of year. No matter; it *looked* inviting. I found myself gliding along the path, lost in runner's nirvana. I told Matt that even though this was just his second marathon, nature and the race director had conspired to give him a grand treat. He would see many wonderful scenes if he continued racing, but there might never be another moment as perfect as this one.

And suddenly it was gone. We came off the trail and returned to asphalt roads, rolling through rich Idaho farmland. The views here were less spectacular, but no less interesting, at least for this city boy. I had been warned by several runners, though, that there would be a big hill coming up shortly at about mile 18, so I girded myself for the worst. There was a hill all right, but it was not a heartbreaker, not in the Boston mold. I threw my mental lasso around the runner in front of me—fitting imagery for this part of the country—and labored up to the crest. With the hill now behind me, I settled in to a steady pace and started to think more about the finish line.

Houses multiplied alongside the road, farmland gave way to stores and short buildings, and I realized that I was on the outskirts of Ashton and nearing the finish line. The streets were quiet as I passed an auto parts store and a thrift shop. Up ahead on my right were grain silos, and I knew the end was at hand. There were some spectators cheering now, as a volunteer steered us through a right turn, and toward Ashton City Park.

As I crossed the finish line, I heard my name being announced—always a nice touch—and was awarded a finisher's medal. Marathon number 89 was over.

But things would soon get even better. Our goody bags contained a coupon, redeemable after the race, for a huckleberry shake from City Drug. I retrieved the coupon and set off for my hard-earned treat. Along the way I passed other runners who had already claimed their prize, and their smiles quickened my step.

City Drug was only a few short blocks away, but it was of another time and place. It was a small storefront shop, featuring a soda counter with stools. An older woman gave me a smile as I came in, and a young boy reached down below the counter and produced a genuine, prepoured huckleberry shake. I didn't even have to say a word; it must have been pretty obvious why I was there.

Stepping out into the street, I took a long pull on the straw, savoring the creamy coolness. As I walked back to the park, I shouted encouragement to the other runners nearing the finish line—"Get the shake! Get the shake!" Back at the park I found the race director, Dave, and thanked him for a top-notch marathon. The last runners were still more than an hour away from finishing—there would be 120 finishers in all—but Dave was already looking to the future. Heady with success, he was hoping to expand the race. "We can accommodate about 500 runners before we have to have any restrictions," he said. It sounded like an explosion of runners, but it would still just amount to a small 5K field back home.

I picked an inviting patch of sun-warmed grass near the covered picnic area and settled down for the awards ceremony. The winning times were 2:51:12 for the men, and 3:12:27 for the women. Very respectable times, but far from the otherworldly ones posted by the world's elite runners at the big races. My own finishing time left me well behind the leaders, but as I watched them claim their prizes, I felt that we were at least still members of the same species.

As the winners of the various age categories were honored, and random prizes distributed—everything from a heart rate monitor to beef jerky—I realized that many of these people knew each other, and had probably known each other for years. The camaraderie among them was palpable. I found myself daydreaming of having lived here, trained here, and raced here, so I could share in their jokes and stories.

Finally, all the awards had been claimed, all the prizes had been distributed, and it was time to go. I showered, gathered my things, and checked out of the Four Seasons Motel, saying good-bye to the owner's young son, who was manning the front desk. I drove back to Little Falls, dropped off the car, and boarded my flight.

Gazing out the window past the thin, wispy clouds to the farm-land far below, I thought about the Mesa Falls Marathon, and the other small towns I had visited for marathons. Tupelo, Mississippi. Fayetteville, Arkansas. Tulsa, Oklahoma. And Wichita, Kansas, so quiet on a Saturday night downtown that I wouldn't have been surprised if the city rolled up their sidewalks after dark. These races all felt like family gatherings, with people working hard to make the events come off smoothly, for no glory other than to have managed to make it happen and to have shown a few hundred runners a good time.

Sometimes, though, things didn't go quite so well, like in Louisville, Kentucky, where a mismeasured course added an unnecessary mile to the race, leaving runners swarming like angry bees at the finish line. There were times when the aid stations were not well-stocked, when there were so few spectators and fellow runners that it seemed to be a race in theory only. But still, there was something to these races, an earnestness that seemed truer to the marathoning spirit than the marketing and spectacle of the big city races. And those huckleberry shakes, of course.

But would I really trade Ashton for the New York City Marathon? No. What is lost in numbers is gained in excitement; there is no phenom-enon as startling as the sight of a huge mass of people running down the street, not in panic, but with joy and determination. But if I had only experienced the Big Race, I would not have a complete understanding of the marathon.

So, my favorite marathon? I still can't tell you. Perhaps I'm too greedy. I want them all.

Soon after returning from Idaho, I had another interesting running adventure in my own backyard. In the green spaces throughout Washington, D.C., creatures stirred, awakening from their seventeen-year slumber. Soon, they would arise in the thousands from their underground lairs, like graveyard zombies, and invade the city, filling the air with a hellishly loud buzz. They were short and squat with thick, greenish bodies and blood-red eyes, and they were called "Brood X." The city seemed transfixed in nervous anticipation, but was powerless to stop them.

Despite their ominous name and hellish appearance, they were, in fact, just insects. Cicadas. And rather than being worried about them, most people seemed intrigued. As zero-hour drew near, the local newspapers themselves became infested with articles about them. We were told where we could expect the highest concentrations, and how to protect trees with netting. There were even recipes on how to prepare them for dinner. But no one told runners what they could expect.

The days flew by, and every morning I stepped outside, only to find ... nothing. As it turned out, not every neighborhood would get a visit from the Brood. Why were they snubbing me? This was expected to be a seminal D.C. event, and I wasn't invited to the party.

I realized that if I wanted to experience these pests, I would actually have to go looking for them. I had read that areas farther northwest that had older trees would be harder hit by the little buggers. So I laced up my running shoes, corralled a running partner, and went north, entering Rock Creek Park near the Carter Baron amphitheater.

We soon came across our quarry. We saw first one, then another cicada laid out on the ground in front of us. There were dozens more nearby. Then we saw one fly right into a parked car. It occurred to me that was the equivalent of failing to notice a skyscraper and walking into it facefirst. These were not bright creatures. We continued our run.

I soon became accustomed to seeing small black clumps whizzing around us. Their style of flying can best described as awkward and clumsy, even out of control. I wondered if perhaps they were screaming in panic as they flew past. Suddenly, a cicada dove straight at me. I ducked to avoid a head-on collision. I looked over to see my running partner twisting and pirouetting herself to avoid contact. It was then that we stopped viewing the cicadas as silly little aerial clowns and more as incoming missiles, and we began to wonder how much a direct hit from one would sting. Luckily, we made it home with that question still unanswered.

A few days later I ran a different route up near Glover Park. Hurtling down Massachusetts Avenue, I saw hundreds of little black corpses on the sidewalk. Revulsion soon tuned to curiosity, which turned to sadness. Seventeen years of waiting, for only a few days of life. Their silly little existence suddenly seemed more precious, making my own life that much more valuable, too. Their ungainly attempts at flight now reminded me of so many runners who trump their own clumsiness with sheer determination, and who, through their efforts, gain a type of grace.

The cicadas no longer seemed to me to be tiny invaders, but instead, in a way, little creatures with whom I could share a strange kinship. Not born myself with a natural runner's body or a smooth stride, I run fearlessly, just like the cicadas seem to fly, knowing that honest sweat has its own grace, and knowing, too, that my days here are numbered. Perhaps we weren't so very different after all.

Of course, my empathy has its limits. If ever I run into the wall of an office building by accident, I'm hanging up my running shoes for good.

## Running Tip #16

### *Mind Games*

- *Stay mindful of what you're doing.* It's like driving: you don't have to hold the steering wheel in a death grip, but you should be calmly aware of both your car and your surroundings.

- *Have a checklist.* Are you landing too heavily? Are you swinging your arms too far? How's your breathing? How's your posture? Become aware of your bad tendencies, and keep an eye out for them.

- *Manage your intensity.* Some runners visualize how strong they'll feel at specific, difficult parts of an upcoming race. Others repeat a supportive phrase like a mantra. I like to visualize catastrophe. It's actually not as crazy as it sounds. If I can accept the worst that could happen on race day, I've conquered my fears, and I can relax and just run. Find out what works for you. Your mind is a puzzle that can be solved, and once you find the right answer, you can achieve your best times.

# There and Back:
# Adventures in South Africa

I sat in the dark theater, gazing up at the image on the screen. It was of a man pumping his arms rhythmically as he ran over brown, unpaved earth. The man was Haile Gebrselassie, the great Ethiopian middle-distance runner, and the movie was *Endurance,* the film that chronicled his rise from poverty in Ethiopia to Olympic gold in Atlanta. The opening scene was of Gebrselassie on a training run, covering the African countryside with long, powerful strides, gliding over rocks and hills with no display of effort. He looked like a running god, and the land looked primeval. This, to me, was Africa.

But Africa was also a land of war, oppression, corruption, and disease. Alongside its great beauty sat great hardship. It was difficult for my mind to encompass the whole of it. I've often imagined the world as being crisscrossed with running trails, interrupted here and there by mountains and oceans. Some of them are paved and measured. Most are not. Some haven't even been discovered yet. But try as might, I couldn't quite fit Africa into my vision of the world; I couldn't imagine racing there.

Clearly, something needed to be done. Stephanie, always up for a good adventure, agreed. I went online, signed up for the Two Oceans Marathon, to take place on March 26, 2005, and booked our trip to South Africa. One way or the other, I was going to sort this out.

Our itinerary would be challenging. We were to fly to Johannesburg, then on to Hoedspruit for a safari, and then down to Cape Town, where the race would be held. All that sounded fine, except that our return flight was booked for the afternoon of race day. Not an ideal plan, but that was the only schedule that met all of the conflicting requirements of our work lives and the available flights and excursions, so that was the way it was going to be. If nothing else, the fear of missing an international flight would be a great incentive to run faster.

The conceit of our age is that we live in a world that is becoming ever smaller. Interconnected economies, e-mail and online services, and fast, relatively cheap flights make almost any part of the globe as close as your next-door neighbor.

Don't you believe it. Africa is still a long way from the United States. From our home in D.C., we made our way to New York for a flight to Johannesburg, with a layover in Dakar, Senegal. The entire adventure would require almost a full twenty-four hours, but instead of moaning about the discomfort of it all, I actually appreciated the difficulty involved. Something magical happens during a long flight to a distant, exotic land. The idea of adventure ferments in your mind until it is fully risen upon arrival, making you hungry for whatever you may discover. This process takes time, and as we boarded our flight at JFK airport, I knew we would have all the time we needed.

That was the emotional argument in favor of a long flight. The physical arguments weighed in against it. I tossed and turned in my seat, bent and straightened my legs in a futile attempt to find a truly comfortable position, all to no avail. There were some bright spots, though; plenty of good movies to watch, and one truly memorable sight—a predawn liftoff from Dakar, with a view of dozens of fishermen slowly heading out to sea in their small boats, hundreds of feet below us, as the dark blue of the sky bled crimson and orange. It was an impossibly beautiful moment. I settled in for the remainder of the flight, contemplating Africa.

Eight hours later, the sun was setting as we touched down in Johannesburg. We would be spending only one short night there before leaving first thing in the morning for another flight to Hoedspruit. As we drove from the airport to our hotel on the edge of town, any guilt I felt about not spending more time in Johannesburg was allayed by our driver, who, while insisting that security was improving downtown, warned us about the prolific and violent street crime. When apartheid ended and movement by nonwhites was no longer restricted, millions of people migrated to the cities with a dream of finding a better job. When those jobs did not materialize, the dispossessed survived as best they could, building shantytowns on the fringes of the city, and, in some cases, preying on those around them. Our driver said that some downtown hotels had closed because of the crime, to which the government responded by installing street cameras.

During the ride, our driver taught us a few basic words of Zulu, one of the nine African languages spoken throughout the country. Most South Africans speak several languages in addition to Afrikaans and English, including Zulu. It was very humbling. Like many Americans, I'm limited to English and a smattering of high school Spanish. Stephanie and I were entranced as he ran through several dialects, occasionally making clucking sounds that no Westerner could emulate. As we drove past some abandoned buildings and gold mines, I wondered at this unique place. *Egoli*, the Zulu name for Johannesburg—City of Gold.

In the morning I made use of the treadmill in our hotel for a quick run, not wanting to get lost on the city streets. On the television was Nelson Mandela, who, even in retirement, is generally looked upon as perhaps the world's foremost moral authority. He was onstage at a concert on Human Rights Day, the national holiday memorializing the murder of sixty-nine pepole in the 1960 Sharpeville massacre. Taking the stage after a performance by Annie Lennox, Mandela said that healthy women were also victims of the AIDS epidemic. AIDS was becoming a disaster of epic proportions in South Africa, fueled by misconceptions about its origin and how to cure it. Some South Africans even believe that the virus can be cured by sleeping with virgins. The day after Mandela's speech, the local newspapers reported that a man with AIDS was arrested for brutally killing his wife, his wife's child, and his wife's mother because his wife stopped sleeping with him.

A few hours later, Stephanie and I boarded a small plane bound for Hoedspruit. After our long journey the day before, we were happy that this flight would only last a single hour. As the plane descended, I nervously scanned the countryside for signs of an airport, but found none. Nevertheless, the plane continued to drop, and then we touched down.

Stepping out into the bright sunshine, I was struck by the unlikeliness of the place. The airport was a tiny military airstrip that was converted to civilian use. The terminal consisted only of a small building outfitted with a couch, several comfortable chairs, and animal prints on the walls. It looked like a room in which you might relax with a drink after a long day traversing the grassy veldt.

After collecting our bags, we stepped through the building to our transport, and immediately saw a waterbuck—a deer-like animal—leap across the road into the bush. We weren't even off the airport grounds and we'd had our first wild animal sighting. This was the Africa of our dreams.

The wildlife preserves of Hoedspruit are large, but not the endless open miles of our imaginations. Fences—some of them electrified—separated the various preserves. These areas are large enough to get lost in, and for even the largest animals to hide. With the beautiful Drakensberg Mountains as a backdrop, we made our way to our campsite within the

Gwalagwala game preserve. This was nothing like the scouting adventures of my youth. These tents are mounted on large wooden platforms, and enclose modern accommodations, including a bed, proper bathroom, and electricity. There was also a treehouse bar in which to meet other travelers, and an open-air dining area.

Our hosts were Dorian and Ann, a couple who had decided later in life that they wanted a change, and gambled on buying untilled farmland and converting it into a game preserve. It soon became apparent, however, that they were still trying to figure out their proper place in this environment. Ann had unwittingly managed to adopt several animals, including a young, wayward warthog, despite concerns that it might not be good for a wild animal to become too accustomed to being in close quarters with humans. Still, the little warthog had a certain charm, and it was fun watching him try to chew the elastic laces on my running shoes. He pulled back the laces several times, only to jump with a start when it snapped out of his mouth. After several attempts, he grunted and turned away, much to our amusement.

After settling in and having lunch, we set out for an afternoon game ride. Early mornings and late afternoons are the best times for viewing animals, when the sun is the least oppressive and the animals are more active. *Not unlike runners,* I thought, as we clambered in to the open Land Rover.

We had scheduled three game rides over the next several days, in search of the African safari Holy Grail—sightings of the Big Five: lion, rhino, elephant, water buffalo, and leopard. We managed to see all except the elusive leopard, and saw many others as well, including giraffe, hyena, cheetah, and impala.

The impala were perhaps the most memorable, leaping as if staying planted on the earth took more effort than getting airborne. Locals referred to the impala as their "McDonald's," which had nothing to do with fast food, but instead refers to the pattern made by the distinctive black streaks running down each of their haunches and their tails, creating nature's version of the Golden Arches.

I wondered what it would be like to have so much power in my legs, to be able to leap so quickly and gracefully. Watching wild animals filled me with a sense of awe, and also revealed the limitations of my own body. Humans are not the fastest, strongest, or most graceful creatures found in nature, and I could only imagine how pitiful even the fastest among us must look to the rest of the animal kingdom. I recalled reading, however, that humans can track and run down game on foot over long distances, due in large part to the amazing shock-absorbing properties of our feet. We might not be the fastest, but as long as we can keep the game in sight, we can eventually overtake it, like the proverbial tortoise beating the hare.

This all reminded me of some trash talk I had recently engaged in with a friend at a local gym. He was younger than I, very fit and athletic, and had just started running. He boasted that he was already a faster runner than I was. I assured him that I could beat him. He told me that he was faster than I was in the 5K. I told him that might be true, but I'd race him in a 10K. He said he could still beat me at that distance. Maybe so, I replied, but if it took a half-marathon, a marathon, or a 50-mile ultramarathon, I would eventually beat him. I could run all those races, and I would eventually win. He was silent after that.

Not everyone among our group seemed enamored with the aesthetic beauty of the animals in quite the same way. One great big strapping fellow—a former rugby player—seemed to look at nature as one big all-you-can-eat smorgasbord. He talked a great deal about the South African taste for meat. From wild buck—especially one type called "kudu"—to crocodile and ostrich, South Africans will eat it all, as long as it once moved. They are carnivores with a capital "C." My wife is no vegetarian, but she was astounded. "Don't you ever eat any salad?" she asked. Winking, our companion said, "When we want vegetables, we eat chicken." I suddenly wondered whether a prerace carb load might be harder to find than I thought.

Managing a game preserve isn't all fun, though, as Dorian told me. He pointed to a young giraffe that was limping. His right hind leg was marred by a gaping wound, and his footprints were marked with spots of blood. He had been attacked by a hyena. As we watched the suffering animal, we wanted to help it, but that is not how things are handled on a game preserve. To maintain the balance of things, the animals must be left alone in all but the most extreme circumstances. The hyenas have to eat also, of course. It seemed cruel, but this was nature's way.

At our last evening there, we sat once again under the stars, drinking South African wine, eating a delicious dinner that did, thankfully, include some fresh vegetables, and compared stories with our fellow travelers. Several of them were South Africans on holiday, and they were open about their feelings about their country and recent events. Their mood seemed hopeful, although they had their doubts about particular politicians. Their criticisms seemed reaffirming, though, because not one of them stated any disillusionment with the overall direction their nation had taken over the previous decade, or even with much of what the current administration was trying to achieve.

Eventually the conversation drifted around to my upcoming challenge, and everyone wished me good luck in the race. The Two Oceans Marathon seemed to be quite well known; even people who were not runners were quite familiar with it. Finally, the dessert was over, the last of the wine had been drunk, and it was time for Stephanie and me to get our things together for our flight out the next morning. We would be departing Hoedspruit for Cape Town, and suddenly the race, which had not seemed real before, loomed large.

Cape Town is a beautiful, wondrous city, embodying much of what is best and worst about South Africa. Nestled between the sheltered waters of Table Bay and the majestic heights of Table Mountain, Cape

Town has a long and checkered past. Phoenicians and Arabs thought it had magnetic powers that would draw ships to their doom along its rocky coast, and the Portuguese explorer Vasca da Gama sighted it as he rounded the Cape of Good Hope in 1498. The town was laid out in 1652 by the Dutch East India Company as a replenishment station for its fleet. The local population mostly succumbed to smallpox brought inadvertently by the colonialists, and the surviving indigenous population mostly worked as poorly treated laborers.

In 1795 and 1806, the British invaded South Africa, and by 1843, it had annexed large parts of the country. Clashes with native Zulus and the rising population of Dutch-speaking farmers, known as Boers, led to the Anglo-Boer Wars of 1880–1881 and 1899–1902. The British crushed the Boers with a scorched-earth policy, burning farms and establishing the world's first concentration camps. Eventually, over 136,000 Dutch Afrikaners were imprisoned in these camps, in which more than 26,000 women and children died from typhoid, dysentery, and neglect.

The Union of South Africa was formed in 1910, and the policy of oppression against the native population reached full fruition in 1948 with the creation of apartheid, a complex system that separated the races by law. Apartheid weathered international boycotts and domestic protest and violence, until President F. W. de Klerk unexpectedly abandoned it in 1990, and began negotiating with Nelson Mandela, his formerly jailed adversary. Mandela's African National Congress then won South Africa's first full and open election, and South Africa's journey from darkness was completed when president-elect Mandela announced that "Never, never, and never again shall it be that this beautiful land will again experience the oppression of one by another."

Cape Town reflects all of this history. From its 300-year-old Castle of Good Hope, to its beautiful architecture and manicured gardens, Cape Town shows the best of its colonial past. But then there is District Six, the vibrant port area that was bulldozed in 1979 and declared "whites-only."

Loud protests followed, and the area was kept barren. Today a museum commemorates the destruction of this neighborhood. And there is also Robben Island, an Alcatraz-like penal colony sitting in the bay, where Mandela and others spent years imprisoned for dedicating their lives to fighting apartheid.

Stephanie and I settled into our hotel room overlooking Greenmarket Square, built in 1710 and still used daily as a popular flea market. One evening, we were serenaded by a free jazz concert held there. From our window we could see the square, nearby churches, and the looming mass of Table Mountain, draped in the morning hours with clouds. Over the next several days we would visit all of these sights, riding a cable car to the mountain top, wandering the through towns and visiting museums. Still, my mind kept turning to the marathon.

The Two Oceans Marathon is actually poorly named; it is not a marathon at all. Rather, it is a 56-kilometer ultramarathon, with a half-marathon option also available. The most striking feature of the ultra is its course profile. Starting with a small hill early on, the race meanders over flat roads for the first 28 kilometers, but then it takes a nasty turn as it makes a precipitous ascent of Chapman's Peak at kilometer 34. It then screams back down over the next 6 kilometers, and, at the point when a regular marathon would be over, begins a steep ascent of Constantia Nek. It's the kind of course profile to strike fear even into the heart of an experienced marathoner.

I was concerned about the race, and decided that seeing the beast might allay my fears. Stephanie and I decided to take a tour of the Cape of Good Hope, and the driver readily agreed to drive along as much of the race course for us as he could. Soon, we were driving up to Chapman's Peak, called simply Chappies by the locals. Even in a microbus I could appreciate the steepness of the climb. After severe rock falls plagued the area, the road up Chappies was closed and the course was altered to skirt around Chappies from 2000 to 2004.

I could see why so many runners were disappointed. The view was amazing. The road hugged the pale orange cliff-side, providing a beautiful view of Hout Bay to the west. Our driver pointed out the 1,560 meters of fencing and the concrete canopy that had been installed as part of the new safety measures that allowed the race to return to Chappies in 2004. The netting looked quite fragile to me, though, and I imagined struggling up this road on race day, conquering Chappies, and pausing to celebrate one of the greatest moments of my running life, only to be clunked on the head by a falling boulder. I made a mental note to remember not to pause here on race day if I could help it.

Finally, Stephanie and I found ourselves at the Cape of Good Hope, the storied tip of Africa, where the rough waters of the Atlantic meet the warm waters of the Indian Ocean. We stared out over the open expanse of water before us, and marveled at how far we had come. Ahead of us still was a visit to a penguin colony at Boulders Beach—yet one more sign that we were far, far from home. But standing at the Cape seemed to be the crowning moment. There was, finally, nowhere farther to go.

After feeling like the race would never come, I suddenly found myself picking up my race packet at the University of Cape Town the day before the start. I meandered through the expo, had a pasta dinner in the hotel restaurant, and then settled back in our hotel room with some good reading: the racing instructions. Among the papers included was a booklet entitled "Information and Statistics." It was an absolute compendium of minutiae about the race. There were 7,830 participants registered in the ultra. There were nearly four times as many male ultra runners as female, though there were 339 husband and wife teams. I was disappointed to see that there was no statistic on divorces caused by racing together.

There were also three runners going for their thirtieth finish, and twenty-four runners who would be celebrating their birthday on race day. The oldest registered runner was seventy-six, and the youngest was nineteen. Sixty-three countries were represented, although only 360 runners were from overseas, and only thirty-three were from the United States. I realized then that the worst I could do as a finisher would be to place thirty-third in my category—not bad for bragging rights back home, as long as there were no follow-up questions about the number of runners.

A few scant hours later, I stood in front of the hotel with some other runners in the predawn darkness, waiting for transport to the starting line at the University of Cape Town. The others were visiting Germans. One, in fact, was here on his honeymoon. I wondered whether he had even bothered to tell his bride that he was racing, or whether he was hoping to finish before she awoke. As the van sped along the highway, we talked about our hopes for the race and offered each other energy bars.

The van dropped us off on the main commercial street near to the University, in the suburb of Newlands. I wished the Germans good luck and joined the throng of runners making their way to the starting line. Despite the darkness, it was already quite warm, and I quickly shed my throwaway long-sleeved shirt. I settled into a spot in the crowd behind the starting line, and listened to the last-minute instructions that bellowed from the speakers. The various countries represented were named, to sporadic cheers and applause, and certain notable runners were introduced. The crowd then sang the traditional African song "Shozaloza."

Finally, the announcements were over, and I felt my body tense as I awaited the start, my finger poised on my watch's start button. The gun roared at precisely 6 A.M. I surged forward with the crowd, buoyed by a familiar wave of adrenaline. The asphalt below my feet, smiling faces and cheers of the onlookers, the sight of the runners around me, and even the smells of the race all seemed familiar. The gap in my worldview quickly closed, and Africa, wonderful and exotic, also became, for me, simply another place to run.

As we streamed along the dark city streets, I thought about my race preparation. I had trained for the Two Oceans Marathon as I had trained for the JFK 50 Miler: by including a full marathon in my final long run. This time it was the Virginia Creeper Marathon, a beautiful race in that state's southwest corner which I ran with my friends Dave and Renata. It was my ninty-sixth marathon.

The Two Oceans Marathon has a unique system for awarding finishers' medals. Rather than dividing the field into elite runners and everyone else, the organizers reward different levels of achievement. Runners breaking the 4-hour barrier in the race earn a silver medal, and those breaking 6 hours earn a bronze. Previously, the race had a 6 hour time limit, but now runners who beat 7 hours earn a blue medal. However, many veteran marathoners still consider 6 hours to be the "official" time limit. Factoring in my recent training, jetlag, and the great unknown of the two ascents, I pegged myself as coming in somewhere between 5:15 and 5:30, placing me solidly in the bronze group. In those first few minutes of the race, I calculated the pace necessary to hit my goal, and settled back into an easy stride.

As the sun broke the darkness, I looked at the runners around me. Although they looked like any race field I would find back in the United States, I quickly noticed one key difference: their conversations. Many spoke in the native tongues of South Africa, and even when their conversation dropped into English, the clipped cadences of Afrikaans or Zulu remained. Despite this language barrier, I still felt our bonds as runners, and enjoyed the voices around me.

Passing the first refreshment station, I realized another novelty of the race: there were no rows of cups, as are found in most other races I've run in the United States and abroad. In Cape Town, volunteers handed out water and sports drink in sealed plastic pouches. I ripped a hole in the pouch with my teeth and squirted the water into my mouth.

Newlands gave way to Kenilworth, which became Plumstead, and the city melted into open spaces and small towns. I spotted the pacer for the 6-hour finishers' group, and I reasoned that as long as I keep that group behind me, I would be certain to have a bronze finisher's medal. I passed them and didn't look back.

Being new to the race, I asked several other runners about the course as we ran, and was introduced to another unusual feature of the course: all runners who persevere through ten editions of the race are awarded a permanent blue number to mark their achievement. For me, this meant that veteran ultramarathoners were easier to locate and probe for words of wisdom. They seemed more than willing to oblige.

We entered the town of Lakeside, and then Muizenberg, which gave us our first views of water. This is False Bay, and beyond it the Indian Ocean, the first of the two oceans for which the race is named. The road fell before us as we passed old stone homes in St. James and Kalk Bay, and then, as we entered Fish Hoek and turned inland, we were greeted by a young couple painted entirely in green, cheering us as we streamed past. The views were beautiful and there was still plenty of energy in my legs. These were the good miles.

As I felt energy surge through me, I spied a runner up ahead holding a banner aloft. I wondered if he could possibly be the pacer for sub-5-hour group. No, it couldn't be. But it was. I caught them and stuck to them like glue. As we ran, I asked the pacer about the South African racing circuit. Although the Two Oceans seemed to be a challenging course, he told me that many runners use it as preparation for the Comrades Ultramarathon that follows several months later in mid-June.

Wow. Using a brutal 56-kilometer race as a training run for a more difficult race? There were definitely some tough runners out here.

We ran through Sun Valley, and entered the town of Noordhoek, at kilometer 28, the halfway point of the race. Craft shops and restaurants lined the road, eventually giving way to trees and parkland. Chappies lay just ahead. Our pacer announced that it was time to go to work.

The Chapman's Peak Drive, the race route, was opened to the public in 1922. A popular tourist and sporting destination, it actually consists of two peaks: "Little Chappies," at the 30 kilometer mark of the race, followed by "Big Chappies" 4 kilometers later.

Stands of trees thinned and then disappeared altogether, and the grass melted away as we began our first ascent. The sun was shining brightly now, but I felt comfortable and strong as we followed the road upward. The incline actually felt like a nice change from the earlier flats, and I was surprised at how good I felt. Soon the pace group crested the first summit, and we eased into a short easy stretch of road before the next peak. Talking to the pacer, I learned that the difficulty with Chappies is often not the actual climb, but rather the quick descent that follows, which can wreak havoc with the quads. But other than keeping proper form and trying not to go too fast, there wouldn't be much I could do about that. After all, I never expected to get through this race without some pain.

My thoughts were interrupted by the pacer's announcement that we would resume climbing around the next curve. Feeling confident after conquering Little Chappies, I surged forward ahead of the pack, and after rounding the corner, was able to see the road ahead as it wound its way to the top of Big Chappies. The ascent was over 2½ kilometers, but the views were even more spectacular than they had been from the van window a few days earlier.

Finally, I was at the top of Chappies. Fear that had been gnawing at me since signing up for the race melted away. The climb of Constantia Nek still loomed ahead, but with 17 kilometers left to go, things were looking very, very good. My legs swallowed the descent without a problem, and I said a silent farewell to Chappies as we entered Hout Bay.

Hout Bay was the site of a battle between the Dutch settlers and a British naval force in September, 1795. The Dutch were victorious in a battle that resulted in little loss of life, and cannons used in that victory still guard the town to this day. The proud residents of "the Republic of Hout Bay" have maintained a tradition of firing a cannon as the lead runners enter the town, though I was too far back of the lead pack at that point to hear anything other than the sound of thousands of feet slapping the asphalt. But the spectators and refreshments along the streets of Hout Bay were still a welcome sight.

At about this time fatigue began to seep into my legs, and my earlier soaring confidence started to leak out. I realized that I would probably not be able to maintain the sub-5-hour pace, but I resolved to stay with the group to the 42.1 kilometer mark. I would not have a sub-5-hour finish this day, but making it to the regulation marathon distance with this pack would be my moral victory.

Time ebbed past as I continued to press forward, clinging to the pace group. Finally, I saw an inflated archway spanning the road up ahead—it was the 42.1 kilometer mark. I had earned my victory in the race-within-a-race. As I crossed the timing mat set up near the distance marker, I fought the urge to consider the race finished. The visual cues all said that I'd completed a marathon, and my body certainly felt like it had finished a marathon. Like trained dogs sensing when it is time to go home, my legs were sure that it was time to downshift into cool down mode. Not yet, I told them. There was one last big challenge immediately ahead: Constantia Nek.

With a climb of 215 meters, Constantia Nek is actually the biggest hill on the course, higher even than Big Chappies. But it's also a completely different hill than Chappies. Gone were the cliffs and commanding bayside views; here, the roadside was thick with trees and dotted with residences. The race organizers, knowing that this was where the most suffering would occur, squeezed refreshment stations closer together here, and spectators lined the roads in groups to cheer us on.

At first, the climb didn't seem bad at all. But just as I started to relax, the road suddenly soared up toward the treetops. I had earlier resolved to run the ascents, but this stretch of road made me break that promise, and I briefly joined those who were walking the worst parts of the climb. The strained faces of the runners—runners in name only at this point — mirrored my own determination. Finally, I could see the top of the hill just ahead, and, like a swimmer reaching for poolside, I surged forward with one last push and crested the summit. Constantia Nek was history. Only 10 kilometers left to go.

With all of the fearsome hills finally behind me, I settled into the final task of finishing the race. I shortened my stride and searched for my last reserves of energy as I ran the rolling hills of Rhodes Drive down to the open, sun-drenched avenues of Kirstenbosch, where the glorious Gardens are found. There was now less than 6 kilometers to go. The bright sunlight pulled sweat from our bodies, but I saw no quitters around me. Up ahead was the sweeping turn known as "Harry's Corner," named for a course marshal who manned that corner for years until his death.

The crowd of spectators thickened as we entered Rondebosch, and with it, the university and its football field, where the finish line waited. Mustering the last of my strength, I sprinted to meet it. My final time was 5 hours 15 minutes, the exact time that I had originally hoped for.

As I slowly moved through the crowd, my newly awarded bronze medal hanging around my neck, someone pressed an application for the New York City Marathon into my hand. I continued moving, grabbing fluids and a goody bag, and made my way to the steps leading out of the university and down to the main thoroughfare, to catch a city bus back to Greenmarket Square. As I sat on the bus, an anomalous figure among the Sunday riders, I considered the race application in my hand. I had traveled so far, had experienced so much, but this piece of paper in my hand shrunk all that, shrunk the world. It was as if I had journeyed to the farthest reaches of the North Pole, beyond the edge of civilization, only to find a note from my family waiting for me. And then I realized what I'd always suspected was true: the world is indeed a matrix of running paths, all connected together, stretching from Haile Gebrselassie's flying feet to Chapman's Peak and over to Central Park in Manhattan. In a few short hours I would board a jet back to the States, but standing there with that paper in my hand, I knew that I was already home.

Only one final thing to resolve, though: did this race belong on my list or not? It was billed as a marathon, so that would seem to settle the issue. But it was not the standard marathon distance; it was about 9 miles longer, so it was an ultramarathon. As much as I would have like to have counted this race toward my 100, I knew that could not be allowed. I had now officially run ninety-six marathons and *two* ultramarathons. End of discussion.

## Running Tip #17

### *Trail Running*

- *Keep your weight over your feet and shorten your stride.* This will allow you to shift your weight quickly if your footing is unstable.
- *Don't zone out.* Running a trail requires focus and concentration, since a sudden misstep can lead to a debilitating injury. But focus isn't fear. Look at trails as puzzles to be solved.
- *Get the right gear.* Trail-running shoes are best because of their thicker outsoles and better traction. Bring a mini first-aid kit and water; there are no fountains in the woods.
- *Be safe.* Trails, even urban ones, are much more isolated than roads. Use common sense: don't run with an mp3 player or in the dark, since you need to be aware of what's around you, and run with a friend if possible.

# Almost There: Marathon Number 99, Wilmington, Delaware

On the morning of May 15, 2005, Dave and I stood in front of Frawley Stadium in Wilmington, Delaware. We were among a small group of people shaking their legs nervously, pacing back and forth, and tying and retying their shoes. I was at another starting line, waiting for the signal that would launch us forward.

We were lucky to be there. Earlier in the morning Dave and I had checked out of our nearby hotel and got in our car for the short drive over to the start. It was about a mile away, a distance that we could easily have jogged or walked, which is exactly what we should have done. Driving on unfamiliar roads, though, we somehow wound up on the entrance ramp to I-95, the major interstate that runs through Wilmington. Peering out the window, I could see people gathering at the starting line as it receded into the distance at 55 miles per hour. I was annoyed, but it wasn't a major problem; we would just get off and turn around.

Except that we couldn't. After getting off the highway at the very next exit, we realized that we weren't near an entrance onto the highway heading back. We had to try our luck on local roads, and ended up having to stop off at a gas station to ask for directions. With scant minutes to spare before the start, I couldn't believe what a mess we had made of things. There was silence in the car as we made our way back, and only after we parked with enough time to walk to the start did we finally relax. Even after all these years of racing, I couldn't take anything for granted.

The prerace dinner had not gone smoothly either. The brochure promised pasta with vegetables and chicken for all runners who attended, which sounded great, but whoever had arranged the meal clearly did not understand the crowd that would be showing up to be fed. A pasta station was set up with chefs cooking up meals to order; a nice touch, but not a very efficient way to feed hundreds of people. As time slipped by, runners grumbled on line and started to fill up on bread and dessert. I managed to finally get some pasta, but it was an unwelcome detour from my prerace regimen.

Despite the setbacks, I felt relaxed at the starting line. I was finally right where I was meant to be, feeling good and loose. It was a warm day, but not a bad one for racing. Clouds lingered from the rain that had blown through overnight, and a light breeze stirred the air. The deputy mayor made a few brief remarks, and a young lady sang "The Star Spangled Banner." And then we were off.

The course was mostly flat, consisting of four loops along the waterfront, the stadium, and an outlet shopping mall. I set out at a comfortable pace, sticking with Dave for a time until he dropped back. I set off on my own, lost in thought, reminiscing about my eighteen years of marathoning. I thought about the ambulances I'd seen out on various racecourses. There is a dark emptiness that marathoners feel anytime they see or hear an ambulance, and I've seen too many of those over the years. I've also seen runners throwing up, lying flat on their backs on the asphalt, and sitting dejectedly on curbs. One friend running the Marine Corps Marathon on an unseasonably hot day made it as far as mile 23 before she collapsed, only to awaken in a medical tent, buried under bags of ice. She recovered fully, but it was a very close call. I thought about how lucky I've been over the years to never have needed those ambulances, and to have escaped major injury. Despite the great demands I had put on my body, it had never broken, and had never given up completely.

I hadn't bothered to look at my watch as I crossed the first two mile markers, which was unusual for me. I suddenly wondered if I could manage to avoid looking at my watch for the entire race. Could I stand not counting the seconds and minutes as they passed? I wanted to be able to do that, to run the race by feel alone, as an experiment in "Zen running." As I finished the first lap, though, I passed beneath the official timing clock, and couldn't help glancing up. Just that quickly, my little experiment was over.

And then came the difficult miles, which every marathoner knows are out there somewhere on the course, the miles that test our will. Four laps in Wilmington were like the four laps of a mile on the track: the first lap is filled with energy and hopefulness; the second lap is for settling into a strong pace and holding it; the third lap is where the pain and doubt set in, when so much running is behind you, but where the finish line is still so far away; and the fourth lap is for just hanging on, where you try to not spoil all the hard work that preceded it.

I ran the race like I was running a hard mile, feeling all the ups and downs of my journey. Each lap on the course had an out-and-back portion, meaning that I was able to see many of the runners in front and behind me. I saw Dave on each lap, as well as the lead runners, striding easily like gazelles. There was a man running in pink tutu; Dave later accused him of lacking the proper respect for the race. I didn't mind—at least it was a distraction.

Finally, I set out on the fourth and final lap. I came upon an older man standing by himself on a street corner, wearing a shirt and tie. He was handing out free bottles of water, and near as I could tell, was not a race volunteer, but just a local resident who thought we needed and deserved to have some support. I took a bottle and thanked him, and then doused myself, feeling the coolness bring strength back to my tired muscles, even if only for a few moments.

Four laps provided enough time for the runners and the race volunteers to come to know each other, even if only in passing. As I passed one volunteer at mile 24, I told him that I hoped he wouldn't take it the wrong way if I said that I was happy not to have to see him again. He laughed and told me to get going.

And then, finally, the finish line was just ahead. As I crossed the line, the official clock overhead read 3:35:07. I had run my 99th marathon 10 minutes and 23 seconds faster than I had run my first one. The Me-That-Is had beaten the Me-That-Was. Someday, I knew, I would no longer be able to beat the Me-That-Was. But that day had not yet come, not in Wilmington.

And now, after all these years and all these miles, there was just one more marathon to go.

## Running Tip #18

### *Eat to Run, Eat to Live*

- *Eat a balanced diet:* 65 percent complex carbohydrates, 25 percent lean protein, 10 percent fat, preferably unsaturated vegetable fat, like olive oil.
- *Avoid processed foods and fried foods, and limit your intake of sweets.*
- *Aim to eat a good variety, especially fruits and vegetables.* The brightest and most colorful pack the biggest punch.
- *Graze.* Have something every two hours or so to avoid hunger and binging.
- *Take a daily multivitamin.* How many of us really have a perfect diet? No one I know. So cover your bases.
- *Don't skip breakfast.* You might lose more fat that way, but your workouts will suffer. With your tank full, you'll train better, race better, and lose excess pounds anyway.
- *Watch your portion size.* You should be able to fit most meals in the palm of your hand.
- *Read food labels.* You might be surprised at what's in there. Generally, if the list of ingredients is more than four or so lines long, it's not really food anymore.
- *Low-fat desserts aren't necessarily low-calorie!* These products often still have lots of sugar, so eat sparingly.

# Marathon Number 100!

Back in 1987, my supply of running gear consisted of a simple pair of running shoes, a cotton T-shirt, and gym shorts. Nearly two decades down the road, my closet looked much different. On the floor were several pairs of running shoes, costing over $100 each, that were ultra-light and packed with all manner of hi-tech wizardry. On an overhead shelf were neatly folded shirts made of space age breathable fabrics, sporting evocative brand names like Gore-Tex, Dri-FIT, and CoolMax. On a rack hung several breathable, wind and water resistant jackets, and on another shelf sat my wrap-around sunglasses that block out UV rays and random ambient light.

Strapped to my wrist was a watch that could count and store up to 100 interval splits, although it was considered a dinosaur because it couldn't also measure my heart rate, or triangulate with orbiting satellites to record my route and speed. Of course, if I wanted to measure my route, there were now several Web sites that allowed me to precisely calculate the distance I ran, indicating elevation changes as well. In a drawer sat my mp3 digital player, although I usually didn't bring that along on my runs, since I feared getting too dependent on it.

My kitchen had undergone some changes as well. Although I still stocked whole-grain cereals, lean meat, fish, low-fat dairy, and unprocessed fruits and vegetables, I also now used engineered food, such as energy bars, sports drinks, and gels.

Change had also come to the races I ran. Online registration had largely replaced the ritual of mailing in a check and a race application, and the electronic timing chip is now used not only in major marathons, but in races of all distances. And the races themselves have grown larger than I ever thought possible. A field of 20,000 marathoners is now common, and the largest races are nearly double that size.

None of these changes had come about overnight, even if it felt that way to me. But as much as both my own life and the world of marathoning had changed over the years, one thing was constant: more than anything else, I just wanted to run.

And so I had. Now, impossibly, improbably, Dave and I were both about to take our final steps toward achieving our long-held dream. One hundred marathons. Over the years, I kept running, trying not to focus too much on that distant goal. So much could have gone wrong, but now it was really about to happen. I suddenly felt more nervous about it than ever. Which race should it be?

I pored over marathon listings, compared different race courses, and contemplated logistics. Finally, Dave and I made our choice. After coming so far, we wouldn't cut any corners now; we were going to run one of the most grueling races in North America: Grandfather Mountain. Set in the Blue Ridge Mountains in the town of Boone, North Carolina, it represented everything I loved about the marathon. It was beautiful, but after starting at 3,333 feet, it climbed almost 1,000 feet to the peak for which it's named. But it wasn't the net elevation gain that made this race so ominous; there were also numerous drops and climbs along the way. The course elevation profile posted on the race Web site looked like a shark's toothy grin. And to top it all off, the final 4 miles to the finish line were almost entirely uphill.

It was a race that was guaranteed to plumb every runner's well of courage and resolve. But to those who made it to the top came bragging rights, and the sense of accomplishment that only comes from facing a dragon and staring it down. I had learned the hard way over the years never to take a marathon for granted; there were simply too many things that could go wrong. But with Grandfather Mountain, even careful preparation might not be enough. If I could conquer this course, I would have truly earned my record.

Dave agreed that this would be a fitting capstone to our 100-marathon quest. Our friend Renata and another marathoner, Greg, committed to joining Dave and me for our milestone adventure.

Our first challenge would be simply getting there. We opted to make the seven-hour drive the day before the race. When we finally arrived at our hotel on the outskirts of town, we dragged our stiff and sore bodies out of our car and acknowledged to each other with silent looks that this was a less-than-ideal way to prepare for a race.

We were quickly distracted by the strange, mournful sound of a hotel guest practicing her bagpipes in the parking lot. It turned out that the Scottish Highland Games were also being held that weekend on Grandfather Mountain. They were the second largest such games in the world, and the marathon was actually being run in cooperation with them; runners who survived the climb would finish with a victory lap around the competition field, and were welcome to stay afterward and watch the rest of the day's events. This was clearly going to be a race to remember, if only I could make it to the finish.

We went to Appalachian State University to pick up our race numbers and official T-shirts, and to scout out the start of the race, which would be on the university's track at Kidd Brewer Stadium. We then spent the rest of the day wandering around downtown.

Boone was clearly a college town, with cafés and coffee shops lining the main street. It had apparently experienced some recent growth, but it still managed to retain much of an older, enduring charm. I wandered into a small barber shop for a haircut. This had become a little tradition of mine; I had originally started getting haircuts on race weekend simply to kill time and get a chore done, but I also got a little psychological boost from the grooming, since a haircut left me feeling lighter, leaner and faster. I also found that getting a haircut is also a great way to get to know a town if you can get the barber talking. The barber shop in Boone proved especially friendly, and I soon knew not just everything about the town, but all about the barber's own family as well. By the time I stepped back out to the street, I felt that I really knew the place.

On race day, we joined a small but determined group of 400 runners. At the sound of the starting horn, we set off for a single lap around the track, and then exited the stadium for a lap of the parking lot. In any other race, I would have been antsy to hit the roads and get to the meat of the race, but here I knew what lay ahead, and I wasn't in any such hurry.

Finally, we left the university grounds. We cruised past a row of fast-food joints and restaurants and ran toward the town of Blowing Rock. From there we turned onto the scenic Blue Ridge Parkway, and began the climb toward Grandfather Mountain. Here, hills were measured in miles, not feet or yards, and the lush green beauty of our surroundings failed to completely distract any of us from the difficulty of our climbing. I found myself pushing off from my backside with each step, as if I were ascending a ladder instead of running a race.

As I pushed on, I fell into conversation with several other runners. There were clearly a lot of race veterans in this crowd. These runners seemed to love the race not despite the hills, but because of them. With each conquered hill, I began to understand why. Year after year, these runners hurl themselves against the mountain, and are enriched by the experience. The hills stripped away all other concerns, and left us focused on achieving one simple goal: making it to the top. In the process, it would reveal our worst or best selves.

The hills came and went with jarring regularity, until I became accustomed to their rhythm, as if I were standing offshore and weathering a steady surge of waves. Suddenly, the road turned into a gravel and dirt path that rose before me like a wall. It looked so utterly preposterous that I laughed out loud, but I had no choice but to grit my teeth, churn my arms, and attack. With each step I became more determined not to stop running. It was as if eighteen years of marathoning were distilled into this one moment, and I needed to prove that my will was stronger than this latest obstacle. I had decided that if I could make it to the top of that hill, I would finish the race and could claim ownership of my dream, but if I failed, it was all a hoax. It would all come down to this.

Having raised the stakes to that level, I couldn't let myself fail. I sucked in great gulps of air and drove my legs and arms. My eyes blurred with effort; I felt like I was climbing this hill more than running it. A voice in the back of my mind told me that it would be okay to stop, but I pushed that aside. The crest of the hill was now just a few steep yards ahead. No matter how much it hurt, I couldn't stop now. After eighteen years of running, I could not let it end here. Push, I told myself. Push!

And then I had done it; I was king of the hill. I still had miles left to go, but I knew the race was effectively over. Whatever lay ahead, it would not, could not, defeat me.

Still, it could hurt. The final few miles were mostly uphill as promised. The very last stretch passed the aid tent where food and drink were available for finishers—a cruel sight for runners who hadn't yet crossed the finish line. The road rose up toward the make-shift arena; it was an incline that earlier would have worried me, but I had come too far now and conquered too much already. I crested Grandfather Mountain, and entered McRae Meadows. Passing through the crowd, I entered the arena for my victory lap on the dirt track, buoyed by the applause and cheers of the spectators. I pulled my form together and asked my tired, sore legs for just one more effort, a burst of speed to give the spectators something to cheer about. Just a few more minutes of agony, and it would all be over. My legs agreed, and they propelled me across around the final curve and across the finish line. I checked my watch: 3 hours, 46 minutes, 25 seconds. Eighteen years after my first marathon, I had finally arrived.

One hundred marathons. It was done.

Dave came in a short time later, and I and cheered him as he, too, crossed the finish line. He had reached his 100-marathon milestone as well. We had run some thirty marathons together; a friendship forged on roads and trails, spanning more race miles together than most runners compile in their entire lives. That crazy idea we had concocted years earlier had somehow come true. Now we grinned, shook hands, and hugged.

Now that my race was over, I felt fatigue, but mostly relief and joy. Not just for having survived one of the toughest races in the country, but to have had the right combination of determination and luck to have reached my goal. Dave and I gobbled down some peanut butter sandwiches, grabbed some drinks, and settled into the stands to watch some of the Highland Games as we waited for Renata and Greg to come into view. On the field, athletes were doing something that could only be described as a telephone-pole toss. Just watching them made my back ache, and I realized that in this crowd, running a marathon probably looked like a tame thing to do.

Finally, our little group was reunited, and we made our way to the Scottish Clan reunion area, where booth displays honored different family lines. I didn't expect to see any tables for Clan Horowitz, but Dave found some distant brethren.

On the long ride home, we had plenty of time to consider what we had achieved. In the coming days, I thought about all those race miles, and tried to wrap my head around the immensity of it. I had raced in fourty-six states, thirteen countries, and four continents (not including my ultramarathon in South Africa). I had run up and down mountains, across deserts and lava fields, through forests, vineyards, and cities. I had met many extraordinary people, and witnessed the very best of human nature. I had, I believed, lived life to the fullest.

But did I remember it all? Such a strange question. I certainly remembered each marathon, but did I remember every minute of each one? No, of course not. My 100 marathons had cumulatively taken about 385 hours to run. That's over sixteen days of non-stop, round-the-clock racing. Who can recall every minute of a single hour, let alone sixteen entire days? But still, I was surprised at how few minutes I did recall. I remembered certain moments from each race when I saw something interesting, or when I crossed the finish line, but all the other moments were lost to me.

I have memories, however, that are untethered to any specific race. I experience random flashbacks of running beneath sun-dappled leaves along a tree-lined street, or past a row of shops, and I can't link those memories with any particular race. It's a bit like finding an old photograph wherein you recognize yourself, but not all of the people around you. You knew them once, but no longer. It's an uncomfortable, disconcerting feeling.

Equally disturbing was a realization that I had midway through a recent race. I suddenly knew that I'd soon forget most of what I was seeing around me. I ran past ordinary office buildings and plain houses, thinking, "I'll forget that one, and that one, and that one, too." It was as if I was erasing my life almost as fast as my mind was recording it. Then I realized that this realization applied not just to my racing, but to our lives in general, since most of our day-to-day experience is lost to us as time goes by. Perhaps that's for the best, since our memories would be a chaotic sea of details if our minds didn't filter out unimportant minutiae.

Still, I wouldn't trade a single minute of this racing life, whether I remembered each of them or not. But what could I do for an encore? The answer was as simple as it was predictable: check the calendar and fill out my next race application. There were four states still remaining for me to conquer to be able to claim having run marathons in them all. Then the Canadian provinces—of which I'd already done three—and then the last three of the seven continents I hadn't yet raced on. Then there were dream race destinations, like the Himalayas and the Machu Picchu trail, and beautiful cities around the globe that boasted breathtaking marathons, like Prague, Madrid, Venice, and London. There would never be a shortage of marathons that could quicken my pulse and capture my imagination.

I thought about an advertising campaign put on not long ago by a major running-shoe company. It featured the slogan "There is no finish line." But rather than finding myself inspired, I was demoralized. Without a finish line, I had no sense of accomplishment, no valid way to measure my journey. Without finish lines, my running would consist of endless miles, as devoid of perspective as the emptiness of space, as empty of joy as boundless time. I need finish lines as much as I need the seasons, a calendar, and a watch. But these finish lines are not ends; they are only a brief rest stop before the next race. I had now crossed one hundred of these finish lines, but the journey wasn't over; I'd already begun planning my next 100.

## Running Tip #19

### The Last Supper

The best race preparation can be undermined by bad eating decisions the night before a race. Don't make that mistake.

- *Eat early.* You don't want to feel bloated at the starting line.
- *Don't over-eat.* Carb-loading doesn't mean carb-gorging. Eat a relatively light meal early, and have a light snack before bedtime.
- *Avoid foods you haven't tried before.* Choose a carb, like pasta, rice, or bread, and a protein, like lean meat, skinless poultry, or low-fat dairy. It doesn't have to be bland, but don't be adventurous.
- *Hydrate!* Avoid alcohol and caffeinated drinks.

# Why Run the Marathon? Bell Lap: Running & Remembrance

In middle-distance races held on a track, race officials let the runners know when they're on their final lap by ringing a bell. This is the bell lap, the lap that determines the winner. It's the lap that counts.

I'm now in the bell lap of my story. I have traveled all over the world, running marathons, celebrating life. Along the way, I've pondered why I ran. I reached my goal; and I've told my story, but I still have one last chapter to write; I still need an answer to that question: why run the marathon?

I thought about a recent trip I'd taken back up to Queens, New York, to visit friends and family. That Saturday morning, I set out on a run. It was early, and after stepping out of the apartment where I'd been raised, I began running down the old familiar streets of my youth, past stores where I held after-school jobs, past school yards where I used to spend long summer days playing handball and stickball. I ran past Alley Pond Park, where my friends and I would occasionally do short runs on a bike trail through the woods. Back then, our 3-mile run seemed like a tremendous achievement.

I left the park and headed west on Union Turnpike, a major thoroughfare that ran past the apartment complex where I lived. Every weekday morning from age twelve through eighteen, I would board the Q44 bus on Union

Turnpike for the 6 mile ride to the train station, where I would take the F train to the N train to the uptown 7, exiting at 96th Street for the short walk to my school. It was an hour-and-a-half commute, but that didn't seem unusual to me. Everyone in New York commutes.

As I ran down the avenue, I thought about my father. He used to take the Q44 bus also, getting off earlier to transfer to another bus to nearby Jamaica Avenue and the clothing store where he worked. After I moved to D.C. and became a runner, I ran along this bus route when I was visiting. I'd try to keep pace with each bus as it passed, looking to see if my father was on board, on his way to work. He always stood toward the back of the bus, a figure in a dark raincoat, looking out the window, leaning in to get a better view, looking for me as I was looking for him, waving at me as I waved back.

My father and I, like many fathers and sons, weren't very close, though I think we both wanted to be. We had difficulty talking with one another, of finding common ground. This chasm grew when I went to college and entered a world that he had no experience with. It would be many years until I began to understand that he showed more character through his daily sacrifice for his family than I would ever learn in school. It is a lesson that I continue to learn. But on those runs back home, I didn't yet understand these things, so the brief morning encounters we had, with me on foot and him peering through the bus window, were one of the few ways we had of connecting.

My parents were actually very proud of my running. Even Dad, who never let on when he approved of anything his children had done, bragged about me to his coworkers, and when I gave him a plaque with mounted photos of me crossing the finish line, he showed it to anyone who would be foolish enough to agree to see it. Dad wasn't an athletic man; in fact, he was often quite overweight. I had the feeling that my running somehow balanced the scales for him, that by producing someone who could accomplish these things, he had shown that it was in him somewhere as well.

Then, in 1988, right after I graduated from law school, I decided that I wanted to go skydiving. It sounded like a fun thing to do. My parents weren't so proud of that decision. They thought me foolish for wanting to throw myself out of a plane after all the hard work I put in to getting through law school. It was all fine and good to run marathons—even if I didn't win any of them, as my dad once pointed out—but at least that was safe. You get tired, you stop. Easy. But what sane person jumps out of a plane?

We never agreed on it, but one sunny day, I did it anyway. It was a static line jump, like in those old World War II movies where paratroopers dove out the door and their chutes opened automatically, except in my case there was no diving. Each of us crawled out to the edge and then slid out the door, hanging onto the strut of the overhead wing, waiting for the signal to let go from the jumpmaster, who sat just inside the door. I was third of three to go, and after sucking in engine fumes as our plane circled, climbing and dropping, I was more than ready to jump. I crawled out and looked up for the instructor's thumbs-up sign. He gave it, and I let go.

I didn't get a free fall, didn't get to assume the arch position that the instructor had us practice earlier. As it turned out, my chute opened almost immediately after I let go of the plane. But I did get some fine gliding time under the canopy, circling left and right as I tugged on the toggles above me.

I slowly drifted down to the target landing spot on the field. I misjudged my distance from the ground, though, so I landed hard and rolled instead of stepping gracefully back onto the earth. Not perfect, but good. And very fun.

I called my parents afterward. I hadn't told them that this was the day I would be jumping; no point in having them spend the day gazing at the clock, wondering if I'd splattered yet. They were relieved that I got through it okay, and that I had gotten it out of my system. Except that I hadn't. My jump was fun, but a free fall, well, that would be something else altogether. I needed just a few more jumps to graduate to that level. It would be easy.

My parents didn't share my enthusiasm. In fact, Dad started a letter-writing campaign against it. Well, he didn't actually write any letters. Instead, he clipped articles on gruesome skydiving accidents and sent them to me, without even attaching a note. Stories like the one about the skydiver who got tangled up in a plane's fuselage and had to cut himself loose from his chute to save the plane, while dooming himself. I wondered where he found these; I had never seen a single one on my own.

I knew that I'd have to deal with this sooner or later, or one of us would crack. I needed a plan.

Here's what I came up with: while Dad was always overweight, he would occasionally add on an extra twenty pounds or so, which he would drop as soon as his coworkers started teasing him about it. He'd gotten big again recently, and wasn't losing weight, despite the teasing. So I offered Dad a deal: no more skydiving if he lost forty pounds and kept it off. There seemed to be no downside there for me; if he agreed, he would either lose the weight, but probably put it back on later, freeing me from my bond, or he wouldn't lose the weight, and would have forfeited his right to campaign against me, since he knew exactly what he had to do to get me to stop. Brilliant.

Dad agreed to the deal. Then he quickly lost the forty pounds. That surprised me, but I was okay with it, because I knew that the game wasn't over yet. Then something unexpected happened; he seemed pale and tired easily, and Mom said that he was getting night sweats. That wasn't part of my plan.

We talked Dad into seeing his doctor, who took blood samples and ordered some tests. I figured Dad's crash diet had left him with some type of anemia, and the doctor said yes, that there was evidence of anemia, but he also said that there was something more. He wanted to take some tests. So Dad took off a week from work and let the doctor poke and prod and stick him. After all that, the doctor announced that he wanted to do a bone-marrow biopsy.

For me, that was the first sign that something might be seriously wrong.

I went up to New York that weekend, right before the biopsy was scheduled to be performed, to spend time with my parents and with my younger sister, Dori. My older sister, Marlene, was abroad traveling, but we were keeping her updated. While I was home, we just relaxed, and spent time poring through old photographs. We found some of Mom and Dad's wedding shots, and laughed at Dad's terrified expression, looking at us across the decades with great big eyes.

I was back at work on Monday when I got a phone call from a neighbor telling me that my dad was ill, and that I needed to come up immediately. I called my mother to find out exactly what was going on, and she could only say, "He's gone, he's gone." Finally, she told me that Dad had just collapsed and died. I jumped on the next flight to New York.

I sat gazing out the window, tears welling in my eyes, waiting for the flight to be over, but wishing that the plane would never land. An elderly woman sitting beside me started up a conversation. More than a decade later, I still wonder whether she somehow guessed what had happened, and was just trying to distract me.

She asked what I did for a living. I told her that I was an attorney. Looking at my hands, callused from working out in the gym, she said, "there's no shame in being a workman, you know."

"Yes," I said. "I know. But I really am an attorney."

After I arrived in New York, I kept wondering what it was the doctor had been testing for. I finally called and asked. Lymphoma, he said. Cancer. He was sure of it, and only ordered the biopsy to confirm it. Dad would have been dead within two years, he said. He was surprised at my dad's sudden death, but he said that perhaps it was for the best.

*My dad dropping dead was for the best.* I rolled that one around in my mind for a while. It was hard to accept, but I knew he was probably right.

But here's what I'm not supposed to tell you: a day or two after I had returned home, I took a late-night walk with my mother. She seemed to want to say something, so I asked her what was on her mind. She told me that on the day Dad died, he had been nervous about the biopsy, and had asked her to lie down with him. Mom paused and looked me in the eyes. "You know what I mean? *Lie down.*" The dime dropped, and I got it.

"Afterward," she continued, "he got up and went into the next room and collapsed." She looked me in the eyes, deadly serious. "Do you think I killed him?"

Good god. Can you imagine? Bad enough to have to think about my parents having sex, but now I had to imagine Mom killing Dad in the sack. *Well,* I thought, *maybe she did. Good for him. Good for her. Good for the both of them! What a great way that would be to go: spend a week at home, have your son come in for a visit, make love to your wife, then go into the next room and check out. That's a pretty sweet deal.*

Of course, I didn't say any of this to my mom. I told her, "Of course not. When it's your time, it's your time, and nothing you did with him could have changed that."

Which might be true. Or perhaps not.

Meanwhile, I was comforted, too, by the realization that my parents had always wanted it to be this way. Not at that exact moment or in that way, but in the scheme of things. Children bury parents; that's how it was supposed to be. Any time we heard about a child dying first, the expression on my parents' faces betrayed pain for the grieving parents that they didn't even know. Looking back, I realized that my parents had, knowingly or not, prepared me for this moment all my life.

I had it in my mind that burying my dad was a very personal thing, and I didn't want a stranger to do it. In Jewish funerals, the immediate family and closest friends each toss a shovelful of dirt on the coffin after it's been lowered down into the earth. After that, workers generally come over and shovel the bulk of the dirt into the grave. It seemed too impersonal to me. Burying my father was my last act of devotion to him, and I wanted to do it myself. My mother and sisters understood, and gave their consent. I then asked my family rabbi if it would be allowed. He warned me that it would be hard work. I smiled, and explained to him that I was in pretty good shape.

And that's how it went. For years afterward, when I ran down Union Turnpike, I couldn't help but glance up at each passing bus, looking to see if my father was on board. I know it makes no sense, but part of me imagined that it would still be possible to see him standing there, waving at me, if only I could run fast enough and catch the right bus. My running would bring him back to me.

I think now about all the other places that I had run over the seasons and the years, the people I met, the person I was, and the person I had become. Running seems to be the thread that connects it all, a line to all that was and all that is; a strip of asphalt thousands of miles long, on which I'd run all the workouts and races of my life.

I wonder what the Runner-That-I-Was would think about the Runner-That-I-Am, and I imagine that if I run really fast, I would be able to fold the years and catch sight of the Me-That-Was. We'd lock eyes in passing, and he'd nod slightly and tip his hand, the runner's greeting that says, "I know you; you are one of us."

My mind floods with the memories of my running in D.C. I recall crossing Key Bridge during a driving rainstorm, and the sweltering heat of the 14th Street Bridge in late summer. I recall the reflection of myself on an office building's gleaming window during a 10K race, and the potholes I've scrambled over, and occasionally stepped into.

I think again about the marathon, and again about the question why. I've lived with the marathon for nearly two decades; it has become a part of my being, my personal culture. It is no longer just something I do; it is a reflection of who I am. The great Czech Olympic champion Emil Zátopek said that if you want to win something, run 100 meters, but if you want to experience something, run a marathon. I've wanted the experience, and I've discovered that each marathon is a life-journey all its own, filled with expectation, disappointment, realization, and, sometimes, triumph. It has become the measure and mirror of my life.

I think again about Burt, my personal training client who passed away. I think about how the muscles we fought so hard to strengthen have now melted from his bones, and that I may be the only one who knows how hard he struggled to improve himself. But I know that Burt labored not just to gain strength and fitness; what Burt gained in the gym was a sense of purpose. His struggles were a demonstration of his character and his faith in the wonder of life. I think, too, about my two team members in Rome, and how we talked about the meaning of the marathon, of the arbitrariness of the number 26.2, of the relative insignificance of finishing times.

Finally, I had my answer. I knew why it was important to run the marathon. The race distance matters, but only because it takes 26.2 miles to strip away the falsehoods and comfortable compromises of daily life. My finishing times matter also, but only as a reflection of my effort. I know that I will eventually lose my speed, and that someday I will get old and die. But during the time I am here, I will find a deeper satisfaction and meaning to my daily routine; I will find a way to connect to the animal that I am, and to make a statement about what kind of person I am, and what I stand for. It doesn't really matter that I will slow and weaken. There is a kind of glory to be found here, a glory earned through sweat and effort, from a stubborn refusal to give less than your best. It is the reward that dwarfs all the medals tucked away in my drawer. It is why I run the marathon.

Here's a story: during the 1968 Olympic Games in Mexico City, the winner of the marathon had already crossed the finish line over an hour earlier when John Stephen Akhwari of Tanzania entered the stadium. Akhwari was limping, and his leg was wrapped in a bloody bandage. Akhwari slowly made his way around the track to the finish line, as the few spectators who remained in the stands applauded his efforts. Afterward, a reporter asked Akhwari why he hadn't just dropped out of the race, since he clearly had no chance of winning. Akhwari paused, and then said, "My country did not send me to Mexico City to start the race. They sent me to finish." It was the greatest last-place finish ever, and perhaps the most succinct expression I'd ever heard of the marathon spirit.

Everyone needs a place to make their stand, to declare their character through their actions, to say "this is who I am and what I believe." For me, that statement begins with a race application and a pair of running shoes. We marathoners are the people who suffer and persevere. That is who we are.

As I write these words, I look over at Stephanie. Soon after we married, we talked about whether we wanted a child. We were both accustomed to an adventurous lifestyle, and we were reluctant and even scared to take on the burden of parenthood. Even if we wanted one, we knew that the odds were against us. We were both forty, which we knew was a problem. Friends our age had gone to extraordinary lengths to conceive, using fertility drugs and in vitro fertilization. We fully expected that would be our lot as well, much as we hoped to avoid it.

We finally decided to try to start a family. Actually, it would be more accurate to say that we decided that we didn't want to *not* have one, which was what we thought would be the result if we put off making a decision any longer. Since we were sure that we would have difficulty getting pregnant anyway, we made an appointment with a clinic. Stephanie showed up for her appointment on time. She'd missed her last period, but she wasn't concerned. These things happen occasionally. The doctor did a few preliminary tests, and then came back with surprising news: we didn't need his services after all. Stephanie was already pregnant.

We were dumbstruck. As Stephanie's belly swelled, the reality of our situation slowly sunk in. In time, we found out that we were going to have a boy, and we began the ritualistic collecting-of-things that all expecting parents go through. I trusted her to decide what we needed; I hadn't even heard of many of the things that she told me were essential, and even holding them in my hands left me with little clear idea of what to do with them.

The one thing I did take responsibility for, though, was the choosing of the jogging stroller. After extensive research, I bought a model that just screamed speed. It looked like it was setting a PR even when it was standing still. I felt ready for our son.

As we got closer to our due date, I thought more about what kind of father I wanted to be, and I began to feel hopelessly ill prepared. How had my father handled it, and his father before him? I hoped that my instincts and basic common sense would carry me through. And I also counted on close supervision by Stephanie.

One thing I did feel confident about, though, was my determination to be a running father. If children really do learn best by example, then my little boy would learn that it's perfectly natural to run on a nice day, and to enter a marathon and finish it. He would watch his old man compete, and see that hundreds and thousands of other dads and moms did the same thing. He would grow up thinking that there was nothing extraordinary or unusual about this, and that he could do it, too, if he wished. He could do anything he wanted, if he did the work.

As I glance over at Stephanie's belly now, I think of the lessons I learned from my father, and I think of how I will some day be regarded by my own son when I'm gone. I hope that he'll recall the passion with which I pursued my dreams, and understand that in my running, I was trying to explain to him my understanding of life, and how to live it. This is the gift I wish to give to my son.

My 100th marathon has now come and gone, less a finish line itself than a marker on a path. More are planned, and after that, more will hopefully follow, stretching into the distance like light posts on an endless highway. As each one comes into view, I will greet it and test myself against it, pushing muscle and sinew against time and distance. If ever I should forget who I am, and what I believe, I only need to run that path, and in my running, I will find my way back to myself, and discover once again who I am.

# Epilogue: Bumps in the Endless Road

In November 2004, a story was reported in the back pages of *The New York Times* that was of great interest to me.[8] Dr. Dennis M. Bramble of the University of Utah and Dr. Daniel E. Lieberman of Harvard had published a paper hypothesizing that ancient humans were physiologically predisposed to be long-distance runners.

The scientists had begun by analyzing the evolution of our physique. As early as two million years ago, humans developed an upright posture, long legs, shorter arms and a narrower ribcage and pelvis. We also lost our fur, which allowed us to develop sweat glands and prevent overheating during intense exertion. We developed a ligament network to keep our heads steady while running, and a muscle and tendon network along the back of our legs, including an Achilles tendon, to store and release great amounts of energy—enough to propel our bodies forward quickly with power. And then there's our highly-developed backside, which stabilizes our midsection during running.

---

8 "Even Couch Potatoes May Have Been Born to Run," by John Noble Wilford, *New York Times*, November 17, 2004.

243

All of these traits are conducive not just to walking, but to long distance running, and apes don't share any of them. Bramble and Lieberman speculated that running would have increased the early humans' chances of survival, as they could cover large areas of African grassland in pursuit of food.

Apparently, then, we are all born to run.

Of course, I knew that already. I was once told that there's a German word, *tatesfruedig,* which roughly means the joy of doing that which you can do well. A cheetah loves to sprint because it is built to sprint, and a monkey loves to climb because it is built to climb. My running wasn't an aberration; it was an expression of my genetic heritage. It was something I was born to do.

So I kept on running. I ran marathons in Montana, Alaska, and North Dakota. In late September, with the birth of my son just days away, I returned to the Marine Corps Marathon yet again. And then, on November 12, 2005, I experienced something more miraculous than a marathon finish line: the birth of Alex Michael, named in honor of my grandfather and Stephanie's dad. I cut his umbilical cord and then later laid my hand across his tiny body. There was no amount of thinking that could compare to the reality I saw before me. It was magical and humbling. I thought about my life, and I felt like I was the luckiest man on earth.

Then things became unhinged. A dear friend of twenty years died of breast cancer. A cousin died from lung cancer. And then hardest of all, I had to watch my mother's health suddenly spiral downward, despite all the treatments recommended by the best doctors we could find. Mom was obese and had diabetes, which I knew was a time bomb waiting to explode, but there was little I could do about it. As a coach and trainer, I felt particularly responsible, but I couldn't force her to save her own life, and after a while, I decided not to spend whatever time we had left together fighting with her over this. But now her problems gained a velocity I never could have imagined: she experienced full renal failure and had to go on dialysis, then she contracted pneumonia twice and a vicious intestinal infection. Fear and various drugs addled her mind, and a foot infection forced her doctors to amputate her leg. The lone bright spot for us was the look on her face when she held tiny Alex in her arms for the first time.

Her health continued to decline. Every time the phone rang, I feared the worst. My sisters and I shuttled Mom between hospitals and nursing homes, and we realized at some point that she would never return to her old apartment. We were still hopeful of her recovery, and had just filed the paperwork to move her into a home that could properly care for her. My sister Marlene was visiting us in D.C. with her two children when we got the phone call from New York. Mom's blood pressure had suddenly plummeted, and she had needed to be resuscitated twice. She now had a tube snaking down her throat, delivering oxygen, and her heart was beating only because she was being fed drugs intravenously. Her doctors wanted to know if we wanted to give them the order to stop resuscitating her. They wanted to know if we were ready to let her die.

Marlene had been on a grand tour of Europe and Asia when Dad fell ill. When she called us from Istanbul, we told her not to worry, but that she should sit still for a while and keep in touch. There was no need to panic, after all. Everything would be okay. And then Dad suddenly died, as you know. Marlene immediately got on a plane heading home, and spent that twelve-hour flight weeping and growing the guilt she would carry forever for not being home when her daddy passed away.

As I looked at Marlene now, I knew that more than anything else, I didn't want Mom to pass away without Marlene being at her bedside. So the answer was no. We would not give a do-not-resuscitate order. We told the doctors to keep the meds flowing. We were on our way.

When we reached the hospital, Stephanie took Alex and Marlene's children back to Marlene's house, where Marlene's husband Jerry was waiting for them. Marlene and I went up to Mom's room in intensive care. Our sister Dori was already there, with red-rimmed eyes. She had been there for hours.

We went right to Mom's bedside. She looked back at us, wide-eyed, gasping for air as a tube hung from her mouth. Her gaze shifted, and I realized that she was looking back and forth across the room. Back and forth, again and again. I wondered if she knew we were there.

We stepped into the hall to speak with the doctors on call. They told us that the only thing keeping Mom alive was the medication they were pumping into her veins to maintain her blood pressure and heartbeat. Mom's body had already begun to shut down; the flow of blood to her remaining leg had virtually stopped. After absorbing this information, we returned to her room. I pulled back the blanket and looked at her right leg. Her foot was already turning black.

My sisters sobbed while they held Mom's hands and stroked her head. I stood at the bedside, waiting. Finally, we looked at each other, and started talking about what needed to be done.

How do you go about stating the obvious when no one wants to hear it? I was a lawyer, so I approached it in a lawyerlike way: I made the case. Mom could not live on her own without these extreme lifesaving measures, and what she had now was not living. Even if she were to somehow revive and not need life support, her remaining leg was rapidly dying, and would need to be removed. Would she be able to survive another amputation? We doubted it.

When we were finished reviewing the situation, we just stood there, not wanting to say what needed to be said. It seemed like we had been led into a Faustian bargain; in exchange for being allowed to be at her mother's bedside at her passing, we had to give the order to let her die. It was an awful responsibility, but as we looked at Mom, the reality sunk in. We realized that we really had no choice at all. It had already happened. We were there to just hold her hand and observe the passage.

We went back out in the hall and summoned the doctors. They told us that if we discontinued the medications, her heart rate would immediately begin to drop. She would probably only start to feel lightheaded, and then gently slip away. After all the months of physical and mental agony she had endured, it seemed only fair that she was at least given a peaceful end.

We had the meds cut off, and my sisters and I stood around her bedside, stroking her face and saying "I love you." I leaned in close to her cheek, kissed her, and whispered, "Be at peace," and then I glanced at the monitor and watched the drop in her heart rate. It fell slowly but steadily, from 119, to 107, to 98. My sisters cried more intensely, and held her hands tightly. Mom still looked up at us wide eyed.

84. 77. 65.

Her cheek felt cold to me, but as soft as it was when I stroked it as a boy. When I was very little I once told her that when she got old, I would get her a facelift. I don't know where I had gotten that idea. I wondered what she thought when I said it.

59. 53. 48. 42.

Her eyes seemed to lose their vitality. I wanted the moment to be over, and I wanted it to never end. I wondered what she was thinking.

36. 28. 19. 12.

Stillness.

After my mother died, I felt numb and detached. Even with Stephanie and Alex beside me, I was shaken by the sudden disappearance of so many people from my life. I didn't know what to do to make it all seem okay, so I relied on the one thing that had always provided me with support when I was troubled: I ran. I raced in Arizona, Florida, Wyoming, and still that was not enough. While Mom was ill, Stephanie and I had made plans to let her mother watch Alex while the two of us went to Mexico for a vacation—and a chance for me to run the Mexico City Marathon. After Mom died, I wasn't sure we should still go, but we decided it would be best for us to stick with our plans. More than anything, we needed some time alone. It was the right choice. We had a wonderful time, even if we missed Alex.

And still I kept running. On October 8, 2006, Dave and I completed the Mt. Rushmore Marathon, crossing the finish line together. We had added the final state to our list, and could now both claim to have run the entire country.

I didn't stop there; I added more and more marathons to my list, running them more frequently than I ever had before. And then I committed the cardinal runner's sin: I ignored pain, thinking it would just go away. It didn't. My body suddenly decided that enough was enough, and grounded me with a series of devastating injuries. Tenderness in my hamstrings, blinding pain in my Achilles tendon, and stabbing pain in my heel. My running came to a screeching halt. I was through.

After a series of X-rays and MRIs, I accepted that I would be off running, and that I would never again run the way I used to. I was allowed to cross-train, and I attacked the bike and weight room with a singled-minded fury, but I missed my running. The weeks passed, and I followed the doctor's orders religiously, but I was still grounded. I kept up a cheerful face for my charity running team and my friends, but I'd never before had to face a setback like this. After all I had just witnessed, I knew that not being able to run was hardly the worst tragedy one could face, but it was still a difficult blow to me. The one crutch that I had consistently relied upon over the years to help me through all my crises was itself in crisis. I felt lost.

In April 2008, I sat in an airport, waiting by a gate for a plane that would take my charity runners and me to Monterey, California for a race along the coast. They would run, but I would not. But I was their coach, and I was committed to helping them achieve their goals. It was all I could do. But in the airport at that moment, I just wanted to sit quietly and read. I didn't want to think about running.

"You ran the Dublin Marathon?"

"Huh?" I said, confused.

"Did you run the Dublin Marathon?" The tall man standing in front of me pointed at my backpack. "It says so on your bag."

"Oh, right. Yeah, I ran that a couple of times. It's a fun race."

"Do you run a lot?"

"Well, not right now, but I used to." And so I told him about my races. Eventually I told him how many I'd run.

"You should write a book."

"Funny you should say that."

"Wait a minute," he said, getting up. "I gotta get someone." He came back with a few people and introduced me. We all sat there and talked running. Races we'd finished, races we'd dreamed of doing, the great moments and the horrible ones. And little by little, I began to feel better.

"Good talking with you," the first man said. "You're an inspiration."

An inspiration. That was funny. They hadn't known how depressed I was just a few minutes earlier. And now like a summer storm, it had blown away. Talking with them, I felt my hope rekindle, and I suddenly knew that these injuries—these terrible but completely common injuries—would pass, and I would solve the puzzle of my body and find a way to run again, to race again. Despite all, the road was not ended and I was not finished. Everything in my life would be all right.

I was still a runner.

# By the Numbers

1 Marine Corps Marathon, Washington, D.C., November 8, 1987—
  3:45:30
2 Marine Corps Marathon, Washington, D.C., November 4, 1990—
  4:08:00
3 New York City Marathon, November 3, 1991—4:11:12
4 Shamrock Marathon, Virginia Beach, March 20, 1993—3:45:33
5 Pittsburgh Marathon, May 2, 1993—4:25:42
6 Columbia Birthday Marathon, Maryland, September 19, 1993—
  3:35:00
7 Northern Central Trails Marathon, Maryland, November 27,
  1993—4:00:17
8 Boston Marathon, April 18, 1994—3:57:38
9 Vermont Marathon, Burlington, May 29, 1994—3:40:33
10 Grandma's Marathon; Duluth, Minnesota, June 19, 1994—
  3:47:38
11 Atlantic City Marathon, New Jersey, October 16, 1994—3:39:52
12 New York City Marathon, November 6, 1994—3:42:33
13 Richmond Marathon, Virginia, November 27, 1994—3:35:38

14 Philadelphia Marathon, November 20, 1994—3:43:44

15 Las Vegas Marathon, February 4, 1995—3:58:26

16 LaSalle Chicago Marathon, October 15, 1995—3:21:28

17 Marine Corps Marathon, Washington, D.C., October 22, 1995—4:27:55

18 Schweizer's Delaware Marathon, December 10, 1995—3:34:12

19 Disneyworld Marathon, Orlando, January 7, 1996—3:26:55

20 *Charlotte Observer* Marathon, North Carolina, February 17, 1996—3:28:48

21 Music City Marathon; Nashville, Tennessee, March 16, 1996—3:38:39

22 Cleveland Marathon, May 5, 1996—3:44:39

23 Mayor's Midnight Marathon, Anchorage, June 22, 1996—3:19:41

24 Marine Corps Marathon, Washington, D.C., October 27, 1996—3:37:46

25 Atlanta Marathon, November 28, 1996—3:32:05

26 Kiawah Island Marathon, South Carolina, December 14, 1996—3:23:47

27 25th Olympiad Memorial Marathon, St. Louis, February 23, 1997—3:48:51

28 Ridge Runner Marathon, West Virginia, June 7, 1997—3:40:57

29 San Francisco Marathon, July 13, 1997—3:32:00

30 East Lyme Marathon, Connecticut, September 28, 1997—3:12:57

31 Detroit International Marathon, Michigan, October 19, 1997—3:08:59

32 Vulcan Marathon; Birmingham, Alabama, November 8, 1997—3:31

33 Mardi Gras Marathon; New Orleans, Louisiana, January 17, 1998—3:45:02

34 Lincoln Marathon, Nebraska, May 3, 1998—3:18:05

35 Heroes Marathon; Madison, Wisconsin, May 24, 1998—3:10:09

36 Sunburst Marathon; South Bend, Indiana, June 6, 1998—3:36:50

37 Pikes Peak Marathon, Colorado, August 16, 1998—6:58:00

38 New Hampshire Marathon, October 3, 1998—3:46:00

39 Louisville Marathon, December 5, 1998—3:30:22

40 Houston Marathon, January 19, 1999—3:25:14

41 The Last Marathon, Antarctica, February 13, 1999—5:10:00

42 Los Angeles Marathon, March 14, 1999—3:27:25

43 Boston Marathon, April 19, 1999—3:09:00

44 *Deseret News* Marathon, Utah, July 24, 1999—3:54:00

45 Tupelo Marathon, Mississippi, September 5, 1999—3:32:13 (19/120)

46 Berlin Marathon, September 26, 1999—3:26:17

47 Marine Corps Marathon, Washington D.C., October 24, 1999— 3:21:15 (with a borrowed number—sorry, Mr. Race Director!)

48 New York City Marathon, November 7, 1999—3:34:51

49 Seattle Marathon, November 28, 1999—3:32:34

50 Jacksonville Marathon, Florida, December 18, 1999—3:24:15

51 Myrtle Beach Marathon, South Carolina, February 5, 2000— 3:15:00

52 B&A Trail Marathon, Maryland, March 12, 2000—3:40:01

53 Boston Marathon, April 17, 2000—3:11:44

54 Portland Marathon, Maine, October 1, 2000—3:22:04

55 Beijing Marathon, October 15, 2000—3:31:01

56 Dublin Marathon, October 30, 2000—3:27:45

57 Honolulu Marathon, December 10, 2000—3:25:37

58 Bermuda Marathon, January 14, 2001—3:23:37 (16/287)

59 Desert Classic Marathon; Phoenix, Arizona, February 18, 2001— 3:44:01

60 Rome Marathon, March 25, 2001—3:49:38

61 Boston Marathon, April 16, 2001—3:19:05

62 Vienna City Marathon, May 20, 2001—3:41:37

63  New Mexico Marathon, September 9, 2001—3:33:00

64  Steamtown Marathon; Scranton, Pennsylvania, October 7, 2001—3:20:14

65  Dublin Marathon, October 31, 2001—4:07:00

66  Athens Marathon, Greece, November 4, 2001—3:23:00

67  Honolulu Marathon, December 9, 2001—3:48:34

68  Rome Marathon, March 24, 2002—3:49:38

69  Paris Marathon, April 7, 2002—3:52:43

70  Toronto Marathon, September 15, 2002—3:28:10

71  Portland Marathon, Oregon, October 6, 2002—3:38:00

72  Amsterdam Marathon, October 20, 2002—4:27:00

73  New York City Marathon, November 3, 2002—3:37:00

74  Marathon in the Parks, Maryland, November 17, 2002—3:57:21

75  Honolulu Marathon, December 8, 2002—3:47:29

76  Miami Tropical Marathon, February 2, 2003—3:16:16

77  Boston Marathon, April 14, 2003—3:22:00

78  Kona Marathon, June 21, 2003—5:21:00

79  Pikes Peak Marathon, Colorado, August 17, 2003—7:24:00

80  Médoc Marathon; Bordeaux, France, September 6, 2003—4:41:18

81  Wichita Marathon, Kansas, October 19, 2003—3:35:47

82  Auckland Marathon, New Zealand, November 2, 2003—3:39:00

83  Tulsa Marathon, November 22, 2003—3:28:00

84  Barbados Marathon, December 7, 2003—4:38:00

85  Hog Eye Marathon; Fayetteville, Arkansas, March 28, 2004—3:43:58

86  Boston Marathon, April 19, 2004—3:34:00

87  Vancouver International Marathon, British Columbia, May 2, 2004—3:25:43

88  Bunco Calgary Marathon, July 11, 2004—3:55:57

89  Mesa Falls Marathon; Ashton, Idaho, August 28, 2004—4:00:42

90  Des Moines Marathon, Iowa, October 17, 2004—3:20:34

91  Marine Corps Marathon, Washington, D.C., October 31, 2004—3:28:33

92  Marathon in the Parks; Montgomery County, Maryland, November 14, 2004—3:45:01

93  White Rock Marathon; Dallas, Texas, December 12, 2004—3:32:58

94  Las Vegas International Marathon, January 30, 2005—3:36:59

95  George Washington Birthday Marathon; Greenbelt, Maryland, February 20, 2005—3:49:40

96  Virginia Creeper, Abingdon, March 13, 2005—3:49:36

97  Ocean City Marathon; Ocean City, Maryland, April 16, 2005—3:53:00

98  Vancouver Marathon, British Columbia, May 1, 2005—3:57:19

99  Coventry Healthcare Delaware Marathon, Wilmington, May 15, 2005—3:35:07

100  Grandfather Mountain Marathon; Boone, North Carolina, July 9, 2005—3:46:00

# Acknowledgments

To borrow a well-used phrase, it takes a village to publish a book, and I was lucky enough to have a particularly great bunch of villagers to help me turn this idea into a reality. First, thanks to my agent, Lauren Abramo, for her support and ever-helpful guidance. Thanks also to Bill Wolfsthal and Sarah Van Bonn at Skyhorse Publishing for their patience and vision, and to Jan Seeley and Rich Benyo of *Marathon & Beyond* for a decade's worth of friendship and encouragement. I still remember the first article query I sent over to Rich: I suggested a word limit, and he e-mailed back that I shouldn't worry about that; I should just write all that I needed to say. It's a freedom I've never taken for granted, and which I hope I haven't abused.

Thanks to Dave Harrell for being a big part of my story, and to Renata Carvalho for running and racing with me and for offering me valuable advice after reading the first draft of this book. Thanks also to my pace team organizers, who have invited me to enjoy a new side of marathoning: Josh Leibman of FunnerRunner and Marathon Memories, and Star and Darris Blackford and the entire Clif Bar Pace Team family.

Finally, a world of thanks to my sisters, Marlene and Dori, and their families, all my friends and colleagues, and especially to my parents, who I wish could have been here to see this.

# About the Author

**JEFF HOROWITZ** is a certified personal trainer and running coach, living in Washington, D.C. He got hooked on marathoning in 1987, and in addition to his own running, he has coached hundreds of others to run their first marathon while raising money for various charities. When he's not busy doing these things, he's also an attorney, columnist, husband, and father to little Alex Michael, who pleased his daddy by quickly learning how to say, "Look, I'm running!" Visit Jeff at www.runtothefinishline.com.